CRC SERIES IN MODERN NUTRITION

Edited by Ira Wolinsky and James F. Hickson, Jr.

Published Titles

Manganese in Health and Disease, Dorothy J. Klimis-Tavantzis

Nutrition and AIDS: Effects and Treatments, Ronald R. Watson

Nutrition Care for HIV-Positive Persons: A Manual for Individuals and Their Caregivers, Saroj M. Bahl and James F. Hickson, Jr.

Calcium and Phosphorus in Health and Disease, John J.B. Anderson and Sanford C. Garner

Edited by Ira Wolinsky

Published Titles

Handbook of Nutrition in the Aged, Ronald R. Watson

Practical Handbook of Nutrition in Clinical Practice, Donald F. Kirby and Stanley J. Dudrick

Handbook of Dairy Foods and Nutrition, Gregory D. Miller, Judith K. Jarvis, and Lois D. McBean

Advanced Nutrition: Macronutrients, Carolyn D. Berdanier

Childhood Nutrition, Fima Lifschitz

Nutrition and Health: Topics and Controversies, Felix Bronner

Nutrition and Cancer Prevention, Ronald R. Watson and Siraj I. Mufti

Nutritional Concerns of Women, Ira Wolinsky and Dorothy J. Klimis-Tavantzis

Nutrients and Gene Expression: Clinical Aspects, Carolyn D. Berdanier

Antioxidants and Disease Prevention, Harinda S. Garewal

Advanced Nutrition: Micronutrients, Carolyn D. Berdanier

Nutrition and Women's Cancers, Barbara Pence and Dale M. Dunn

Nutrients and Foods in AIDS, Ronald R. Watson

Nutrition: Chemistry and Biology, Second Edition, Julian E. Spallholz, L. Mallory Boylan, and Judy A. Driskell

Melatonin in the Promotion of Health, Ronald R. Watson

Nutritional and Environmental Influences on the Eye, Allen Taylor

Laboratory Tests for the Assessment of Nutritional Status, Second Edition, H.E. Sauberlich

Advanced Human Nutrition, Robert E.C. Wildman and Denis M. Medeiros

Handbook of Dairy Foods and Nutrition, Second Edition, Gregory D. Miller, Judith K. Jarvis, and Lois D. McBean

Nutrition in Space Flight and Weightlessness Models, Helen W. Lane and Dale A. Schoeller

Eating Disorders in Women and Children: Prevention, Stress Management, and Treatment, Jacalyn J. Robert-McComb
Childhood Obesity: Prevention and Treatment, Jana Parizkova and Andrew Hills
Alcohol and Substance Abuse in the Aging, Ronald R. Watson
Handbook of Nutrition and the Aged, Third Edition, Ronald R. Watson
Vegetables, Fruits, and Herbs in Health Promotion, Ronald R. Watson
Nutrition and AIDS, 2nd Edition, Ronald R. Watson

Forthcoming Titles

Nutritional Anemias, Usha Ramakrishnan
Advances in Isotope Methods for the Analysis of Trace Elements in Man, Malcolm Jackson and Nicola Lowe
Handbook of Nutrition for Vegetarians, Joan Sabate and Rosemary A. Ratzin-Tuner
Tryptophan: Biochemicals and Health Implications, Herschel Sidransky
Handbook of Nutraceuticals and Functional Foods, Robert E. C. Wildman
The Mediterranean Diet, Antonia L. Matalas, Antonios Zampelas, Vasilis Stavrinos, and Ira Wolinsky
Handbook of Nutraceuticals and Nutritional Supplements and Pharmaceuticals, Robert E. C. Wildman
Inulin and Oligofructose: Functional Food Ingredients, Marcel B. Roberfroid
Micronutrients and HIV Infection, Henrik Friis
Nutrition Gene Interactions in Health and Disease, Niama M. Moussa and Carolyn D. Berdanier

Vegetables, Fruits, and Herbs in Health Promotion

Edited by
Ronald R. Watson, Ph.D.

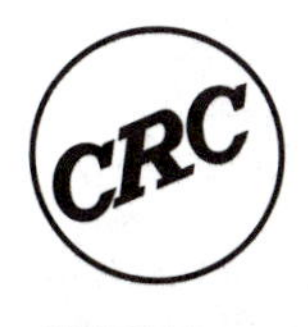

CRC Press
Boca Raton London New York Washington, D.C.

Library of Congress Cataloging-in-Publication Data

Vegetables, fruits, and herbs in health promotion / edited by Ronald R. Watson.
p. cm. — (Modern nutrition)
Includes bibliographical references and index.
ISBN 0-8493-0038-X (alk. paper)
1. Vegetables in human nutrition. 2. Fruit. 3. Herbs — Therapeutic use. 4. Functional foods. 5. Phytochemicals — Health aspects. 6. Health promotion. I. Watson, Ronald R. (Ronald Ross) II. Modern nutrition (Boca Raton, Fla.)

QP144.V44 V425 2000
613.2'8 — dc21 00-033730

Direct all inquiries to CRC Press LLC, 2000 N.W. Corporate Blvd., Boca Raton, Florida 33431.

International Standard Book Number 0-8493-0038-X
Library of Congress Card Number 00-033730
Printed in the United States of America 1 2 3 4 5 6 7 8 9 0
Printed on acid-free paper

Series Preface

The CRC Series in Modern Nutrition is dedicated to providing the widest possible coverage of topics in nutrition. Nutrition is an interdisciplinary, interprofessional field par excellence. It is noted by its broad range and diversity. We trust the titles and authorship in this series will reflect that range and diversity.

Published for a scholarly audience, the volumes in the CRC Series in Modern Nutrition are designed to explain, review, and explore present knowledge and recent trends, developments, and advances in nutrition. As such, they also appeal to the educated general reader. The format for the series varies with the needs of the author and the topic, including, but not limited to, edited volumes, monographs, handbooks, and texts.

Contributors from any bona fide area of nutrition, including the controversial, are welcome.

We welcome the contribution *Vegetables, Fruits, and Herbs in Health Promotions*, edited by Ronald R. Watson. There has been a recent explosion of interest in the therapeutic value of vegetables and herbs in our diet. This book brings together experts writing on very timely subjects. As such, it furthers our appreciation of the benefits of vegetables and some herbs in our diets in health promotion.

Preface

Diet and nutrition are vital keys to controlling morbidity and mortality from chronic diseases affecting humankind. The multitude of biomolecules in dietary vegetables play a crucial role in health maintenance. They should be more effective than a few nutrients in supplements. For decades, it has been appreciated that oxidative pathways can lead to tissue damage and contribute to pathology. Fortunately, nature has provided us with mechanisms found predominately in plants to defend against such injury. Antioxidant nutritional agents have consequently attracted major attention and rightfully deserve to be studied carefully for possible beneficial roles. One of the main reasons for the interest in antioxidant agents in dietary vegetables, and their products, is their virtually complete lack of harmful side effects. This stands in stark contrast to many drugs that are promoted and studied for possible disease-preventive activity.

The subject of foods and nutritional agents in disease prevention is often associated with strong emotional responses. How could agents that have a near absence of any side effects be health promoting in patients with disease or cancer? Studies have been conducted by respected scientists in a number of important disease entities, ranging from cancer and heart disease to eye disease. These have included general health maintenance such as infection prevention in the elderly.

The long-recognized role of vegetables in cancer prevention is expanded with the understanding of carcinogenesis. Constituents with anticancer activities, phytochemicals, are described in prevention. Bioavailability of important constituents plays a key role in their effectiveness. Their role as well as that of whole vegetables in gastrointestinal disease, heart disease, and old age are defined. Each vegetable contains thousands of different biomolecules, each with the potential to promote health or retard disease and cancer. By use of vegetable extracts as well as increased consumption of whole plants, people can dramatically expand their exposure to protective chemicals and thus readily reduce their risk of multiple diseases. Specific foods, tomatoes, raw vegetables, and Japanese vegetables and byproducts are novel biomedicines with expanded understanding and use. Damage due to UV irradiation is the major cause of skin cancer and skin damage in most American adults. Herbal and dietary vegetables are becoming better understood and are now used in prevention of skin damage and cancer, as well as for eye disease. While vegetables and their products are readily available, there are important legal questions relating to marketing of foods with health claims. Use of specific dietary materials has reduced disease for centuries and a prime example, the Mediterranean diet, is described along with a developing understanding of its mechanisms of action. Use of vegetables and their specific constituents is the most readily available approach to health promotion in the hands of the general public.

The National Cancer Institute reports that only 18% of adults meet the recommended intake of vegetables. While Americans eat 4.1 portions of vegetables, approaching the desired 5 portions per day, much of this is peeled potatoes with little nutritional or biological benefits. Unfortunately, 40%, rather than 25%, of calories come from fat and sugar added to foods. Increased vegetable consumption and use of their extracts should dramatically reduce major dietary risk factors for cancer and heart disease. Thus, greater consumption of a variety of vegetables and fruits will lower use of meat, margarine, sugar, and fat. A better understanding of the role of vegetables and fruits in health promotion will encourage research for altered lifestyles, thus decreasing disease and cancer while lengthening longevity.

Editor

Ronald R. Watson, Ph.D., has edited 50 books, including 22 on the effects of various dietary nutrients in adults, the elderly, and AIDS patients. He initiated and directed the Specialized Alcohol Research Center at the University of Arizona College of Medicine for 6 years. The main theme of this National Institute of Alcohol Abuse and Alcoholism (NIAAA) Center grant was to understand the role of ethanol-induced immunosuppression with increased oxidation and nutrient loss on disease and disease resistance in animals.

Dr. Watson is a member of several national and international societies concerned with nutrition, immunology, and cancer research. He has directed a program studying ways to slow aging using nutritional supplements, funded by the Wallace Genetics Foundation for 22 years. Currently, he is the principal investigator on an NIH grant studying the role of alcohol to exacerbate heart disease in a model of AIDS, including tissue antioxidants. He has recently completed studies on immune restoration and DNA protection in the elderly using extracts of fruits and vegetables. His research group recently completed studies on the use of carotenoids and bioflavonoids to protect skin from ultraviolent irradiation in sunlight.

Dr. Watson attended the University of Idaho, but graduated from Brigham Young University in Provo, UT with a degree in chemistry in 1966. He completed his Ph.D. degree in 1971 in biochemistry at Michigan State University. His postdoctoral education was completed at the Harvard School of Public Health in Nutrition and Microbiology, including a two-year postdoctoral research experience in immunology. He was Assistant Professor of Immunology and did research at the University of Mississippi Medical Center in Jackson from 1973 to 1974. He was an Assistant Professor of Microbiology and Immunology at the Indiana University Medical School from 1974 to 1978 and an Associate Professor at Purdue University in the Department of Food and Nutrition from 1978 to 1982. In 1982, he joined the faculty at the University of Arizona in the Department of Family and Community Medicine. He is also a research professor in the University of Arizona's newly formed College of Public Health. He has published 450 research papers and review chapters.

Contributors

James W. Anderson
Dept. of Medical Services
VA Medical Center
Lexington, KY

Michael Roland Clemens
Medizinische Abteilung I
Krankenänstalt Mutterhaus
der Borromaerinnen
Trier, Germany

Winston J. Craig
Professor of Nutrition
Andrews University
Berrien Springs, MI

Cindy D. Davis
USDA
Grand Forks Human Nutrition
Research Institute
Grand Forks, ND

Hubert T. Greenway
Scripps Clinic
La Jolla, CA

Iman A. Hakim
Research Asst. Professor
University of Arizona
Tucson, AZ

Tammy J. Hanna
Dept. of Medical Services
VA Medical Center
Lexington, KY

Tuneo Hasegawa
Professor
Grad. School of Health
and Welfare
Yamaguchi Prefectural University
Yamaguchi, Japan

Ingrid Hoffmann
Institute/Ernaehrungswissenschaft
Giessen, Germany

Bronwyn G. Hughes
Dept. of Microbiology
Brigham Young University
Provo, UT

Paul M. Hyman
Hyman, Phelps, & McNamara
Washington, D.C.

Walt Jones
Pure-Gar
Chatsworth, CA

Marge Leahy
Ocean Spray Cranberries
Lakeville, MA

Jeongmin Lee
College of Public Health
University of Arizona
Tucson, AZ

Claus Leitzmann
Professor of Nutrition
Institute/Ernaehrungswissenschaft
Giessen, Germany

Kimberly A. Moore
Dept. of Medical Services
VA Medical Center
Lexington, KY

Satoru Moriguchi
Professor
Grad. School of Health
and Welfare
Yamaguchi Prefectural University
Yamaguchi, Japan

Byron K. Murray
Dept. of Microbiology
Brigham Young University
Provo, UT

Kim L. O'Neill
Dept. of Microbiology
Brigham Young University
Provo, UT

Piergiorgio Pietta
ITBA-CAN
Segrate, Italy

Marisa Porrini
Dept. of Food Science
and Technology
Division of Human Nutrition
University of Milan
Milan, Italy

Steven G. Pratt
Scripps Memorial Hospital
La Jolla, CA

B.S. Ramakrishna
Dept. of Medicine
Salmaniya Medical Center
Manama, Bahrain

Patrizia Riso
Dept. of Food Science
and Technology
Division of Human Nutrition
University of Milan
Milan, Italy

Belinda M. Smith
Dept. of Medical Services
VA Medical Center
Lexington, KY

Stephen W. Standage
Dept. of Microbiology
Brigham Young University
Provo, UT

Martin Starr
Ocean Spray Cranberries
Lakeville, MA

Tomoko Taka
Professor
Grad. School of Health
and Welfare
Yamaguchi Prefectural University
Yamaguchi, Japan

Etor E. K. Takyi
Nutrition Unit
Noguchi Memorial Institute
for Medical Research
University of Ghana
Legon, Ghana

Ali Reza Waladkhani
Medizinische Abteilung I
Krankenänstalt Mutterhaus
der Borromaerinnen
Trier, Germany

Ronald R. Watson
College of Public Health
University of Arizona
Tucson, AZ

John A. Wise
Natural Alternatives, International
San Marcos, CA

Yuko Yamamoto
Professor
Grad. School of Health
and Welfare
Yamaguchi Prefectural University
Yamaguchi, Japan

Acknowledgments

This work is the result of research by Ronald Ross Watson over many years studying the effects of nutrient mixtures, hormones, and plant extracts on immune functions. These studies have been graciously supported by the Wallace Genetics Foundation, Inc. In addition, recent studies using extracts of fruit and vegetables to restore immune functions were supported by NSA and Natural Alternatives International, increasing interest in editing the literature. The editorial office and functions were supported by donations from Ross Laboratories, Henkel Corporation, and NSA, with encouragement and support from Dr. Robert Hesslink, Dr. Steven Wood, and Dr. Richard Staack. These contributions were vital to the editorial efforts and eventual completion of this book and are much appreciated. The editorial assistant, Jessica Stant, was key to bringing the book together. All these people and groups contributed critically to the climate of encouragement and excitement about the role of fruits and vegetables in health promotion, leading to this book.

Contents

Section I

Vegetables and Health

1 Effect of Dietary Phytochemicals on Cancer Development

Ali Reza Waladkhani and Michael R. Clemens

CONTENTS

ABSTRACT

Fruits, vegetables, and common beverages as well as several herbs and plants, each having a variety of pharmacological properties, have been shown to be rich sources of microchemicals with the potential to prevent human cancers. Several epidemiological studies have suggested that microchemicals present in our diet could be the most desirable agents for the prevention and/or intervention of human cancer incidence and mortality due to stomach, colon, breast, esophagus, lung, bladder, and prostate cancer. Also, the consumption of vegetables and fruits often is lower in those who subsequently develop cancer. There are many biologically plausible reasons why consumption of plant foods might slow or prevent the appearance of cancer. The specific mechanisms of action of most phytochemicals in cancer prevention are not yet clear, but appear to be varied. Phytochemicals can inhibit carcinogenesis by induction of phase II enzymes and inhibiting phase I enzymes, scavenge DNA reactive agents, suppress the abnormal proliferation of early preneoplastic lesions, and inhibit certain properties of the cancer cell.

0-8493-0038-X/97/$0.00+$.50

1.1 INTRODUCTION

Fruits, vegetables, and common beverages as well as several herbs and plants with diversified pharmacological properties have been shown to be rich sources of microchemicals with the potential to prevent human cancers.[1,2] About 30 classes of chemicals shown to have cancer-preventive effects that may have practical implications in reducing cancer incidence in human populations have been described.[3] Several epidemiological studies, supported by long-term animal tumor experiments, etc., have suggested that microchemicals present in our diet could be the most desirable agents for the prevention and/or intervention of human cancer incidence and mortality due to stomach, colon, breast, esophagus, lung, bladder, and prostate cancer.[4] Also, a diet rich in fruits and vegetables is associated with reduced risk for a number of common cancers. Food chemists and natural product scientists have identified hundreds of phytochemicals that are being evaluated for the prevention of cancer. These include the presence in plant foods of such potentially anticarcinogenic substances as carotenoids, chlorophyll, flavonoids, indoles, isothiocyanates, polyphenolic compounds, protease inhibitors, sulfides, and terpenes (Table 1.1). The specific mechanisms of action of most phytochemicals in cancer prevention are not yet clear, but appear to be varied. Considering the large number and variety of dietary phytochemicals, their interactive effects on cancer risk may be extremely difficult to understand. Phytochemicals can inhibit carcinogenesis by induction of phase II enzymes while inhibiting phase I enzymes, scavenge DNA reactive agents, suppress the abnormal proliferation of early preneoplastic lesions, and inhibit certain properties of the cancer cell (Figures 1.1 and 1.2).[6,7]

This chapter will help to elucidate the current knowledge on dietary phytochemicals in cancer prevention.

TABLE 1.1
Some Dietary Sources of Phytochemicals[5]

Phytochemical	Food Source
Carotenoids	Apricot, peach, nectarine, orange, broccoli, cabbage, spinach, pea, pumpkin, carrot, tomato
Flavonoids	Green tea, black tea, citrus fruits, onion, broccoli, cherry, wheat, corn, rice, tomatoes, spinach, cabbage, apples, olives, red wine, soy products
Polyphenols	Grapes, strawberry, raspberry, pomegranate, paprika, cabbage, walnut
Protease Inhibitors	Soy bean, oats, wheat, peanut, potato, rice, corn
Sulfide	Cabbage, chives, allium, onion, garlic
Terpenes	Grapefruit, lemon, lime, orange, lavender, mint, celery seed, cherry

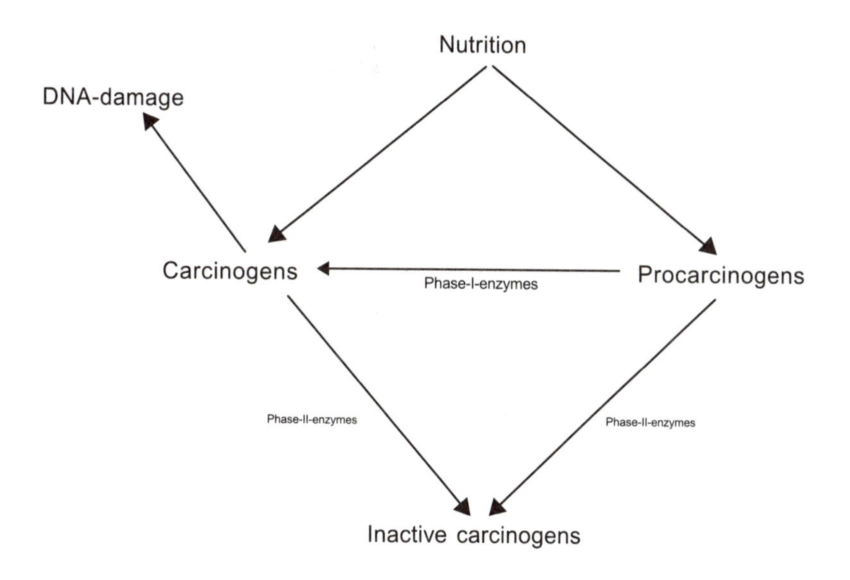

FIGURE 1.1 Effect of phase I and phase II enzymes.[6]

1.2 CAROTENOIDS

Carotenoids are a diverse group of over 600 structurally related compounds synthesized by bacteria and plants. The dietary carotenoids undergo a series of metabolic conversions, extracellularly in the lumen of the intestine and intracellularly in the intestinal mucosa.[8] Many carotenoids have the ability to quench singlet oxygen and thus function as antioxidants. Evolving evidence suggests that carotenoids may modulate processes related to mutagenesis, cell differentiation, and proliferation, independent of their role as antioxidants or precursors of vitamin A.[9,10] They also act on the differentiation and growth control of epithelial cells[11,12] and inhibit 1,2-diglyceride-induced growth and protease secretion.[13] Epidemiological data[14] show that increased consumption of beta carotene-rich foods and higher blood levels of β-carotene are associated with a reduced risk of lung cancer (Table 1.2).

1.3 CHLOROPHYLL

Chlorophyll is the ubiquitous pigment in green plants. Chlorophyllin, the food-grade derivative of chlorophyll, has been used historically in the treatment of several human conditions, with no evidence of human toxicity.[16] The potential carcinogenic activity of chlorophyll is of considerable interest because of its relative abundance in green vegetables widely consumed by humans. Chlorophyll and chlorophyllin have been shown to exert profound antimutagenic behavior against a wide range of potential

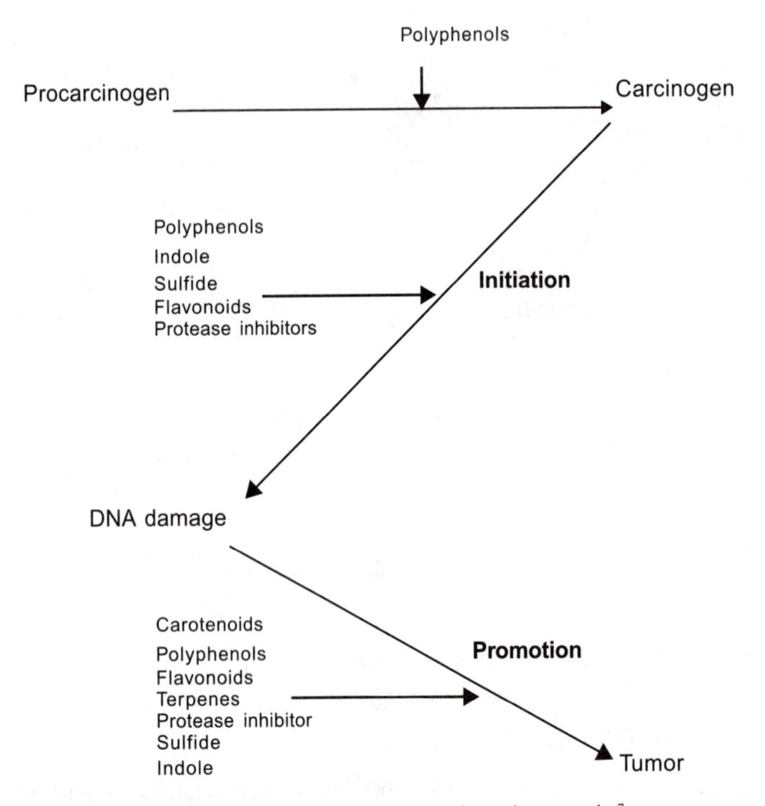

FIGURE 1.2 Relationship between phytochemicals and carcinogenesis.[7]

TABLE 1.2
Biological Behavior of Some Carotenoids[15]

Carotenoid	Anticarcinogenic activity	Inhibition of Lipid peroxidation
β-Carotene	++++	++
Canthaxanthin	++++	+++
Lutein	+	+++
α-Carotene	++	+
Lycopene	+	++

Note: weak = +, middle = ++, strong = +++, very strong = ++++.

human carcinogens.[17,18] In spectrophotometric studies mutagen-inhibitor interaction (molecular complex formation) was identified. *In vivo*, chlorophyllin reduced hepatic aflatoxin B1-DNA adducts and hepatocarcinogenesis when the inhibitor and carcinogen were co-administered in the diet.[19] Also, the formation of a chlorophyllin:aflatoxin B(1) complex reduced systemic aflatoxin B(1) bioavailability.[20] Vibeke et al.[21] indicated that the chlorophyllin dosage required to give an overall protection against aflatoxin B1-induced hepatocarcinogenesis was less than 1500 ppm in animal experiments. By comparison, the reported concentration of chlorophyll in spinach isolates is in the range of 1500 to 600,000 ppm, depending on agronomic conditions.[22]

Further, chlorophyllin possesses free-radical scavenging properties. Recent studies suggest that chlorophyllin effectively protects plasmid DNA against ionizing radiation independent of DNA repair or other cellular defense mechanisms.[23]

Chlorophyll-related compounds pheophytin a and b have been recently identified as antigenotoxic substances in the nonpolyphenolic fraction of green tea.[24] They have potent suppressive activities against tumor promotion in mouse skin.[25]

1.4 FLAVONOIDS

Flavonoids are a group of polyphenolic compounds ubiquitously found in fruits and vegetables. The family includes monomeric flavanols, flavanones, anthocyanidins, flavones, and flavonols. In addition to their free-radical scavenging activity[26] flavonoids have multiple biological activities,[27] including vasodilatory,[28] anticarcinogenic, anti-inflammatory, antibacterial, immune-stimulating, anti-allergic, antiviral, and estrogenic effects, as well as being inhibitors of phospholipase A2, cyclooxygenase, lipoxygenase,[27,29,30] glutathione reductase,[32] and xanthine oxidase.[32]

Flavonoids are known to be good transition metal chelators; most lipid peroxidation inhibition assays measure a combination of transition metal (usually iron) chelation and radical scavenging. In animal experiments cyanidanol-3 led to a strong inhibition of lipid peroxidation.[33] Also, some flavonoids might regenerate the reducing agent, ascorbate.[34]

Increased levels of estrogens in blood and urine are high-risk markers for breast cancer.[35,36] In a large, prospective, case-control study there was a significant relationship between serum estrogen levels and the risk for breast cancer in women in New York.[36] Goldin et al.[37] reported 44% lower blood levels of estrogen and androgens in Asian women who emigrated to the U.S. from areas of low breast cancer risk, when compared to Caucasian Americans, who have a higher risk for breast cancer. Another studies indicated a 36% lower plasma estrogen level in women in rural China when compared to women in Britain, where breast cancer is more common.[38] Among premenopausal women in Singapore, breast cancer risk was inversely related to soy protein intake.[39] These epidemiological observations are supported by results of animal studies. Also, soy feeding is protective against experimentally induced mammary and other organ cancers.[40] Soy contains significant amounts of the isoflavones daidezein and genistein.[41] They may act as antiestrogens by competing with endogenous estrogens for receptor binding, and this may reduce estrogen-induced stimulation of breast cell proliferation[42] and breast tumor formation (Table 1.3).

TABLE 1.3
Some Dietary Sources of Flavonoids[43]

Flavonoid	Food Source
Flavanol	
Epicatechin	
Catechin	
Epigallocatechin	Green and black teas
Epicatechin gallate	Red wine
Epigallocatechin	
Flavanone	
Naringin	Peel of citrus fruits
Taxifolin	Citrus fruits
Flavonol	
Kaempferol	Endive, leek, broccoli, radish, grapefruit, black tea,
Quercetin	onion, lettuce, broccoli, cranberry, apple skin, berries, olive, tea, red wine
Myricetin	Cranberry, grapes, red wine
Flavone	
Chrysin	Fruit skin
Apigenin	Celery, parsley
Anthocyanidins	
Malvidin	Red grapes, red wine
Cyanidin	Cherry, raspberry, strawberry, grapes
Apigenidin	Colored fruit and peels
Phenyl propanoids	
Ferulic acid	Wheat, corn, rice, tomatoes, spinach, cabbage, asparagus
Caffeic acid	White grapes, white wine, olives, olive oil, spinach, cabbage, asparagus, coffee
β-Coumaric acid	White grapes, white wine, tomatoes, spinach, cabbage, asparagus
Chlorogenic acid	Apples, pears, cherries, plums, peaches, apricots, blueberries, tomatoes, anise

1.5 INDOLES

In ancient times, cruciferous vegetables were cultivated primarily for medicinal purposes.[44] The biologically active compound is glucobrassicin, a secondary plant metabolite that is abundant in cruciferous vegetables.[45] Glucobrassicin undergoes autolysis during maceration to indole-3-carbinol, which is known to undergo acid-condensation in the stomach following ingestion. Incubation of indole-3-carbinol under conditions that mimic the acid conditions in the stomach results in the production of multimeric derivatives of indole-3-carbinol.[46] *In vitro* acid-condensation of indol-3-carbinol may include cyclic and noncyclic tetramers, pentamers, and hexamers.[47,48]

Rabbits fed on cabbage leaves survived a lethal dose of uranium.[49] A series of 3-substituted indoles: indole-3-carbinol, 3-indoleacetonitrile, and 3,3'-diindolylmethane, are inhibitors of induced cancer.[50] Animals fed diets high in cruciferous vegetables and then exposed to various carcinogens expressed lower tumor yields and increased survival rates.[51,52] Indole-3-carbinol administration is known to induce cytochrome P450 and glutathione *S*-transferase activities, resulting in increased metabolic capacity toward chemical carcinogens.[53] These properties of indole-3-carbinol are considered to contribute to the known anticarcinogenic properties of this compound, as well as to the reduced risk of cancer associated with diets rich in cruciferous vegetables.[54] Evidence from an epidemiological case-control study of diet and cancer also suggested that consumption of cruciferous vegetables are associated with a decreased incidence of cancer.[55]

Oligomeric acid-condensation derivatives of indol-3-carbinol inhibit P-glycoprotein-mediated cellular efflux by acting as competetive inhibitors of the pump by overloading its capacity to transport cytotoxic therapeutic agents from the cell.[56] So, inhibition of P-glycoprotein transport results in an increase in cellular accumulation of cytotoxic chemotherapeutic agents, thus increasing the efficacy of these agents.

1.6 ISOTHIOCYANATES

Organic isothiocyanates are widely distributed in plants. In addition to their characteristic flavors and odors, isothiocyanates have a variety of other pharmacological and toxic activities. Gluconasturtiin is a common isothiocyanate. Upon chewing of watercress, gluconasturtiin is hydrolyzed to phenylethyl isothiocyanate. It is responsible for the sharp taste of this vegetable. The consumption of 30 g of watercress will release a minimum of 2–5 mg of phenylethyl isothiocyanate (PEITC).[57] In smokers the consumption of watercress increases urinary excretion of NNK (4-methylnitrosamino-1-3-pyridyl-1-butanone) metabolites.[58] NNK is a potent pulmonary carcinogen in rodents. It is believed to be one of the causes of lung cancer in smokers.[59] NNK requires metabolic activation by α-hydroxylation to express its carcinogenic activity. The metabolic activation of NNK generates reactive intermediates that form a variety of DNA adducts that are involved in carcinogenesis. Inhibition of the α-hydroxylation pathways and other oxidative metabolic pathways of NNK by PEITC cause increased excretion of metabolites in urine.[58] Dietary administration of nontoxic doses of PEITC decreases NNK metabolic activation and lung tumor induction.[60] Recent studies indicate that dietary isothiocyanates have remarkable chemopreventive efficacy in the N'-nitrosonornicotine-induced esophageal tumor model.[61]

1.7 POLYPHENOLIC COMPOUNDS

The polyphenolic components of higher plants may act as antioxidants or as agents of other mechanisms contributing to anticarcinogenic or cardioprotective action.[43] Ellagic acid, a polyphenol generated from ellagitannins, is a most promising chemopreventive for reduction of risk of human cancers and it could potentially be introduced in human intervention trials.[62] Studies of the mechanism of action of ellagic acid have concluded that it could inhibit phase I enzymes involved in the activation of procarcinogens.[63] Ellagic acid induces hepatic glutathione *S*-transferase, a phase

II enzyme responsible for the detoxification of some carcinogen-generated electrophiles.[64] Ellagic acid may also scavenge oxygen radicals involved in oxidative destruction of membrane lipids and involved in tumor promotion.[65] Studies have shown that green tea affords cancer chemopreventive effects in a variety of animal model systems.[66] Green tea polyphenols have also been demonstrated to inhibit ornithine decarboxylase induction caused by tumor promoters in mouse skin and other tissues.[67,68] Epigallocatechin gallate (EGCG) is extracted from the leaves of the plant *Camellia sinensis*. A heavy drinker of green tea may consume 1 g/day.[69] EGCG, at 1 to 10 μM, reduced inflammation-induced generation of mutagenic peroxynitrite radicals and nitrite.[70] Two epidemiological studies indicate that people who consume tea regularly may have a decreased risk of prostate cancer.[71] EGCG has been shown to cause growth inhibition and regression of human prostate and breast tumors in athymic nude mice.[72]

Curcumin is a phenolic compound widely used as a spice and coloring agent in food. Curcumin possesses potent antioxidant, anti-inflammatory, and antitumor promoting activities. Previous studies have shown that topical application of curcumin inhibits TPA (12-*o*-tetradecanoylphorbol-13-acetate) epidermal DNA synthesis, tumor promotion in mouse skin, and edema of mouse ears.[73] In mice, dietary administration of 5000 to 20,000 ppm curcumin reduced the incidence of intestinal tumors.[74] Further, curcumin induced apoptotic cell death in promyelocytic leukemia HL-60 cells at concentrations as low as 3.5 μg/ml;[75] recent studies demonstrated an inhibitory effect of dietary curcumin when administered continuously during the initiation and postinitiation phases.[76,77] Administration of curcumin may retard growth and/or development of existing neoplastic lesions in the colon.[76]

1.8 PROTEASE INHIBITORS

A variety of studies have made it clear that protease inhibitors (PI) can inhibit transformation *in vitro*, as well as development of both benign and malignant lesions *in vivo*.[78,79] The content of two prominent PI (Bowman-Birk inhibitor BBI and Kunitz trypsin inhibitor KTI) varies considerably with species of soy,[80] and PI content of several soy protein isolates can vary by as much as 20-fold. In many models, dietary administration of exogenous PI is effective in reducing cancer incidence.[78,79] Also, their ability to diminish the occurrence of a variety of cancers in organs where the inhibitor is not present points to an indirect role for PI.[79] Recent studies indicate that BBI and BBI concentrate prevent and suppress malignant transformation *in vitro* and carcinogenesis *in vivo*, without toxicity.[81] Further, BBI concentrate could be a useful agent for the potentiation of radiation- and cisplatin-mediated cancer treatment without significant adverse effects on surrounding normal tissues.[82]

A number of clinically important PI are found in serum, including α2-protease inhibitor, α2-macroglobulin, α1-antichymotrypsin, α1-acid glycoprotein, etc. Many of these PI are referred to as acute-phase reactants and are active against serine proteinases.[83] Other potentially important effects of dietary PI may occur via hormonal modulation and inactivation of trypsin and chymotrypsin in the duodenum. For example, potato carboxypeptidase inhibitor is an antagonist of human epidermal growth factor. It competed with epidermal growth factor for binding to epidermal growth factor receptor and inhibited EGFR activation and cell proliferation induced by this growth factor. Potato carboxypeptidase inhibitor suppressed the growth of several human pancreatic adenocarcinoma cell lines, both *in vitro* and in nude mice.[84] A number of studies have documented, for instance, that dietary PI stimulates secretion of pancreatic enzymes, presumably via modulation of cholecystokinin levels.[85] Cholecystokinin release is of additional interest because cholecystokinin acts as a cocarcinogen in various models.[86]

Among other effects, PI block release of oxygen radicals and H_2O_2 from polymorphonuclear leukocytes and activated macrophages,[87] which may protect DNA from oxidative damage or from single-strand breaks. Hydroxyl radicals also appear to be involved.[88] Further, PI inhibit influx of polymorphonuclear leukocytes.[87]

1.9 SULFIDES

Sulfides have been shown to inhibit a variety of tumors induced by chemical carcinogenesis. In rat liver, supernatant ajoene and diallyl sulfide affected aflatoxin B1 metabolism and DNA binding by inhibiting phase I enzymes, and may therefore be considered as potential cancer chemopreventive agents.[89] In mice the oral application of diallyl sulfide suppressed the activity of ornithine decarboxylase.[90] In the murine model, topical application of diallyl sulfide and diallyl disulfide (DAS), oil-soluble constituents of garlic and onions, significantly inhibited skin papilloma formation from the ninth week of promotion and significantly increased the rate of survival.[91]

Animal studies indicate that dietary intake of DAS has chemopreventive potential during the time corresponding to the initiation phase on 2-amino-1-methyl-6-phenylimidazo[4,5-b]pyridine-induced mammary carcinogenesis.[92] Upon examining specific P450 enzymes, the 7-pentoxyresorufin-*O*-dealkylase (PROD) activity, which was low in untreated rat liver microsomes, was greatly increased by DAS, reaching a plateau of 100-fold increase at 24 to 48 h. Subsequent studies indicated that this increase in PROD activity was due to the induction of the CYP 2B1 gene at the transcriptional level.[93] On the other hand, the P450 2E1-dependent *N*-nitrosodimethylamine demethylase activity was lowest (20% of the control) at 15 h and gradually returned to the control level after 2 days. DAS has also been shown to slightly decrease 16β-testosterone hydroxylase activity.[94]

1.10 TERPENES

Monoterpenoids are commonly produced by plants and found in many fruits and vegetables. Pharmacokinetic studies in dogs and rats revealed that oral administration of perillyl alcohol is rapidly absorbed from the gastrointestinal tract and metabolized to perillic acid and dihydroperillic acid.[95,96] Several monoterpenes induce phase II enzymes.[97] With regard to the mode of the chemopreventive action of perillyl alcohol, monoterpenes exhibit a diverse array of metabolic, cellular, and molecular activities, including inhibition of activation of carcinogen metabolism, inhibition of cellular proliferation, and the induction of differentiation and apoptosis.[98,99] Limonene has been studied in animal models as an anticarcinogen.[100] Limonene caused regression of DMBA-induced mammary tumors.[101] Limonene is also capable of inhibiting the development of upper digestive tract carcinomas in *N*-nitrosodiethylamine-treated mice.[102] In humans, the three metabolic derivatives detected in plasma after single oral doses of limonene 100 mg/kg are perillic acid, dihydroperillic acid, and limonene-1,2-diol.[103] The metabolic precursors to perillic acid and dihydroperillic acid are likely perillyl alcohol and perillyl aldehyde, both of which have potent antiproliferative activities in cell culture systems.[104–106] Limonene impairs DNA synthesis in the human-derived myeloid leukemia cell line THP-1 and in the lymphoid leukemia cell line RPMI-8402 in a concentration-dependent manner.[106] In addition, *d*-limonene inhibits carcinogen activation to produce an inhibitory effect in carcinogenesis. Animal studies indicated that *d*-limonene administered in the diet at the 1 to 5% levels inhibited both DMBA- and MNU-induced rat mammary carcinogenesis in female rats.[107]

1.11 CONCLUSION

Review of the epidemiological data, including both cohort and case-control studies of all cancer sites as well as a variety of animal studies, strongly suggest that plant foods have preventive potential and that consumption of vegetables and fruits is lower in those who subsequently develop cancer. Other data suggest that foods high in phytoestrogens are plausibly associated with a lower risk of sex hormone-related cancers.

REFERENCES

1. Boone, C. W., Bacus, J. W., Bacus, J. V., Steele, V. E., and Kelloff, G. J., Properties of intraepithelial neoplasia relevant to the development of cancer chemopreventive agents, *J. Cell Biochem. Suppl.*, 28, 1, 1997.
2. Goodman, G. E., The clinical evaluation of cancer prevention agents, *Proc. Soc. Exp. Biol. Med.*, 216, 253, 1977.
3. Wattenberg, L. W., An overview of chemoprevention: current status and future prospects, *Proc. Soc. Exp. Biol. Med.*, 216, 133, 1997.
4. Ames, B. N., Gold, L. S., and Willett, W. C., The status and prevention of cancer, *Proc. Natl. Acad. Sci. USA*, 92, 5258, 1995.
5. Waladkhani, A. R. and Clemens, M. R., Effect of dietary phytochemicals on cancer development, *Int. J. Mol. Med.*, 1, 747, 1998.
6. Sipes, I. G. and Gandolfi, A. J., Biotransformation of toxicants, in *Toxicology — the Basic Science of Poisons*, Amdur, M. O., Doull, J., and Klassen, C. D., Eds., McGraw-Hill, New York, 1993, 88.
7. Wattenberg, L. W., Chemoprevention of cancer by naturally occurring and synthetic compounds, in *Cancer Chemoprevention*, Wattenberg, L. W., Lipkin, M., Boone, C. W., and Kelloff G. J., Eds., CRC Press, Boca Raton, FL, 1992, 19.
8. Goodman, D. S. and Blaner, W. S., Biosynthesis, absorption, and hepatic metabolism of retinol, in *The Retinoids*. Vol. 2, Sporn, M. B., Roberts, A. B., and Goodman D. S., Eds., Academic Press, Orlando, FL, 1984, 1.
9. Levy, J., Bosin, E., Feldman, B., Giat, Y., Munster, A., Danilenko, M., and Sharoni, Y., Lycopene is a more potent inhibitor of human cancer cell proliferation than either α-carotene or β-carotene, *Nutr. Cancer*, 24, 257, 1995.

10. Matsushima-Nishiwaki, R., Shidoji, Y., Nishiwaki, S., Yamada, T., Moriwaki, H., and Muto, Y., Suppression by carotenoids of microcystin-induced morphological changes in mouse hepatocytes, *Lipids*, 30, 1029, 1995.
11. Phillips, R. W., Kikendall, J. W., Luk, G. D., Willis, S. M., Murphy, J. R., Maydonovitch, C., Bowen, P. E., Stacewicz-Sapuntzakis, M., and Wong, R. K., Beta-carotene inhibits rectal mucosal ornithine decarboxylase activity in colon cancer patients, *Cancer Res.*, 53, 3723, 1993.
12. Sporn, M. B. and Roberts, A. B., Role of retinoids in differentiation and carcinogenesis, *Cancer Res.*, 43, 3034, 1983.
13. Kahl-Rainer, P. and Marian, B., Retinoids inhibit protein kinase C-dependent transduction of 1,2-diglyceride signals in human colonic tumor cells, *Nutr. Cancer*, 21, 157, 1994.
14. Ziegler, R. G., Mayne, S. T., and Swanson, C. A., Nutrition and lung cancer, *Cancer Cause Control*, 7, 157, 1996.
15. Wolf, G., Retinoids and carotenoids as inhibitors of carcinogenesis and inducers of cell-cell communication, *Nutr. Rev.*, 50, 270, 1992.
16. Young, R. W. and Beregi J. S., Use of chlorophyllin in the care of geriatric patients, *J. Am. Geriatr. Soc.*, 28, 48, 1980.
17. Lai, C., Butler, M. A., and Matney, T. S., Antimutagenic activities of common vegetables and their chlorophyll content, *Mutat. Res.*, 77, 245, 1980.
18. Negishi, T., Arimoto, S., Nishizaki, C., and Hayatsu, H., Inhibitory effect of chlorophyll on the genotoxicity of 3-amino-1-methyl-5H-pyrido[4,3-b]indole (Trp-P-2), *Carcinogen*, 10, 145, 1989.
19. Dashwood, R., Negishi, T., Hayatsu, H., Breinholt, V., Hendricks, J., and Bailey, G., Chemopreventive properties of chlorophylls towards aflatoxin B1: a review of the antimutagenicity and anticarcinogenicity data in rainbow trout, *Mutat. Res.*, 399(2), 245, 1998.
20. Breinholt, V., Arbogast, D., Loveland, P., Pereira, C., Dashwood, R., Hendricks, J., and Bailey, G., Chlorophyllin chemoprevention in trout initiated by aflatoxin B(1) bath treatment: An evaluation of reduced bioavailability vs. target organ protective mechanisms, *Toxicol. Appl. Pharmacol.*, 158(2), 141, 1999.
21. Vibeke, B., Hendricks, J., Pereira, C., Arbogast, D., and Bailey, G., Dietary choloro-phyllin is a potent inhibitor of aflatoxin B1 hepatocarcinogenesis in Rainbow Trout, *Cancer Res.*, 55, 57, 1995.
22. Khalyfa, A., Kermasha, S., and Alli, I., Extraction, purification and characterization of chlorophyll from spinach leaves, *J. Agric. Food Chem.*, 40, 215, 1992.
23. Kumar, S. S., Chaubey, R. C., Devasagayam, T. P., Priyadarsini, K. I., and Chauhan, P. S., Inhibition of radiation-induced DNA damage in plasmid pBR322 by chlorophyllin and possible mechanism(s) of action, *Mutat. Res.*, 425(1), 71, 1999.
24. Okai, Y. and Higashi-Okai, K., Potent suppressing activity of the nonpolyphenolic fraction of green tea (*Camellia sinensis*) against genotoxin-induced umu C gene expression in *Salmonella typhimurium* (TA 1535/pSK 1002)--association with pheophytins a and b, *Cancer Lett.*, 120(1),117, 1997.
25. Higashi-Okai, K., Otani, S., and Okai, Y., Potent suppressive activity of pheophytin a and b from the non-polyphenolic fraction of green tea (*Camellia sinensis*) against tumor promotion in mouse skin, *Cancer Lett.*, 129(2), 223, 1998.
26. Kandaswami, C. and Middleton, E., Free radical scavenging and antioxidant activity of plant flavonoids, *Adv. Exp. Med. Biol.*, 366, 351, 1994.
27. Ho, C. T., Chen, Q., Shi, H., Zhang, K. Q., and Rosen, R. T., Antioxidative effect of polyphenol extract prepared from various Chinese teas, *Prev. Med.*, 21, 520, 1992.

28. Duarte, J., Perez-Vizcainom, F., Utrilla, P., Jimenez, J., Tanargo, J., and Zarzuelo, A., Vasodilatory effects of flavanoids in rat aortic smooth muscle. Structure-activity relationships, *Gen. Pharmacol.*, 24, 857, 1993.
29. Middleton, E. and Kandaswami, C., Effects of flavonoids on immune and inflammatory functions, *Biochem. Pharmacol.*, 43, 1167, 1992.
30. Lindahl, M. and Tagesson, C., Selective inhibition of groups by phospholipase A2 by quercetin, *Inflammation*, 17, 573, 1993.
31. Elliot, A. J., Scheiber, S. A., Thomas, C., and Pardini R. S., Inhibition of glutathione reductase by flavonoids. A structure-activity study, *Biochem. Pharmacol.*, 44, 1603, 1992.
32. Chang, W. S., Lee, Y. J., Lu, F. J., and Chiang, H. C., Inhibitory effects of flavonoids on xanthine oxidase, *Anticancer Res.*, 13, 2165, 1993.
33. Clemens, M. R. and Remmer, A., Volatile alkanes produced by erythrocytes: an assay for in vitro studies on lipid peroxidation, *Blut*, 45, 329, 1982.
34. Van Acker, S. A. B. E., van den Berg, D. J., Tromp, M. N. J. L., Griffioen, D. H., van Bennekom, W. P., van der Vijgh, W. J. F., and Bast, A., Structural aspects of antioxidant activity of flavonoids, *Free Rad. Biol. Med.*, 20, 331, 1996.
35. Bernstein, L., Yuan, J. M., Ross, R. K., Pike, M. C., Hanisch, R., Lobo, R., Stanczyk, F., Gao, Y. T., and Henderson, B. E., Serum hormone levels in premenopausal Chinese women in Shanghai and white women in Los Angeles: results from two breast cancer case-control studies, *Cancer Cause Control*, 1, 51, 1990.
36. Toniolo, P. G., Levitz, M., Zeleniuch-Jacquotte, A., Banerjee, S., Koenig, K., Shore, R. E., Strax, P., and Pasternack, B. S., A protective study of endogenous estrogens and breast cancer in postmenopausal women, *J. Natl. Cancer Inst.*, 87, 190, 1995.
37. Goldin, B. R., Adlercreutz, H., Gorbach, S. L., Woods, M. N., Dwyer, J. T., Conlon, T., Bohn, E., and Gershoff, S. N., The relationship between estrogen levels and diets of Caucasian American and Oriental immigrant women, *Am. J. Clin. Nutr.*, 44, 945, 1986.
38. Key, T. J. A., Chen, J., Wang, D. Y., Pike, M. C., and Boreham, J., Sex hormones in women in rural China and in Britain, *Br. J. Cancer*, 62, 631, 1990.
39. Lee, H. P., Gourley, L., Duffy, S. W., Esteve, J., Lee, J., and Day, N. E., Risk factors for breast cancer by age and menopausal status: a case-control study in Singapore, *Cancer Cause Control*, 3, 313, 1992.
40. Messina, M. J., Persky, V., Setchell, K. D. R., and Barnes, S., Soy intake and cancer risk: a review of the in vitro and in vivo data, *Nutr. Cancer*, 21, 113, 1994.
41. Price, K. R. and Fenwick, G. R., Naturally occurring oestrogens in foods: a review, *Food Addit. Contam.*, 2, 73, 1985.
42. Martin, P. M., Horwitz, K. B., Ryan, D. S., and McGuire, W. L., Phytoestrogen interaction with estrogen receptors in human breast cancer, *Endocrinology*, 103, 1860, 1978.
43. Rice-Evans, C. A., Miller, N. J., and Paganga, G., Structure-antioxidant activity relationships of flavonoids and phenolic acids, *Free Rad. Biol. Med.*, 20(7), 933, 1996.
44. Fenwick, G. R., Heaney, R. K., and Mullin, W. J., Glucosinolates and their breakdown products in food and food plants, *Crit. Rev. Food Sci. Nutr.*, 18, 123, 1983.
45. McDanell, R., McLean, A. E. M., Hanley, A. B., Heaney, R. K., and Fenwick, G. R., Chemical and biological of indole glucosinates (glucobrassicins): a review, *Food Chem. Toxicol.*, 26, 59, 1986.
46. DeKruif, C. A., Marsman, J. W., Venekamp, J. C., Falke H. E., Noordhoek, J., Blaauboer, B. J., and Wortelboer, H. W., Structure elucidation of acid reaction products of indole-3-carbinol: detection in vivo and enzyme induction in vivo, *Chem. Biol. Interact.*, 80, 303, 1991.

47. Bradfield, C. A. and Bjeldanes, L. F., High performance liquid chromatographic analysis of anticarcinogenic indoles in Brassica oleracea, *J. Agric. Food Chem.*, 35, 46, 1987.
48. Dunn, S. E. and LeBlanc, G. A., Hypochlosterolemic properties of plant indoles, *Biochem. Pharmacol.*, 47, 359, 1994.
49. Eisner, G., Über die lebensrettende Wirkung von Pflanzenteilen und daraus isolierten Säften bei der tödlich verlaufenden, subakuten Uranvergiftung, *Biochem. Z.*, 232, 218, 1931.
50. Bradfield, C. A. and Bjeldanes, L. F., Structure-activity relationships of dietary indoles. A proposed mechanism of action modifiers of xenobiotic metabolism, *J. Toxicol. Environ. Hlth.*, 21, 311, 1987.
51. Boy, J. N., Babish, J. G., and Stoewsand, G. S., Modification by beet and cabbage diets of aflatoxin B1-induced rat plasma α-foetoprotein elevation, hepatic tumorigenesis, and mutagenicity of urine, *Food Chem. Toxicol.*, 20, 47, 1982.
52. Wattenberg, L. W., Inhibition of neoplasia by minor dietary constituents, *Cancer Res.*, 43, 2448s, 1983.
53. Morse, M. A., LaGreca, S. D., Amin, S. G., and Chung, F. L., Effects of indole-3-carbinol on lung tumorigenesis and DANN methylation induced by 4-(methylnitrosamino)-1-butanone (NNK) and on the metabolism and disposition of NNK in A/J mice, *Cancer Res.*, 50, 1613, 1990.
54. Marchand, L. L., Yoshizawa, C. N., Kolonel, L. N., Hankin, J. H., and Goodman, M. T., Vegetable consumption and lung cancer risk: a population based case-control study in Hawaii, *J. Natl. Cancer Inst.*, 81, 1158, 1989.
55. Graham, S., Results of case-control studies of diet and cancer in Buffalo, NY, *Cancer Res.*, 43, 2409s, 1983.
56. Christensen, J. G. and LeBlanc, G. A., Reversal of multidrug resistance in vivo by dietary administration of the phytochemical indole-3-carbinol, *Cancer Res.*, 56, 574, 1996.
57. Chung, F. L., Morse, M. A., Eklind, K. I., and Lewis, J., Quantitation of human uptake of the anticarcinogen phenethyl isothiocyanate after a watercress meal, *Cancer Epidemiol. Biomark. Prev.*, 1, 383, 1992.
58. Hecht, S. S., Chemoprevention by isothiocyanates, *J. Cell Biochem.*, 22, 195, 1995.
59. Hecht, S. S. and Hoffmann, D., The relevance of tobacco-specific nitrosamines to human cancer, *Cancer Surv.*, 8, 273, 1989.
60. Morse, M. A., Amin, S. G., Hecht, S. S., and Chung, F. L., Effects of aromatic isothiocyanates on tumorigenicity. O-methylguanine formation, and metabolism of the tobacco-specific nitrosamine 4-(methylnitrosamino)-1-(3-pyridyl)-1-butanone in A/J mouse lung, *Cancer Res.*, 49, 2894, 1989.
61. Stoner, G. D., Adams, C., Kresty, L. A., Amin, S. G., Desai, D., Hecht, S. S., Murphy, S. E., and Morse, M. A., Inhibition of N'-nitrosonornicotine-induced esophageal tumorigenesis by 3-phenylpropyl isothiocyanate, *Carcinogen*, 19(12), 2139, 1998.
62. Kelloff, G. J., Malone, W. F., Boone, C. W., Sigman, C. C., and Fay, J. R., Progress in applied chemoprevention research, *Semin. Oncol.*, 17, 438, 1990.
63. Mandal, S., Shivapurkar, N. M., Galati, A. J., and Stoner, G. D., Inhibition of N-nitrosobenzylmethylamine metabolism and DANN binding in cultured rat esophagus by ellagic acid, *Carcinogen*, 9, 1313, 1988.
64. Das, M., Bickers, D. R., and Mukhtar, H., Effect of ellagic acid on hepatic and pulmonary xenobiotic metabolism in mice: studies on the mechanism of its anticarcinogenic action, *Carcinogen*, 6, 1409, 1985.
65. Osawa, T., Die, A., Su, J. D., and Namiki, M., Inhibition of lipid peroxidation by ellagic acid, *J. Agric. Food Chem.*, 35, 808, 1987.

66. Yang, G., Liao, J., Kim, K., Yurkow, E. J., and Yang, C. S., Inhibition of growth and induction of apoptosis in human cancer cell lines by tea polyphenols, *Carcinogen*, 19, 611, 1998.
67. Hu, G., Han, C., and Chen J., Inhibition of oncogene expression by green tea and (-)-epigallocatechin gallate in mice, *Nutr. Cancer*, 24, 203, 1995.
68. Yamane, T., Takahashi, T., Kuwata, K., Oya, K., Inagakme, M., Kitao, Y., Suganuma, M., and Fujiki, H., Inhibition of N-methyl-N-nitrosogaunidine-induced carcinogenesis by (-)-epigallocatechin gallate in the rat glandular stomach, *Cancer Res.*, 55, 2081, 1995.
69. WHO International Agency for Research on Cancer, Tea. IARC Monogr., *Evalu. Carcinog. Risks Hum.*, 51, 207, 1991.
70. Chan, M. M. Y., Ho, C. T., and Huang, H. I., Effects of three dietary phytochemicals from tea, rosemary, and tumeric on inflammation-induced nitrite production, *Cancer Lett.*, 96, 23, 1995.
71. Kinlen, L. J., Willows, A. N., Goldblatt, P., and Yudkin, J., Tea consumption and cancer, *Br. J. Cancer*, 58, 397, 1988.
72. Liao, S., Umekita, Y., Guo, J., Kokontis, J. M., and Hiipakka, R. A., Growth inhibition and regression of human prostate and breast tumors in athymic mice by tea epigallocatechin gallate, *Cancer Lett.*, 96, 239, 1995.
73. Huang, M. T., Lysz, T., Ferraro, T., Abidi, T. F., Laskin, J. D., and Conney, A. H., Inhibitory effects of curcumin on in vitro lipoxygenase and cyclooxygenase activities in mouse epidermis, *Cancer Res.*, 51, 813, 1991.
74. Huang, M. T., Lou, Y. R., Ma, W., Newmark, H., Reuhl, K., and Conney, A. H., Inhibitory effect of dietary curcumin on forestomach, duodenal, and colon carcinogenesis in mice, *Cancer Res.*, 54(22), 5841, 1994.
75. Kuo, M. L., Huang, T. S., and Lin, J. K., Curcumin, an antioxidant and anti-tumor promoter, induces apoptosis in human leukemia cells, *Biochim. Biophys. Acta*, 1317(2), 95, 1996.
76. Kawamori, T., Lubet, R., Steele, V. E., Kelloff, G. J., Kaskey, R. B., and Rao, C. V., Chemopreventive effect of curcumin, a naturally occurring anti-inflammatory agent, during the promotion/progression stages of colon cancer, *Cancer Res.*, 59, 597, 1999.
77. Pereira, M. A., Grubbs, D. J., Barnes, L. H., Li, H., Olson, G. R., Eto, I., Juliana, M., Whitaker, L. M., Kelloff, G. J., Steele, V. E., and Lubet, R. A., Effects of the phytochemicals, curcumin and quercetin, upon azoxymethane-induced colon cancer and 7,12-dimethylbenz[a]anthracene-induced mammary cancer in rats, *Carcinogen*, 17, 1305, 1996.
78. Kennedy, A., Prevention of carcinogenesis by protease inhibitors, *Cancer Res.*, 54, 1999s, 1994.
79. Troll, W., Frenkel, K., and Wiesner, R., Protease inhibitors as anticarcinogens, *J. Natl. Cancer Inst.*, 73, 1245, 1984.
80. Eldridge, A. and Kwolek, W., Soybean isoflavones: Effect of environment and variety on composition, *J. Agric. Food Chem.*, 31, 394, 1983.
81. Kennedy, A. R., The Bowman-Birk inhibitor from soybeans as an anticarcinogenic agent, *Am. J. Clin. Nutr.*, 68(Suppl. 6), 1406S, 1998.
82. Zhang, L., Wan, X. S., Donahue, J. J., Ware, J. H., and Kennedy, A. R., Effects of the Bowman-Birk inhibitor on clonogenic survival and cisplatin- or radiation-induced cytotoxicity in human breast, cervical, and head and neck cancer cells, *Nutr. Cancer*, 33(2), 165, 1999.
83. Clawson, G. A., Protease inhibitors and carcinogenesis: a review, *Cancer Invest.*, 14(6), 597, 1996.

84. Blanco-Aparicio, C., Molina, M. A., Fernandez-Salas, E., Frazier, M. L., Mas, J. M., Querol, E., Aviles, F. X., and de Llorens, R., Potato carboxypeptidase inhibitor, a T-knot protein, is an epidermal growth factor antagonist that inhibits tumor cell growth, *J. Biol. Chem.*, 273(20), 12370, 1998.
85. Ware, J. H., Wan, X. S., Rubin, H., Schechter, N. M., and Kennedy, A. R., Soybean Bowman-Birk protease inhibitor is a highly effective inhibitor of human mast cell chymase, *Arch. Biochem. Biophys.*, 344(1), 133, 1997.
86. Howatson, A., The potential of cholecystokinin as a carcinogen in the hamster-nitrosamine model, in *Nutritional and Toxicological Significance of Enzyme Inhibitors in Foods*, Friedman, M., Ed., Plenum Press, New York, 1986, 109.
87. Goldstein, B., Witz, G., Amoruso, M., and Troll, W., Protease inhibitors antagonize the activation of polymorphonuclear leukocyte oxygen consumption, *Biochem. Biophys. Res. Commun.*, 88, 854, 1979.
88. Troll, W., Prevention of cancer by agents that suppress oxygen radical formation, *Free Rad. Res. Commun.*, 12-13, 751, 1991.
89. Tadi, P. P., Lau, B. H., Teel, R. W., and Herrmann, C. E., Binding of aflatoxin B1 to DNA inhibited by ajoene and diallyl sulfide, *Anticancer Res.*, 11(6), 2037, 1991.
90. Baer, A. R. and Wargovich, M. J., Role of ornithine decarboxylase in diallyl sulfide inhibition of colonic radiation injury in the mouse, *Cancer Res.*, 49(18), 5073, 1989.
91. Dwivedi, C., Rohlfs, S., Jarvis, D., and Engineer, F. N., Chemoprevention of chemically induced skin tumor development by dially sulfide and diallyl disulfide, *Pharmacolog. Res.*, 9(12), 1668, 1992.
92. Suzui, N., Sugie, S., Rahman, K. M., Ohnishi, M., Yoshimi, N., Wakabayashi, K., and Mori, H., Inhibitory effects of diallyl disulfide or aspirin on 2-amino-1-methyl-6-phenylimidazo[4,5-b]pyridine-induced mammary carcinogenesis in rats, *Jpn. J. Cancer Res.*, 88(8), 705, 1997.
93. Pan, J., Hong, J. Y., Ma, B. L., Ning, S. M., Paranawithana, S. R., and Yang, C. S., Transcriptional activation of P-450 2B1/2 genes in rat liver by diallyl sulfide, a compound derived from garlic, *Arch. Biochem. Biophys.*, 302, 337, 1993.
94. Brady, J. F., Wang, M. H., Hong, J. Y., Xiao, F., Li, Y., Yoo, J. S. H., Ning, S. M., Fukuto, J. M., Gapac, J. M., and Yang, C. S., Modulation of rat hepatic microsomal monooxygenase activities and cytotoxicity by diallyl sulfide, *Toxicol. Appl. Pharmacol.*, 108, 342, 1991.
95. Haag, J. D. and Gould, M. N., Mammary carcinoma regression induced by perillyl alcohol, a hydroxylated analog of limonene, *Cancer Chemother. Pharmacol.*, 34, 477, 1994.
96. Phillips, L. R., Malspeis, L., and Supko, J. G., Pharmacokinetics of active drug metabolites after oral administration of perillyl alcohol, an investigational antineoplastic agent, to the dog, *Drug Metab. Dispos.*, 23, 676, 1995.
97. Zheng, G. Q., Zhang, J., Kenny, P. M., and Lam, L. K. T., Stimulation of glutathione S-transferase and inhibition of carcinogenesis in mice by celery seed oil constituents, in *Food Phytochemicals for Cancer Prevention*, I., Huang, M., Osawa, T., Ho, C., and Rossen, R. T., Eds., American Chemical Society, Washington, D.C., 1994, 230.
98. Mills, J. J., Chari, R. S., Boyer, I. J., Gould, M. N., and Jirtle, R. L., Induction of apoptosis in liver tumors by the monoterpene perillyl alcohol, *Cancer Res.*, 55, 979, 1995.
99. Morse, M. A., and Toburen, A. L., Inhibition of metabolic activation of 4-(methylnitrosamine)-1-(3-pyridyl)-1-butanone by limonene, *Cancer Lett.*, 104, 211, 1996.

100. Elegbede, J. A., Elson, C. E., Quershi, A., Tanner, M. A., and Gould, M. N., Inhibition of DMBA-induced mammary cancer by the monoterpene d-limonene, *Carcinogen*, 5, 661, 1984.
101. Elegbede, J. A., Elson, C. E., Tanner, M. A., Quershi, A., and Gould, M. N., Regression of rat primary mammary tumors following dietary d-limonene, *J. Natl. Cancer Inst.*, 76, 323, 1986.
102. Wattenberg, L. W., Sparnns, V. L., and Barany, G., Inhibition of N-nitrosodiethylamine carcinogenesis in mice by naturally occurring organosulfur compounds and monoterpenes, *Cancer Res.*, 49, 2689, 1989.
103. Crowell, P. J., Elson, C. E., Bailey, H. H., Elegbede, A., Haag, J. D., and Gould, M. N., Human metabolism of the experimental cancer therapeutic agent d-limonene, *Cancer Chemother. Pharmacol.*, 35, 31, 1994.
104. Ruch, R. J. and Sigler, K., Growth inhibition of rat liver epithelial tumor cells does not involve RAS plasma membrane association, *Carcinogen*, 15, 787, 1994.
105. Schulz, S., Buhling, F., and Ansorge, S., Prenylated proteins and lymphocyte proliferation: inhibition by d-limonene and related monoterpenes, *Eur. J. Immunol.*, 24, 301, 1994.
106. Hohl, R. J. and Lewis, K., RAS expression in human leukemia is modulated differently by lovastatin and limonene, *Blood*, 80, 299a(Abstr.), 1992.
107. Gould, M. N., Prevention and therapy of mammary cancer by monoterpenes, *J. Cell Biochem.*, 522, 139, 1995.

2 Bioavailability of Carotenoids from Vegetables versus Supplements

Etor E. K. Takyi

CONTENTS

2.1 INTRODUCTION

Carotenoids are the widely distributed, naturally occurring pigments responsible for the yellow, orange, and red colors of fruits, roots, flowers, fish, invertebrates, and birds. They also occur in algae, bacteria, molds, and yeast. In higher plants, they occur in the photosynthetic tissue, the choloroplast, where their color is masked by that of the more predominant green chlorophyll.

The *basic* structure is a symmetric, linear, 40-carbon *tetraterpene*, built from eight five-carbon *isoprenoid* units, in such a way that the order is reversed at the center of the molecule. This basic skeleton could be modified in various ways, such as hydrogenation, dehydrogenation, cyclization, double-bond migration, chain short-

0-8493-0038-X/97/$0.00+$.50

TABLE 2.1
Characteristics of Common Food Carotenes and Xanthophylls[1]

Name	Characteristics	Vitamin A Activity (%)[2]
	CAROTENES	
Phytofluene	Acyclic, colorless	—
Lycopene	Acyclic, red	0
δ-carotene	Monocyclic (1β-ring), red-orange	42
β-carotene	Bicyclic (2β pt-rings), orange	100
α-carotene	Bicyclic (1β pt-ring, 1∈-ring), yellow	53
	XANTHOPHYLLS	
β-cryptoxanthin	Bicyclic (2β-rings), orange	57
α-cryptoxanthin	Bicyclic (1β, 1∈-ring), yellow	—
Zeaxanthin	Bicyclic (2β-rings), yellow-orange	0
Lutein	Bicyclic (1β, 1∈-rings), yellow	0
Violazanthin	Bicyclic, yellow	0
Astaxanthin	Bicyclic (2β-rings), red	0

Note: Unless otherwise stated, the carotenoids are in *trans* form.

ening or extension, rearrangement, isomerization or a combination of these processes, resulting in a great diversity of structures.[1]

There are basically two types of carotenoids; those containing hydrocarbon (e.g., carotene) and those containing oxygen (e.g., x*anthophylls*). Both types of carotenoids may be acyclic (no ring), monocyclic (one ring), or bicyclic (two rings).

The distinctive building feature of carotenoids is an extensive conjugated double-bond system, which consists of alternating double and single carbon-carbon bonds, usually referred to as the polyene chain. This portion of the molecule (chromophore) is responsible for the ability of carotenoids to absorb light in the visible region of the spectrum. At least seven conjugated double bonds are needed for the carotenoids to impart color; phytofluene, with five such bonds, is colorless (Table 2.1). The color deepens as the conjugated system increases, thus lycopene (11 double bonds) is red.

Cyclization causes some limitations; hence even though β-carotene and α-carotene have the same number of conjugated double bonds (11) as lycopene, they are orange and orange-red, respectively. The intensity of food color depends on which carotenoids are present, their concentrations, physical states, as well as the presence or absence of any other plant pigments, such as chlorophyll.

2.2 LOCALIZATION OF CAROTENOIDS

Carotenoids are hydrophobic, lipophilic substances and are virtually insoluble in water. They dissolve in fat solvents such as alcohol, acetone, ethyl ether, and chloroform. Carotenoids are readily soluble in petroleum ether and hexane, while xanthophylls dissolve best in methanol and ethanol.

In plants and animals carotenoids occur as crystals or amorphous solids, in solution in lipid media, in colloidal dispersion, or combined with protein in an aqueous layer. Specifically, in green leaves, β-carotene molecules are organized in pigment-protein complexes located in cell chloroplasts. In fruits, the molecules are found in lipid droplets and chromoplasts.

The formation of carotenoid-protein complexes allows the carotenoids to have access to an aqueous environment, stabilizes the carotenoid, and changes its color. For example, in invertebrates such as crabs, shrimps, and lobsters, the carotenoid astaxanthin appears as blue, green, or purple carotenoprotein complexes. Upon cooking, denaturation of the protein releases the astaxanthin, revealing a red color.[1]

2.3 IMPORTANCE OF CAROTENOIDS

The important physical and chemical properties of carotenoids are depicted in Figure 2.1. It is necessary to highlight the physical-chemical properties of carotenoids since these ultimately confer the multifaceted functions and actions upon them.

The polyene chain is the cause of the instability of carotenoids, including their susceptibility to oxidation and geometric isomerization (change in geometry around a double bond). Heat, light, and acids promote isomerization of trans-carotenoids, their usual configuration in nature, to the cis-form. Oxidation, the major cause of carotenoid loss, depends on available oxygen, the carotenoid involved, and is stimulated by light, heat, peroxides, metals such as iron, and enzymes, while inhibited by antioxidants such as tocopherols (vitamin E) and ascorbic acid (vitamin C).

Oxidation therefore leads to complete loss of activity while isomerization leads to reduced activity. During isomerization, the carotenoid molecules fold back and change from the naturally occurring trans (linear) form to the cis (folded) form. The conditions necessary for the isomerization and oxidation of carotenoids are likely to exist in home preparations, industrial processing, and during storage of foods. The consequences are loss of color, vitamin A activity, and other biological activities. Furthermore, degradation of carotenoids has also been associated with the development of an off-flavor in foods such as in dehydrated carrot and sweet potato flakes.[3]

Many biological functions and actions have been and continue to be attributed to carotenoids. The more important of these functions are depicted in Figure 2.2. Of the more than 600 carotenoids now known, about 50 could be precursors of vitamin A, based on structural considerations. Vitamin A is provided in our diet as preformed vitamin A (retinyl ester, retinol, retinal, 3-dehydroretinol, and retinoic acid) from foods of animal origin such as liver, milk and milk products, fish and meat (liver and organelles), or as carotenoids, generally from plant sources, that can be biologically converted to vitamin A. Globally about 60% of dietary vitamin A is estimated to come from plant foods,[4] however, due to the prohibitive cost of animal foods, the dietary contribution of provitamin A could rise to 80 to 90% in developing countries.

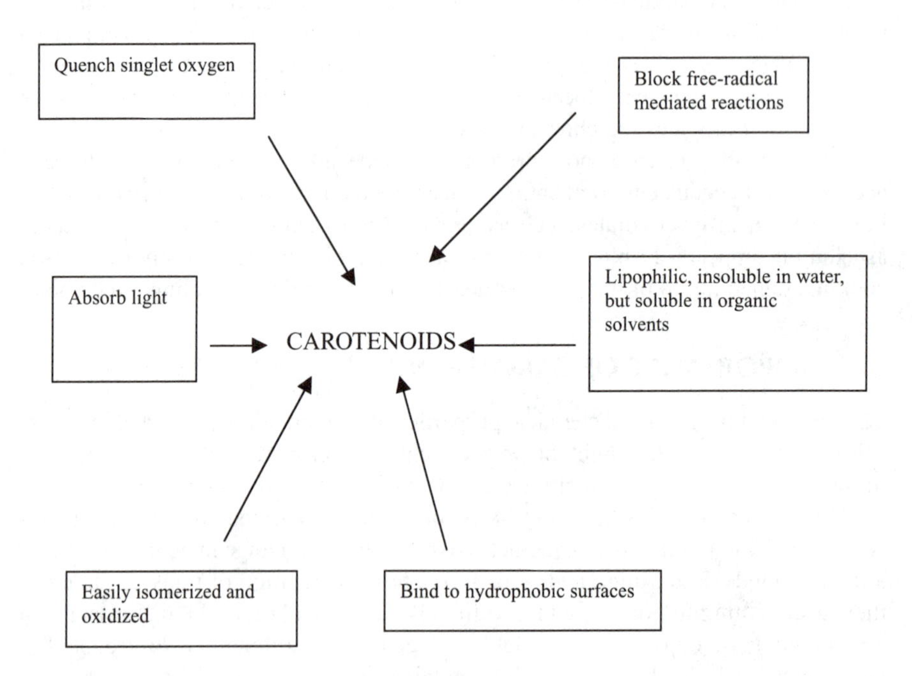

FIGURE 2.1 Important physical and chemical properties of carotenoids.[1]

In developed countries, vitamin A deficiency (VAD) has been largely eliminated, except in people who suffer from lipid malabsorption which interferes with the absorption of fat-soluble vitamins such as vitamin A. While the absence of VAD is largely due to the consumption of vitamin A-fortified foods, there is growing interest in fruits and vegetables because of a negative association between their consumption and the incidence of cancers[5] and coronary heart diseases.[6] This negative association could be due to the carotenoids and/or other antioxidants, both of which normally exist in fruits and vegetables.[7] Thus, carotenoids are important dietary components because of their provitamin A activity as well as their possible roles in the prevention of degenerative diseases.

Provitamin A carotenoids have the advantage of being converted to vitamin A only when vitamin A is needed in the body, thus avoiding potential toxicity due to excesses. On the other hand, many factors influence the absorption and utilization of provitamin A carotenoids, thus the bioavailability of carotenoids is variable and difficult to appraise.

The relative biopotencies (vitamin A activity) of only a few forms of provitamin A have been determined by rat assays (Table 2.1). In terms of biological activity and widespread occurrence, the most important provitamin A carotenoid is β-carotene. Virtually all carotogenic plant foods analyzed to date contain β-carotene as a major or minor constituent. β-Carotene is a potent provitamin A carotenoid to which 100% activity is assigned (Table 2.1). The activity of the other provitamin A carotenoids are ranked on the activity of β-carotene (Table 2.1).

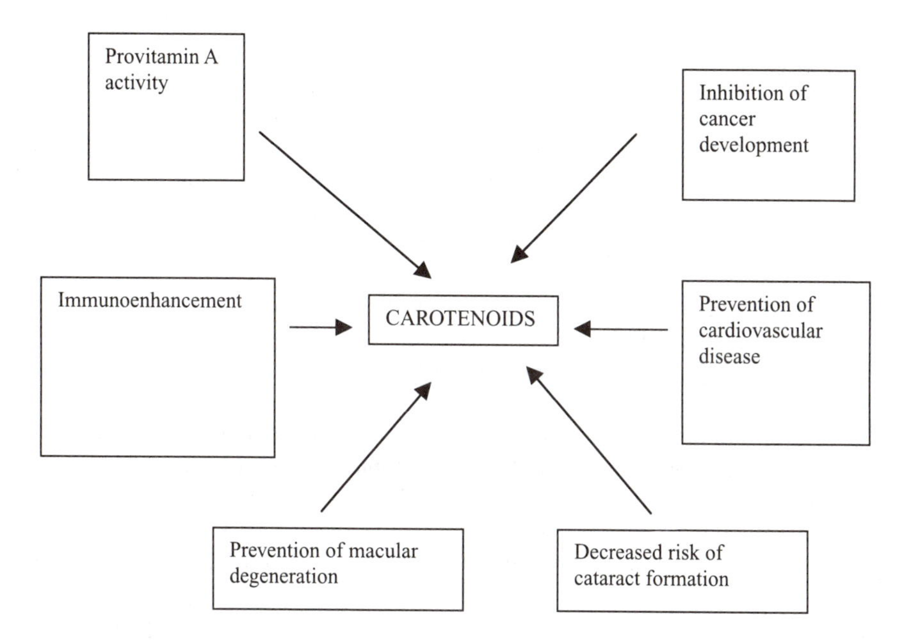

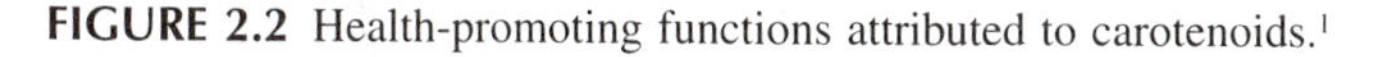
FIGURE 2.2 Health-promoting functions attributed to carotenoids.[1]

Carotenoids have also been associated with enhancement of the immune system and decreased risk of degenerative diseases such as cancer, cardiovascular disease, age-related macular degeneration, and cataract formation.[8-16] These functions are attributed to the antioxidant property of carotenoids through deactivation of free radicals and singlet oxygen quenching.[17-19]

The ability of carotenoids to quench singlet oxygen is related to the conjugated double bond system. Those having nine or more double bonds give maximum protection.[20] The acyclic provitamin A-inactive lycopene was more effective than bicyclic β-carotene;[21] canthaxanthin and astaxanthin, both with conjugated keto groups, were better antioxidants than β-carotene and zeaxanthin.[22]

2.4 IMPORTANT FOOD SOURCES OF PROVITAMIN A

Surveys conducted in different countries show that in terms of provitamin A carotenoid content, the most important sources are dark green leafy vegetables, red palm oil, palm fruits, carrot, orange, sweet potatoes, mature squashes and pumpkins, and other yellow/orange tropical fruits.

2.4.1 Leafy Vegetables

In many countries in the developing world, dark green leafy vegetables are the most common and relatively abundant sources of provitamin A carotenoids. Due to their relative ease of cultivation and their availability practically all year round (except in arid and semi-arid areas, where their availability is seasonal and limited to the short rainy seasons only), they are an inexpensive and accessible source of provitamin A carotenoids.

For most of the developing countries which lie in subtropical and tropical areas, β-carotene is essentially the most important source of vitamin A activity, with α-carotene and α- or β-cryptoxanthin reported occasionally at relatively low levels. However, the β-carotene content of leafy vegetables varies markedly.

Based on the β-carotene content in leafy vegetables, Begum and Pereira[23] classified Indian leafy vegetables into three groups thus:

- Those with a high β-carotene level: 46 to 74 μg/g leaf
- Those with a moderate β-carotene level: 25 to 39 μg/g leaf
- Those with a low β-carotene level: 12 to 23 μg/g leaf

Seasonal variations were noted but no consistent pattern could be seen, with some of the leaves being higher in β-carotene content in the summer and others in the colder months. Recently, analyses using HPLC showed higher results — ranging from 20 to 197 μg/g.[24]

Leafy vegetables have been analyzed by HPLC in several other countries.[25] In Malaysia, of 27 leaves examined 3 had a β-carotene level between 114 and 136 μg/g and 16 contained between 30 and 93 μg/g β-carotene.[26] The commonly consumed green leaves in Bangladesh had β-carotene content between 54 to 100 μg/g[27] while three of the leaves analyzed in Taiwan had β-carotene levels of 70, 92, and 105 μg/g, respectively.[28] The highest level of β-carotene found in leaves analyzed in Napal was 58 μg/g,[29] 187 μg/g from Japan,[30] 40 μg/g from Ghana,[31] 60 μg/g from Brazil,[1] while all 78 Australian leaves had <30 μg/g β-carotene.[32]

2.4.2 Root Crops

Carrot (*Daucus carota*) and yellow-to-orange sweet potatoes (*Ipomoea batatas*) are available throughout the world and are important, rich sources of carotenoids, even though their concentrations vary widely from one locality to another.[1] The average β-carotene level ranged from 36[33] to 182 μg/g,[34] while the average for α-carotene varied from 5.3 μg/g in Finland[35] to 106 μg/g in the U.S.[34]

Dark-orange carrots, consisting mainly of β-carotene and α-carotene, ranged from 63 to 584 μg/g.[1] The carotene content of sweet potatoes varied from 0.2 to 218 μg/g.[36] Japan has established a strong sweet potato breeding program[37] due to the fact that the sweet potato is tolerant to typhoons, droughts, pests, and diseases, and is important as a source of starch and vitamins, including β-carotene.

2.4.3 Fruits

Even though fruits generally have lower provitamin A carotenoids than leafy vegetables, they are usually more readily accepted by both children and adults and their provitamin A content is believed to be more bioavailable.[37,38] Tropical and subtropical fruits have an advantage over temperate fruits in that they are more carotenogenic compared to temperate fruits in which the anthocyamin pigments (noncarotenogenic) predominate. Popular tropical fruits such as mango and papaya are important sources of provitamin A in developing countries. The β-carotene content of mangoes varied from 0.6 mg/g in Thailand[39] to 29 μg/g in India.[40] Papaya also represents important sources of both β-carotene and β-cryptoxanthin (having only one half the bioactivity of β-carotene).[1] Red-fleshed Brazilian papayas analyzed by HPLC contained 1.2 ± 0.3 μg/g β-carotene and 6.7 ± 0.9 μg/g β-cryptoxanthin.[41]

2.4.4 Palm Oil

Crude red palm oil, obtained from the mesocarp of the oil palm (*Elaeis guineensis*) is considered the world's richest plant source of provitamin A carotenoids.[41] The provitamin A content of oil from varieties of *E. guineensis* and *E. oleifera*, ranged from 142 to 1854 μg/g for α-carotene and 377 to 2483 μg/g for β-carotene. Palm fruits are especially important not only because of their high provitamin A content, but also because of the co-occurrence of fat, which results in higher bioavailability of provitamin A most probably due to higher absorption.

In Brazil, the palm fruit *buriti* is the richest source of provitamin A carotenoids, having a β-carotene content of 360 μg/g, an α-carotene content of 80 μg/g, and a gamma-carotene content of 37 μg/g. In most carotenogenic fruits, ripening is accompanied by enhanced carotenoid biosynthesis, which considerably raises the levels of carotenoids, including provitamin A carotenoids. However, in fruits that remain green when ripe and in those that owe their color to anthocyamins, the small amounts of carotenoids tend to decrease during ripening. Also carotenogenesis may continue in intact fruits, fruit vegetables, and root crops after harvest, but in leaves and some other vegetables degradation prevails during post-harvest storage, especially at elevated temperatures and under conditions favorable to wilting.[1]

2.5 FACTORS AFFECTING THE BIOAVAILABILITY OF CAROTENOIDS IN VEGETABLES

Bioavailability is defined as the proportion of carotenoids ingested that is absorbed and converted to vitamin A in the body. Bioconversion is the proportion of bioavailable carotenoids converted to vitamin A. Both absorption and conversion are affected by many complex factors. This chapter presents a summary of the factors which affect the bioavailability of carotenoids.

Early studies which investigated the bioavailability of dietary carotenoids concluded that purified carotene in oil is more bioavailable than carotene from leafy vegetables and carrots, and that grinding and homogenizing foods increase carotene bioavailability. de Pee et al.[38] have developed a mnemonic word "Slamanghi," to describe factors which influence the bioavailability of carotenoids (β-carotene). In this chapter two more factors have been added. The list is discussed briefly below.

S = Species of carotenoids — The vitamin A activity of β-carotene has been set on a weight basis, as one-fourth to one-tenth of that of retinol, depending on the amount of β-carotene in a meal, while that of other provitamin carotenoids has been set at one-twelfth. This appears to be an oversimplification since several stereoiso-

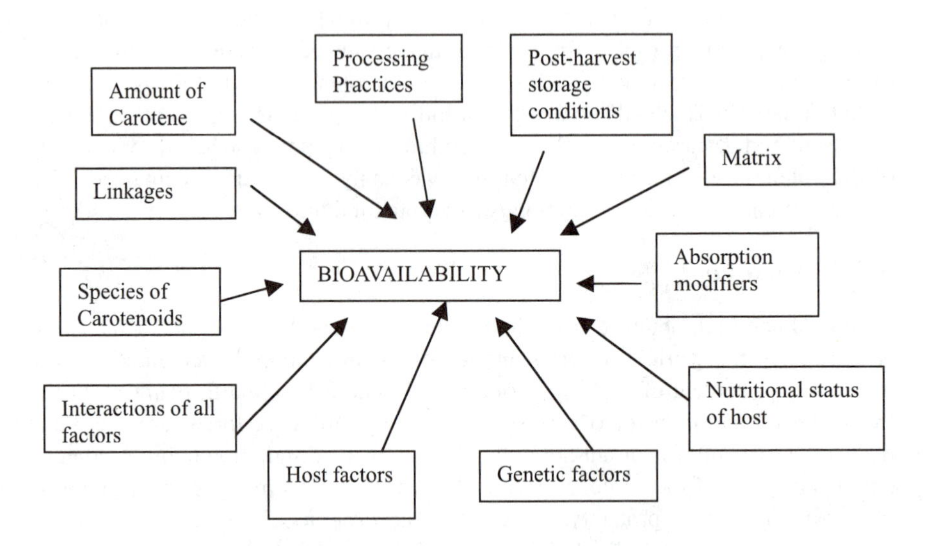

FIGURE 2.3 Factors affecting the bioavailability of dietary carotenoids.

mers exist for each carotenoid and trans-isomers have higher provitamin A activity than cis-isomers. Many factors, such as heat, light, pH, and cooking cause isomerization, leading to the production of species with lower provitamin A activity.

L = Linkages at molecular levels — Some carotenoids such as β-cryptoxanthin exist in plants in both esterified and nonesterified forms. There may be differences in the bioavailability of these two forms.

A = Amount of Carotene — Carotenoids are absorbed through passive diffusion and the proportion absorbed decreases as the amount of carotenoids in a meal increases. FAO/WHO guidelines propose that the amount of dietary β-carotene equivalent to 1 mg retinol is 4, 6, or 10 mg, depending on whether the amount of β-carotene in a meal is <1 mg, $1 - 4$ mg, or >4 mg, respectively. Also the presence of some carotenoids in a medium might inhibit the absorption of other carotenoids.

M = Matrix — The matrix in which the carotenoids is embedded in foods seems to be a very important determinant of its bioavailability. As stated earlier, in green leaves carotenoids are organized in pigment-protein complexes located in cell chloroplasts. In other vegetables and fruits, they are located in the chromoplasts of cells, often found in lipid droplets or bound to protein. To become bioavailable, the carotenoid must be freed from its ligands and other matrixes. The cells must first be disrupted by a process such as homogenization. Releasing the carotenoid from a pigment-protein complex is more difficult than freeing it from a lipid droplet. Thus, carotenoids in a fat matrix are more bioavailable than from vegetables and fruits. Cooking and reduction of particle size by grinding or homogenization can reduce matrix effects. However, since a substantial destruction of the matrix, e.g., through cooking, could also destroy the carotenoids, a compromise must be made between maximal destruction of the matrix effect and minimum destruction and/or isomerization of carotenoids.

A = Absorption modifiers — Since the mucosal cells absorb β-carotene from lipid micelles, the diet should contain a sufficient amount and the right type of fat for micelle formation. Unsaturated fats are more efficient than saturated fats. While the absorption of vitamin A is not significantly affected by its food sources or by the amount ingested, or by gastrointestinal infections,[42] the absorption of dietary carotenoids, on the other hand, is affected by a large number of factors. These include the chemical nature, physical binding within the food, presence of dietary fat, conjugated bile salts, pancreatic enzymes in the intestinal lumen, the presence of other food components that inhibit their absorption (such as fiber, pectin, cellulose, and chlorophyll), the amount ingested, the relative size of the food particles ingested, and food preparation practices that disrupt the food to different degrees. Systemic and parasitic infections reduce carotenoid absorption. Also vitamin A deficiency enhances, whereas protein deficiency reduces, the conversion of β-carotene to vitamin A. Other factors include the amount of vitamin E, the zinc status, and nonprovitamin A carotenoids such as lycopene. Most of these factors are present in appreciable amounts in vegetables.

N = Nutrient status — Even though the absorption of carotenoids is not influenced by carotene status or vitamin A status because absorption occurs through passive diffusion, conversion of carotene to retinol is influenced by serum retinol concentration. An adequate serum retinol level has an inhibiting effect on the enzyme that cleaves carotene into retinol. Also, by improving an impaired zinc status the vitamin A status can also improve since some enzymes involved in vitamin A metabolism are zinc dependent. Protein and iodine status should also be adequate in order to ensure that metabolism of carotene and retinol is normal.

G = Genetics — The bioconversion of β-carotene to retinol is mediated by a cleavage enzyme and there is evidence that some people have a genetic defect which renders them unable to convert β-carotene to retinol. Others have an inherited fat malabsorption, low enzymatic digestion, or poor synthesis of thyroid hormones, proteolytic enzymes, and/or bile salts, which ultimately affect the metabolism of carotenoids and/or vitamin A.

H = Host-related factors — The age of an individual could be an important factor in the bioavailability of carotenoids. Infants handle carotenoids differently from adults or the elderly. Gastrointestinal infections such as *Helicobacter pylori* and parasites (*Giardia lamblia, Ascaris lumbricoides*, and hookworm) can cause maldigestion, malabsorption, and excessive loss of dietary carotenoids.

I = Interactions — All the factors discussed can interact with one another to affect carotenoid availability.

Processing practices — Processing of β-carotene-rich foods can actually make the nutrient more available than it would be if the foods were left raw. For example, the bioavailability of carotenoids in raw carrots can be as low as 1%; mild heating greatly enhances digestibility. Some of the carotenoids in leafy vegetables are bound up in protein complexes, which cooking releases. Blanching — the brief (1 to 3 min) exposure of food to boiling water, steam, or hot air — does not reduce the carotene content appreciably and may make it more bioavailable.

Post-harvest storage — A lot of physiological and biochemical processes take place during post-harvest storage. The type and extent of these processes depend on the storage conditions, such as the temperature and the presence or absence of light and oxygen. An ideal storage condition could lead to carotenoid products with increased bioavailability when the products are finally consumed.

In summary, the bioavailability of carotenoids is influenced by complex and varied factors and is difficult to predict. Even conditions such as the species of leafy vegetables, soil in which the leaves were cultivated, climate, age, and post-harvest storage conditions can affect bioavailability. Thus, one needs caution in extrapolating results from one leaf to another, or even from the same type of leafy vegetable grown in different seasons, since seasonal variations could influence the type and extent of carotenoid-protein complex formation.

2.6 RESEARCH STUDIES

Many research studies have been carried out to determine whether the consumption of dark green leafy vegetables, as the sole source of provitamin A, could raise the serum retinol status of individuals to acceptable levels. While some of the studies showed that serum retinol levels are raised after consumption of the vegetables,[31,41] others showed no significant rise.[42-45]

Though it is true that some of the studies suffer from poor experimental design, the disparities in the results could be due to how well the factors which affect the bioavailability of provitamin A carotenoids have been met in a particular experimental design. It is reasonable to believe that the more factors that are met in a particular study, the more pronounced is the response of serum retinol levels.

de Pee et al.[45] investigated in the Bogor District, West Java, Indonesia the effect of an additional daily portion of dark green leafy vegetables on the vitamin A and iron status in women with low hemoglobin concentration (<130 g/l) who were breast-feeding children 3 to 17 months old.

In the study, 5 days a week for 12 weeks a group of women ($n = 57$) received a stir-fried vegetable; a second group ($n = 62$) received as a supplement a wafer enriched with β-carotene, iron, vitamin C, and folic acid; and a third group ($n = 56$) received a nonenriched wafer. The vegetable-supplemented and the enriched-wafer groups consumed 3.5 mg β-carotene, 5.2 and 4.8 mg iron, and 7.5 and 4.4 g fat, respectively. In the β-carotene-supplemented group (wafer group) there were increases in the serum retinol (mean increase 0.32 μmol/l (95% CI 0.23 to 0.46), breast milk retinol, 0.59 μmol/l (95% CI 0.35–0.84), and serum β-carotene 0.73 μmol/l (95% CI 0.59–0.88). These figures were significantly greater than in the other two groups in which the only changes were small increases in breast milk retinol in the control-wafer group (0.16 μmol/l, 95% CI 0.02–0.30) and in serum β-carotene in the vegetable group, 0.03 μmol/l (95% CI 0–0.06).

It was concluded that a daily portion of dark green leafy vegetables did not improve vitamin A status, whereas a similar amount of β-carotene from a simpler matrix produced a profound improvement.

Takyi[31] carried out a similar study in northern Ghana in which 519 preschool children were randomly assigned to 5 feeding groups and fed once daily for 12 weeks. Two groups were fed 400 RE of dark green leafy vegetable plus and minus

10% fat (groups 1 and 2, respectively), a third group was fed on a home diet containing 10 RE, while the fourth supplemented group was given 400 RE of synthetic β-carotene plus fat, and a fifth group was fed on dark green leafy vegetables (400 RE) after the children were dewormed with mebendazole (Table 2.2).

Relative to the baseline serum retinol value, consumption of dark green leafy vegetables (*Manihot* sp. and *Ceiba* sp.) with fat (10%) significantly ($p < .05$) enhanced the serum retinol; consequently, the percentage of children with adequate retinol status increased from 28.2 to 48.2% after feeding.

The details of the diets are shown in Table 2.2. On the stew basis, there were significant differences in both the change in the retinol level as a result of feeding and the efficiency of each stew in enhancing retinol status. Diets 4 and 5, representing the β-carotene-supplemented group and the dewormed group, respectively, gave similar values. When the percentage efficiency of the stews were computed, the supplemented group (group 4) gave the highest value followed by the dewormed group (group 5). However, analysis of the efficiency values using the chi-square test showed that there were no significant differences between these two groups. This unequivocally demonstrates the extreme importance of deworming in carotenoid bioavailability and further strengthens the recommendation of Jafal et al.[44] that food-based intervention in vitamin A–deficient areas could be successful, but other interventions, such as increasing dietary fat intake and anthelmintic treatment should be considered along with increasing the consumption of β-carotene, for maximum results.

The differences in response to feeding with dark green leafy vegetables in the two studies could be due to the following: (1) de Pee et al.[48] used a leafy vegetable supplement consisting of cassava leaves, water spinach (*Ipomea* sp.), spinach (*Amaranthus* sp.), and carrot (*Daucus* sp.), while (2) Takyi[31] used cassava and kapok (*Ceiba* sp.) leaves. Apart from the cassava leaf, which is common to both studies, the other leaves were different. The bioavailability of provitamin A carotenoids will differ due to the different varieties/species used, as well as differences in the climatic conditions during cultivation. It is known that the provitamin A content of leaves varies markedly because of the cultivar used, growth conditions, and stage of maturity. Carotenoid content increases with age up to a limit[46] and then declines slightly.[47] Second, de Pee et al[48] used stir-fried leaves in feeding while Takyi[31] used leaves which were first pounded in a wooden mortar and then homogenized in a high-speed homogenizer. As discussed earlier, provitamin A carotenoids are in the form of pigment-protein complexes located in the chloroplast of cells. These are indeed complex, strong ligands, needing strong sheering forces to break up and liberate the provitamin A carotenoid molecules from the ligands and other matrixes to make them bioavailable. While pounding followed by high-speed homogenization is considered effective in achieving this, it is not known if stir-frying could achieve similar results. In addition, it is known that frying (excessive heat) could destroy and/or cause isomerization of trans-provitamin A carotenoids into their less active cis-isomers (13-*cis* β-carotene and 9-*cis* β-carotene).

These isomers are about 50% as active as their trans-isomers. Indeed the authors reported that the level of cis-isomers of β-carotene in the supplemented leafy vegetable diet was 30 to 35%, compared to a raw tissue level of 15%. Third, de Pee fed

TABLE 2.2
Characteristics of the Various Stews Fed to Children in Saboba, Northern Ghana

Feeding Group	Composition of Stew	Change in Serum Retinol (post-feeding value – baseline value) (μmol/l)	% Efficiency
1	DVL (400 RE) + dry fish + 10% fat + onion + tomatoes	0.15	26.5[c]
2	DVL (400 RE) + dry fish + onion + tomatoes	0.14	23.4[b]
3	Home-type stew (10 RE) + dry fish + onion + tomatoes	0.02	48.1[a]
4	β-carotene (400 RE) + dry fish + 10% fat + onion + tomatoes	0.22	44.1[d]
5	DVL (400 RE) + dry fish + 10% fat + onion + tomatoes + mebendazole	0.22	38.8[d]

Note: In each group, the condiments were made into stews using a minimum of groundnut oil and served with the main carbohydrate meal of either rice, yam, gari and beans, or gari. The dry fish did not contain any vitamin A. The leafy vegetable was either cassava or kapok leaves. These were fed on alternate days. DVL = dark green leafy vegetable; the fat used was shea butter, a local fat widely used in cooking. The efficiency of each of the five stews in enhancing the vitamin A status of the children was determined by subtracting the retinol level at baseline from the values after feeding and dividing the difference by the retinol level at baseline. Values within each column with the same superscript letter were not significantly different.

the leafy supplements for 5 days per week for 12 weeks while Takyi fed it for 7 days per week for 12 weeks. Perhaps it is necessary to feed the subjects for a longer period in order to effect increases in the serum retinol levels. Fourth, preschool children were used in the study by Takyi while de Pee et al. studied lactating women. It can be expected that there will be qualitative and quantitative differences in the manner in which these two groups respond to ingested carotenoids. It is expected that there will be a higher increment in serum retinol level in preschool children than in lactating women since the physiological demands of the former group will be less than that of the latter group. Fifth, there is no indication as to the iodine status of subjects in the de Pee et al. study, while Takyi sought to increase iodine status in his subjects by using iodized salt in food preparation. It is known that an adequate iodine status is necessary for conversion of β-carotene to vitamin A in humans.

Furthermore, the fat content of meals fed by Takyi was 10%, compared to 7.8% used by de Pee et al. The 10% fat content significantly enhanced ($p<.05$) the bioavalability of carotenoids (group 1) compared to the nonfat group (group 2, Table 2.2).

2.7 RECOMMENDATIONS

Carotenoids are affected chiefly by exposure to air, light, excessive heat, or presence of acids. They are therefore vulnerable during food processsing, storage, and cooking, unless certain precautions are taken. These precautions can be summarized as follows. Protect β-carotene-rich foods from light, particularly sunlight; store them in a manner which excludes light and air and in the cold; cook them with the least amount of water and heat, in the shortest time possible, or use a microwave oven; and cook in closed containers. If they must be preserved by drying, use solar drying, away from direct sunlight.

2.8 CONCLUSIONS

The bioavalability of provitamin A carotenoids in humans can be compared to that of β-carotene (supplement) if the factors which affect the bioavailability are met. These conditions, even though numerous, can be achieved in homes and public feeding programs through concerted and conscious effort. All that is necessary is the willingness of all those involved in the production, harvesting, storage, transportation, and diet preparation of leafy vegetables to realize and ensure that we maintain a dietary approach as the most reliable, natural, and sustainable means of alleviating vitamin A deficiency and degenerative diseases in both the developed and the developing world.

ACKNOWLEDGMENTS

Parts of this chapter were obtained from OMNI publications. These were studies produced with funds from the Office of Health and Nutrition, Bureau for Global Programs, Field Support and Research, U.S. Agency for International Development, under the terms of Contract No. HRN-C-00-93-00025-08. Other parts came from the research of the following: S. de Pee, Jakartar, Indonesia and The Vitamin A Sieve.

REFERENCES

1. Rodriguez-Amaya, D.B., Carotenoids and Food Preparation: The retention of provitamin A carotenoids in prepared, processed, and stored foods. USAID/OMNI publication, 1997.
2. Bauernfeind, J.C., Carotenoid vitamin A precursors and analysis in foods and feeds, *J. Agric Food Chem.*, 20, 456, 1972.
3. Falconer, M.E., Fishwick, M.J., Land, D.G., and Sayer, E.R., Carotene oxidation and off-flavor development in dehydrated carrot, *J. Sci. Food Agric.*, 15, 857, 1964.
4. Simpson, K.L., Relative value of carotenoids as precursors of vitamin A, *Proc. Nutr. Soc.* 42, 7, 1983.
5. Byers, T. and Perry, G., Dietary carotenoids, Vitamin C and vitamin E as protective antioxidants in human cancers, *Annu. Rev. Nutr.*, 12, 139, 1992.

6. Manson, J.E., Gaziano, J.M., Jonas M.A., and Hennekens, C.H., Antioxidants and cardiovascular disease: a review, *J. Am. Coll. Nutr.*, 12, 426, 1993.
7. Rowe, P.M., Beta-carotene takes a collective beating, *Lancet,* 347, 249, 1996.
8. Mathews-Roth, M.M., Carotenoids and cancer prevention — experimental and epidemiological studies, *Pure Appl. Chem.* 57, 717, 1985.
9. Mathews-Roth, M.M., Recent progress in the medical applications of carotenoids, *Pure Appl. Chem.*, 63, 147, 1991.
10. Matus, Z., Deli, J., and Szaboles, Carotenoid composition of yellow pepper during ripening: Isolation of β-cryptoxanthin 5,6-epioxide, *J. Agric. Food Chem.,* 39, 1907, 1991.
11. Merchandes, A.Z. and Rodrigues-Amaya, D.B., Comparism of normal-phase and reversed-phase gravity-flow column methods for provitamin A determination, *Chromatographia*, 28, 249, 1989.
12. Merchandes, A.Z. and Rodrigues-Amaya, D.B., Carotenoid composition and vitamin A value of some native Brazilian green leafy vegetable, *Int. J. Food Sci. Technol.*, 25, 213, 1990.
13. Merchantes, A.Z. and Rodrigues-Amaya, D.B., Carotinoid composition of leafy vegetables in relation to some agricultural variables, *J. Agric. Food Chem.,* 39, 1094, 1991.
14. Merchantes, A.Z. and Rodrigues-Amaya, D.B., Composition of carotinoids in two mango cultivars and mango juice obtained by HPLC. Paper presented at the 10th Int. Symp. Carotinoids, Ttrondheim, 1993.
15. Minazzi-Rorigues, R.S. and Penteado, M.V.C., Carotinoides com atividede pro-vitaminica A em hortalicas folhosas, *Rev. Farm. Bioquim. Univ. S. Paula*, 25, 39, 1989.
16. Minquez-Mosquera, M. I. and Gandul-Rogas, B., Mechanisms and kinetics of carotinoid degradation during processing of green table olives, *J. Agric. Food Chem.,* 42, 1551, 1994.
17. Burton, G.W., Antioxidant action of carotinoids, *J. Nutr.,* 109, 111, 1989.
18. Bushway, R.J., Determination of α and β-carotene in some raw fruits and vegetables by high-performance liquid chromatography, *J. Agric. Food Chem.,* 34, 409, 1986.
19. Bushway, R.J. and Wilson A.M., Determination of α and β-carotene in fruits and vegetables by high-performance liquid chromatography, *Can. Inst. Food Sci. Technol. J.*, 15, 165, 1982.
20. Foote, C.S., Chang, Y.C., and Denny, R.W., Chemistry of singlet oxygen X. Carotenoid quenching parellels biological protection, *J. Am. Chem. Soc.,* 92, 532, 1970.
21. Di Mascio, P., Kaiser, P.S., and Sics, H., Lycopene as the most efficient biological carotenoid singlet oxygen quencher, *Arch. Biochem. Biophys.*, 274, 532, 1989.
22. Terao, J., Antioxidant activity of β-carotene-related carotenoids in solution, *Lipids*, 24, 659, 1989.
23. Begum, A. and Pereira, S.M., The beta-carotene content of Indian edible green leaves, *Trop. Geogr. Med.*, 29, 47, 1977.
24. Bhaskaraachary, K., Sankar Rao, D., Deosthale, Y.G., and Reddy, V., Carotene content of some common and less familiar foods of plant origin, *Food Chem*., 25, 189, 1995.
25. Delia, B. and Rodriquez-Amaya, D.B., Carotenoids and food preparation: The retention of Provitamin A carotenoid in prepared, processed and stored foods, p. 20, John Snow, Inc/OMNI Project, 1997.
26. Tee, E.S. and Lim, C.L., Carotenoid composition and content of Malaysian vegetables and fruits by the AOAC and HPLC methods, *Food Chem*., 41, 309, 1991.
27. Wahed, M.A., Mahalanabis, D., and Sack, R.B., Preparing and preserving green leafy vegetables for poor communities in Bangladesh, in *Empowering Vitamin A Foods*, Eds. E. Wasantwistut and G. A. Attig, Bangkok Institute of Nutrition, 1995.

28. Chen, B.H., Chuang, J.R., Lim, J.H., and Chiu, C.P., Quantification of provitamin A compounds in chinese vegetables by high-performance liquid chromatography, *J. Food Prot.*, 50, 51, 1993.
29. Vaidya, Y., Vitamin A food production and use in Napal, in *Empowering Vitamin A Foods*, Eds. E. Wasantwisut and G.A. Attig, Bankok Institute of Nutrition, 1995.
30. Izaki, Y., Yoshida, K., Hidada, K., and Toda, K., Chlorophylls, carotenes and tocopherols in green vegetables and their relationships, *J. Jpn. Soc. Nutr. Food Sci.*, 39, 485, 1986.
31. Takyi, E.E.K., Children's consumption of dark green, leafy vegetables with added fat enhances serum retinol, *J. Nutr.*, 129, 1549, 1999.
32. Wills, R.B.H., Composition of Australian fresh fruit and vegetables, *Food Technol. Aus.,* 39, 523, 1987.
33. Bushway, R.J., Yaing, A., and Yamani, A.M., Comparison of alpha- and beta-carotene content of supermarket versus roadside stand produce, *J. Food Qual.,* 9, 437, 1986.
34. Khachik, F. and Beecher, G.R., Application of a C45–β-carotene as an internal standard for the quantification of carotenoids in yellow/orange vegetables by liquid chromatography, *J. Agric. Food Chem.*, 35, 732, 1987.
35. Heinonen, M.I., Ollilainen, V., Linkola, E.K., Varo, P.T., and Koivistoinen, P.E., Carotenoids in Finnish foods, vegetables, fruits and berries, *J. Agric Food Chem.*, 37, 655, 1989.
36. Almeida–Muradian, L.B. and Penteado, M.V.C., Carotenoids and provitamin A value of some Brazilian sweet potato cultivars (Ipomoea batatas Lam), *Rev. Farm. Bioquin. Univ. S. Paulo,* 28, 145, 1992.
37. Olson, J.A., The bioavailability of dietary carotenoids, paper presented at the XVII IVACG Meeting, Guatemala, 1996.
38. de Pee, S., West, C.E., Muhilal, and Hautrast, J.G.A., Carotene-rich fruits and vegetables: Their capacity to improve vitamin A status of children in West Java. Paper presented at the XVII IVACG Meeting, Guatemela, 1996.
39. Speek, A.J., Saiechua, S., and Schreurs, W.H.P., Total carotenoid and carotene contents of Thai vegetables and the effect of processing, *Food Chem.*, 27, 245, 1988.
40. Reddy, V.K., Vijayaroghavan, K., Bhaskarachary, K., and Rami, M., Carotene-rich foods: the Indian experiences, in *Empowering Vitamin A Foods*, Eds. E. Wasantwisut and G.A. Attig, Bangkok, Institute of Nutrition, 1995.
41. Kimura, M., Rodriguez-Amaya, D.B., and Yokoyama S.M., Cultivar differences and geographic effects on carotenoid composition and vitamin A value of papaya, *Lebensm. Wiss. Technol.*, 24, 415, 1991.
42. Choo, Y., Palm oil carotenoids, *Food Nutr. Bull.*, 15, 130, 1994.
43. Reddy, V., Raghuramul N., and Arunjyoti, Absorption of vitamin A by children with diarrhoea during treatment with oral rehydration solution, *Bull. WHO*, 64, 721, 1986.
44. Jafal, F., Melheim, M.C., Agns, Z., Sanjur, D., and Habicht, J.P., Serum retinol concentration are affected by food sources of β-carotene, fat intake and anthelmintic drug treatment, *Am. J. Clin. Nutr.*, 68, 623, 1998.
45. Brown, E.D., Micozzi, M.S., and Craft, N.E., Plasma carotenoids in normal men after a single ingestion of vegetables or purified β-carotene, *Am. J. Clin. Nutr.*, 49, 1258, 1989.
46. Micozzi, M.S., Brown, E.D., and Edwards, B.K., Plasma response of children to short-term chronic intake of selected foods and β-carotene supplements in men, *Am. J. Clin. Nutr.*, 55, 1120, 1992.
47. Bwax, J., Quam de Serrano, J. and Ginliano, A. et al., Plasma response of children to short-term chronic β-carotene supplementation, *Am. J. Clin. Nutr.*, 59, 1369, 1994.

48. de Pee, S., West, C.E., Muhilal, Karyadi, D., and Hautvast, J.G.A.L., Lack of improvement in vitamin A status with increased consumption of dark green leafy vegetables, *Lancet*, 346, 75, 1995.
49. Ramos, D.M.R and Rodriguez-Amaya, D.B., Determination of vitamin A values of common Brazilian leafy vegetables, *J. Micronutr. Anal.*, 3, 147, 1987.
50. Lee, C.Y., Changes in the carotenoid content of carrot during growth and post-harvest storage, *Food Chem.*, 20, 285, 1986.

3 Japanese Vegetable Juice, Aojiru, and Cellular Immune Response for Health Promotion

Satoru Moriguchi, Tomoko Taka, Yuko Yamamoto, and Tuneo Hasegawa

CONTENTS

3.1 INTRODUCTION

In Japan the life style-related diseases such as cancer, heart disease, cerebrovascular disease, diabetes, hyperlipemia, and hypertension have increased in recent years. Among these diseases the first cause of death is cancer. About 50 years ago most Japanese men and women died from stomach cancer. However, as shown in Figure 3.1 the rate of death from stomach cancer dramatically decreased and the rates of death from lung and colon cancers steadily increase every year in both men and women.[1-3] For lung cancer, it has been suggested that smoking is one of the risk factors[4-6] and the World Health Organization (WHO) proposes a world without smoking as the goal of 21st century. The Ministry of Welfare in Japan has also stated that smoking is injurious to health. On the other hand, the increase in colon cancer appears to be related to the change of food style in Japan. Immediately after World War II, the Japanese lived on rice and took the most energy from carbohydrate and sodium chloride (NaCl). This food style was closely associated with the increased incidence of stomach cancer.[7,8] The higher intake of rice is linked to the higher intake of NaCl, which is thought to be one risk factor of stomach cancer.[9] However, the

0-8493-0038-X/97/$0.00+$.50

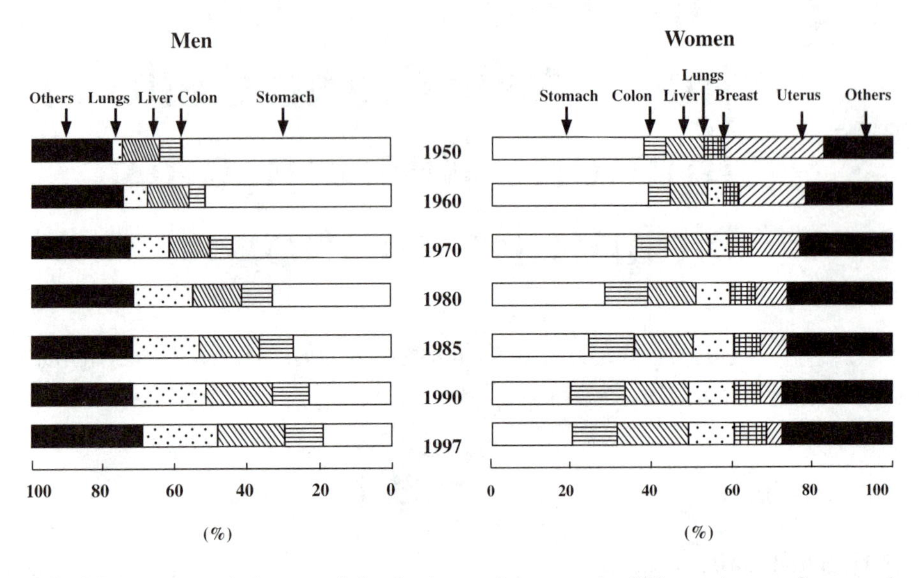

FIGURE 3.1 Annual changes of the death rate for cancer in different tissues of men and women in Japan from 1950 to 1997. (Data adapted from the special edition of *J. Health Welfare Stat.*, 46, 1999.)

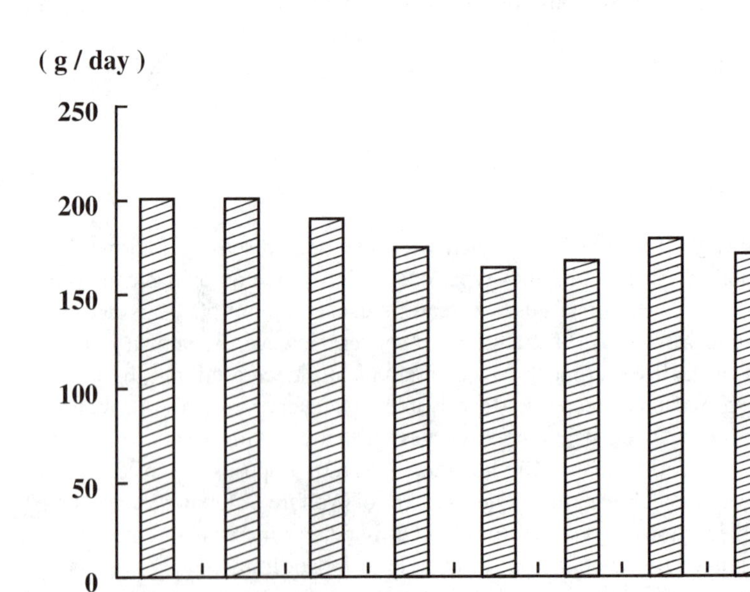

FIGURE 3.2 Annual changes of vegetable intake in Japan from 1975 to 1994. (Data adapted from the special edition of *J. Health Welfare Stat.*, 46, 1999.)

traditional Japanese food style of today has changed into the Western style, which supports the increased intake of animal protein and fat, and results in the increased ratio of fat energy and the decreased ratio of carbohydrate energy. This change of food style in Japan causes a decreased intake of vegetable (Figure 3.2) and rice, which is associated with a decreased intake of dietary fiber. As shown in Figure 3.3, the daily intake of dietary fiber in Japanese decreased to about 15 g/day in 1980 from 20 g/day in 1955. This decrease seems to be related to the increased incidence and death rate of colon cancer in Japan. To reduce the incidence of colon cancer, Japanese have to eat more vegetables and rice to increase the intake of dietary fiber and vitamins such as vitamin A, E, C, and β-carotene.

In this chapter we discuss the effect of Japanese vegetable juice, Aojiru, on growth and peristalsis, and on cellular immune functions such as lymphocytes, macrophages, and natural killer cells (NK) in rats.

3.2 JAPANESE VEGETABLE JUICE: AOJIRU

Aojiru is named from its color and a juice prepared from kale, which is a plant akin to cabbage. As shown in Table 3.1, the main component of Aojiru is water (about 95%). The content of Ca in Aojiru is equal to that of one bottle of milk. The contents of vitamins A and C are equivalent to five and three tomatoes, respectively. Two bottles of Aojiru (180 ml) supply the daily recommended dietary allowance (RDA) for vitamins and minerals. At present 40,000 households periodically purchase and drink Aojiru. Figure 3.4 summarizes the beneficial effects of Aojiru on health promotion. The figures are the percent of the replies to questionnaire sent to 1582 subjects who drink Aojiru daily. As shown in Figure 3.4, Aojiru has the greatest effect on constipation (20.7%), followed by the common cold (13.3%), and hypertension (12.6%). Although many people have experienced the beneficial effects of Aojiru, there has been no scientific evidence to explain the action of Aojiru on health promotion until now. Next, we tried to investigate whether Aojiru can enhance cellular immune functions in rats. In addition, to clarify the effect of Aojiru on constipation, changes in fecal weight have been measured.

TABLE 3.1
Ingredients of Aojiru (100 g)

Protein (mg)	1313
P (mg)	30
K (mg)	289
Ca (mg)	146
Mg (mg)	23
Carotenoids (mg)	1.05
Vitamin A (IU)	580
Vitamin C (mg)	196
Vitamin E (mg)	0.4
Fiber (mg)	200
Water (%)	94.8

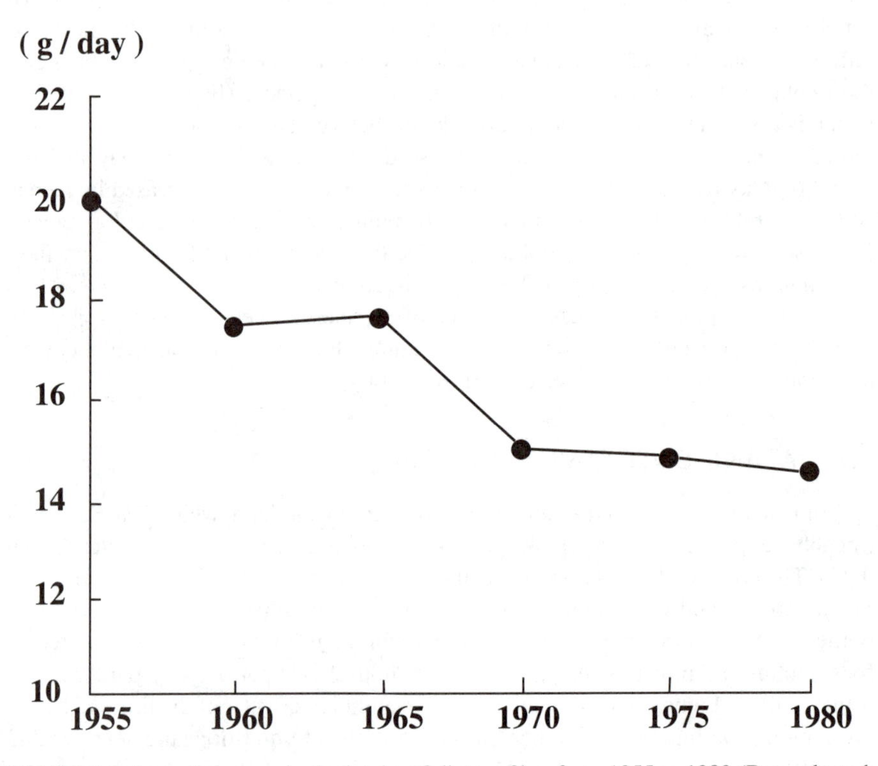

FIGURE 3.3 Annual changes in the intake of dietary fiber from 1955 to 1980 (Data adapted from the special edition of *J. Health Welfare Stat.*, 46, 1999.)

3.3 EFFECT OF AOJIRU ON GROWTH AND PERISTALSIS

As it is difficult for rats to drink the same proportional amount of Aojiru as do human, male rats, four weeks old, were fed a diet containing freeze-dried Aojiru as shown in Table 3.2. After 11 weeks they were sacrificed under anesthesia with pentobarbital (0.1 ml/ 100g BW) and their spleens were used for several immune assays. The daily food intake of rats was not significantly different between the control and freeze-dried Aojiru-supplemented groups throughout the experiment. The weight gain in rats fed the freeze-dried Aojiru-supplemented diet was also not significantly different from that of rats fed the control diet. A high intake of Aojiru (3% of diet) did not induce adverse effects on the growth of rats. In addition, the fecal weight was higher in rats fed the freeze-dried Aojiru-supplemented diet compared to that of rats fed the control diet in the first half of the experiment (Figure 3.5). This result may explain why Aojiru has a beneficial effect on constipation, as shown in Figure 3.4. Although we tried to measure the elapsed time between stools of rats fed the control or freeze-dried Aojiru-supplemented diet by using India ink, we failed to find the feces with India ink. Because the feces of rats fed the freeze-dried Aojiru-supplemented diet was colored dark green, it was hard to distinguish the color of their feces from that of India ink. The increase in fecal weight from rats fed the freeze-dried Aojiru-supplemented diet suggests that the elapsed

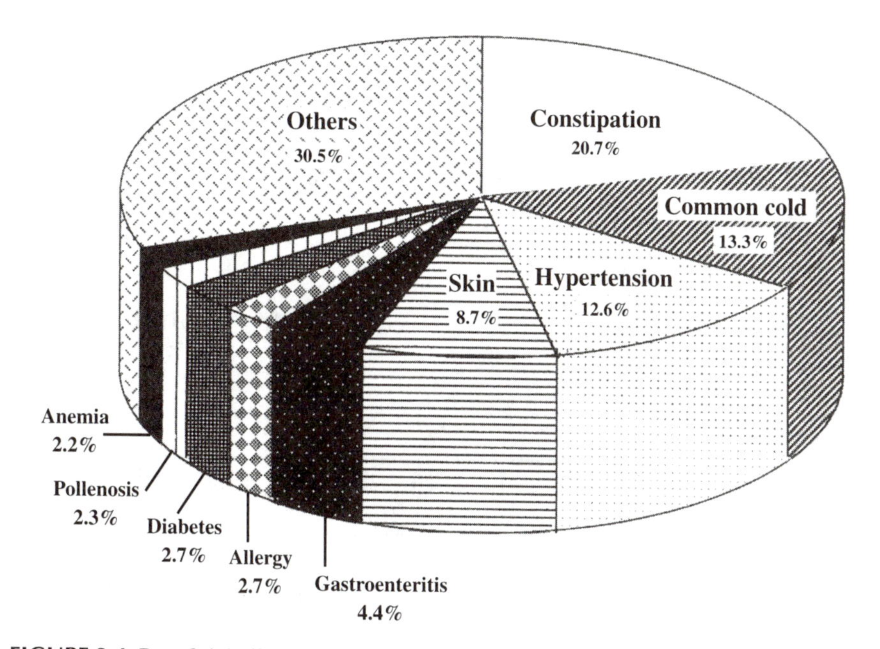

FIGURE 3.4 Beneficial effects of Aojiru on health promotion. Figures are percents of replies to the questionnaire sent to 1,582 persons drinking Aojiru daily.

TABLE 3.2
Composition of Experimental Diets

Ingredients	Control (g)	Aojiru (g)
Casein	20	20
α-Cornstarch	57	57
Sucrose	10	10
Corn oil	8	8
Mineral mix	4	4
Vitamin mix	1	1
Freez-dried Aojiru	–	3
Total	100	103

time between stools is shortened by the intake of Aojiru. However, in the latter half of the experiment there was no significant difference in the fecal weight between control and the freeze-dried Aojiru-supplemented diets (data not shown). This evidence may indicate that the beneficial effect of Aojiru on constipation is induced at an early stage of Aojiru intake. It is known that a higher intake of dietary fiber is in inverse correlation with the incidence and the mortality of colon cancer,[10-12] which is associated with the increased fecal weight and the shortened time between stools.[13-15] As shown in Table 3.1, the content of fiber in Aojiru (100 g) is not much higher compared to those of other vegetables. The increased fecal weight induced by Aojiru intake appears to be due not only to fiber, but also to other factors including the

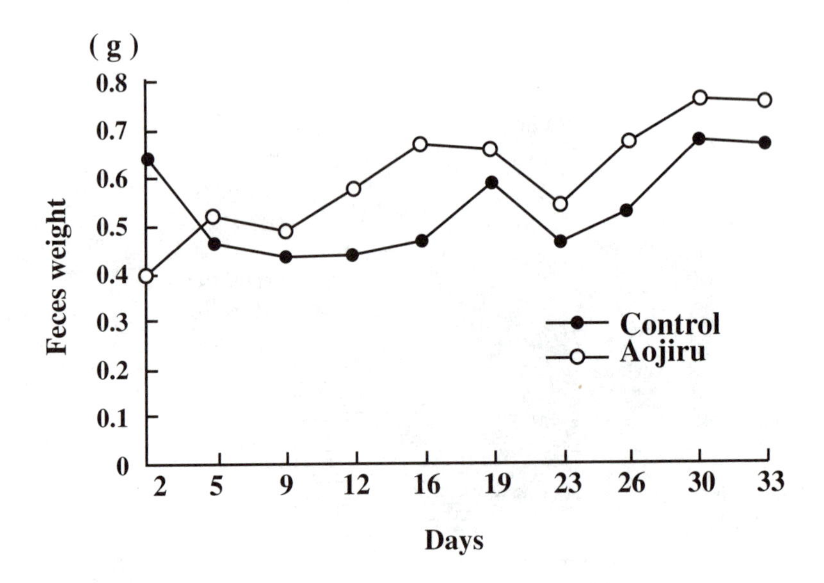

FIGURE 3.5 Changes of the fecal weight in rats fed a control diet or freeze-dried Aojiru-supplemented diet.

viscosity and expansibility. Further study needs to focus on the mechanism by which Aojiru increases fecal weight.

3.4 EFFECT OF AOJIRU ON LYMPHOCYTE AND MACROPHAGE FUNCTIONS

The number of splenocytes was higher in rats fed the freeze-dried Aojiru supplemented diet ($5.16 \pm 0.81 \times 10^8$ cells/g spleen) compared to rats fed the control diet ($4.12 \pm 0.40 \times 10^6$ cells/g spleen). There was no significant difference in number of alveolar macrophages (AM), collected by tracheopulmonary lavage, between both experimental groups (Control: $8.39 \pm 0.75 \times 10^5$ cells/100 g BW; Aojiru: $8.45 \pm 0.94 \times 10^5$ cells/100 g BW).

For the function of splenic lymphocytes, we measured proliferation of lymphocytes following *in vitro* stimulation with PHA (10 μg/ml) or Con A (5 μg/ml) for 72 h. Proliferation of lymphocytes was assessed by using a colorimetric method (MTT test).[16,17] The results were represented as a stimulation index (SI), which was calculated by comparing the absorbance of samples stimulated by mitogens with the absorbance of a sample cultured with medium. Although there was no significant difference in PHA stimulation between both the control and Aojiru groups, proliferation of splenic lymphocytes with Con A was higher in rats fed the freeze-dried Aojiru-supplemented diet (2.47 ± 0.36) than that of control rats (2.16 ± 0.30). This result may indicate that Aojiru activates macrophage function.

In general, macrophages are capble of two types of phagocytosis: nonspecific and specific phagocytosis via receptors for Fc or C3 existing on their membranes.

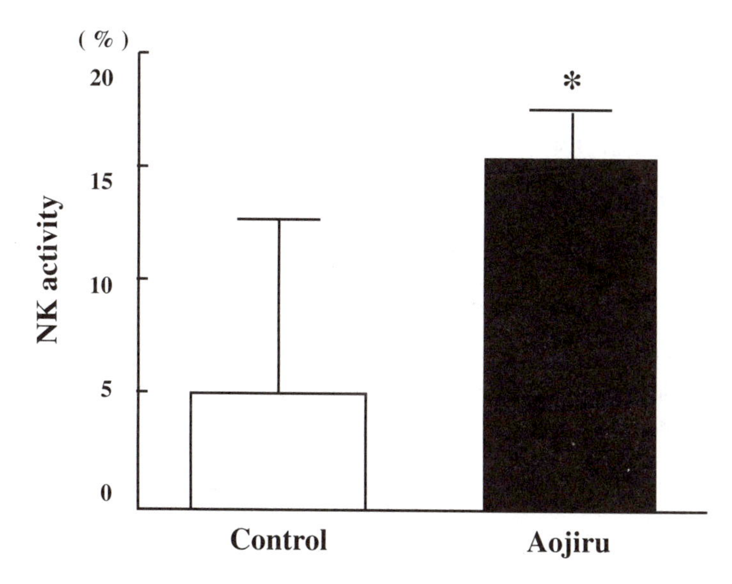

FIGURE 3.6 Natural killer cell (NK) activity of splenocytes from rats fed a control diet or freeze-dried Aojiru-supplemented diet.

And it is known that specific phagocytosis is significantly higher than nonspecific phagocytosis. In this experiment, both phagocytosis types were assayed by using sheep red blood cells (SRBC) and opsonized SRBC (SRBC coated with anti-SRBC antibody), respectively. Phagocytic activity of AM was measured by absorbance at 395 nm, which is an optimum wavelength for SRBC dissolved with 0.1 *N* NaOH. Although nonspecific phagocytosis of AM against SRBC (untreated with antibody or C3) was higher in rats fed the freeze-dried Aojiru diet (0.074 ± 0.028) than that of control rats (0.059 ± 0.032), it was not significant. In addition, phagocytosis of AM against opsonized SRBC (specific phagocytosis) was also slightly higher in rats fed the freeze-dried Aojiru diet (0.148 ± 0.032) compared to that of control rats (0.134 ± 0.058). These results may support the hypothesis that Aojiru activates macrophage function.

3.5 EFFECT OF AOJIRU ON NATURAL KILLER CELL (NK) ACTIVITY

The second beneficial effect of Aojiru is to protect against the common cold. In this study we tried to investigate the function of natural killer cells (NK), which play an important role in protecting the body from bacterial and viral infections, and in excluding transformed cells and suppressing carcinogenesis.[18-20] Splenocytes were used as effector cells and YAC-1 cells; T-cell lymphoma induced by Moloney virus[21] were used as target cells. In this study the effector/target cell ratio was 200 to 1. As shown in Figure 3.6, NK activity of splenocytes from rats fed the freeze-dried Aojiru-supplemented diet was about three times higher ($p < .05$) than that of control rats.

This evidence may support the protective action of Aojiru against the common cold. However, the mechanism by which Aojiru enhances NK activity remains to be elucidated.

3.6 CONCLUSION

In this chapter we described the beneficial effects of the Japanese vegetable juice, Aojiru, on health promotion by using the results of our recent experiments in rats. The evidence obtained in our experiment has strongly supported the beneficial effect of Aojiru, whose mechanism of action remains to be clarified. What is the material enhancing cellular immune function? How does Aojiru activate NK function? Although there still remains several questions to be resolved in the future, this study seems to be definitely worthwhile for providing scientific evidence to explain personal experiences on the beneficial effect of Aojiru.

ACKNOWLEDGMENT

The authors wish to thank Ms. K. Yoshioka and Ms. S. Yamashita for their technical assistance.

REFERENCES

1. Ajiki, W. and Yamamoto, S., Cancer statistics digest. Rectal cancer incidence in Japan, *Jpn. J. Clin. Oncol.*, 29, 408, 1999.
2. Hirohata, T. and Kono, S., Diet/nutrition and stomach cancer in Japan *Int. J. Cancer*, 10, 34, 1997.
3. Tominaga, S. and Kuroishi, T., An ecological study on diet/nutrition and cancer in Japan, *Int. J. Cancer*, Suppl. 10, 2, 1997.
4. Levi, F., Lucchini, F., Negri, E., and La Vecchia, C., Worldwide patterns of cancer mortality, *Eur. J. Cancer Prev.*, 8, 381, 1999.
5. Speizer, F.E., Colditz, G.A., Hunter, D.J., Rosner, B., and Hennekens, C., Prospective study of smoking, antioxidant intake, and lung cancer in middle-aged women, *Cancer Causes Control,* 10, 475, 1999.
6. Enstrom, J.E., Smoking cessation and mortality trends among two United States populations, *J. Clin. Epidemiol.*, 52, 813, 1999.
7. Watanabe, H., Uesaka, T., Kido, S., Ishimura, Y., Shiraki, K., Kuramoto, K., Hirata, S., Shoji, S., Katoh, O., and Fujimoto, N., Influence of concomitant miso or NaCl treatment on induction of gastric tumors by N-methyl-N'-nitro-N-nitrosoguanidine in rats, *Oncol. Rep.*, 6, 989, 1999.
8. Ishii, H., Tatsuta, M., Baba, M., Hirasawa, R., Sakai, N., Yano, H., Uehara, H., and Nakaizumi, A., Low-protein diet promotes sodium chloride-enhanced gastric carcinogenesis induced by N-methyl-N'-nitro-N-nitrosoguanidine in Wistar rats, *Cancer Lett.*, 141, 117, 1999.
9. Honjo, S., Kono, S., and Yamaguchi, M., Salt and geographic variation in stomach cancer mortality in Japan, *Cancer Causes Control*, 5, 285, 1994.
10. Freeman, H.J., Role of high fiber foods in the prevention of colorectal neoplasia, *Can. J. Gastroenterol.*, 13, 379, 1999.

11. Lipkin, M., Reddy, B., Newmark, H., and Lamprecht, S.A., Dietary factors in human colorectal cancer, *Annu. Rev. Nutr.*, 19, 545, 1999.
12. Jeanteur, P., Dietary fibre intake and colon cancer, *Bull. Cancer,* 86, 611, 1999.
13. Cummings, J.H., Bingham, S.A., Heaton, K.W., and Eastwood, M.A., Fecal weight, colon cancer risk, and dietary intake of nonstarch polysaccharides, *Gastroenterology,* 103, 1783, 1992.
14. Levy, R.D., Segal, I., Hassan, H., and Saadia, R., Stool weight and faecal pH in two South African populations with a dissimilar colon cancer risk, *S. Afr. J. Surg.*, 32, 127, 1994.
15. Zoran, D.L., Turner, N.D., Taddeo, S.S., Chapkin, R.S., and Lupton, J.R., Wheat bran diet reduces tumor incidence in a rat model of colon cancer independent of effects on distal luminal butyrate concentrations, *J. Nutr.*, 127, 2217, 1997.
16. Verhulst, C., Coiffard, C., Coiffard, L.J., Rivalland, P., and De Roeck-Holtzhauer, Y., In vitro correlation between two colorimetric assays and the pyruvic acid consumption by fibroblasts cultured to determine the sodium laurylsulfate cytotoxicity, *J. Pharmacol. Toxicol. Methods*, 39, 143, 1998.
17. Wagner, U., Burkhardt, E., and Failing, K., Evaluation of canine lymphocyte proliferation: comparison of three different colorimetric methods with the ^{3}H-thymidine incorporation assay, *Vet. Immunol. Immunopathol.*, 70, 151, 1999.
18. Cooley, S., Burns, L.J., Repka, T., and Miller, J.S., Natural killer cell cytotoxicity of breast cancer targets is enhanced by two distinct mechanisms of antibody-dependent cellular cytotoxicity against LFA-3 and HER2/neu, *Exp. Hematol.,* 27, 1533, 1999.
19. Hirose, K., Nishimura, H., Matsuguchi, T., and Yoshikai, Y., Endogenous IL-15 might be responsible for early protection by natural killer cells against infection with an avirulent strain of Salmonella choleraesuis in mice, *J. Leukocyte. Biol.*, 66, 382, 1999.
20. Baraz, L., Khazanov, E., Condiotti, R., Kotler, M., and Nagler, A., Natural killer (NK) cells prevent virus production in cell culture, *Bone Marrow Transplant.*, 24, 179, 1999.
21. Galili, N., Devens, B., Naor, D., Becker, S., and Klein, E., Immune responses to weakly immunogenic virally induced tumors. 1. Overcoming low responsiveness by priming mice with a syngeneic in vitro tumor line or allogeneic cross-reactive tumor, *Eur. J. Immunol.*, 8, 17, 1978.

4 Tomatoes and Health Promotion

Patrizia Riso and Marisa Porrini

CONTENTS

4.1 INTRODUCTION

The consumption of fruits and vegetables has been recognized as being important for good health, giving rise to the need to identify the specific compounds that could impart such a benefit. Particular attention has been given to substances such as vitamin C, vitamin E, thiols, β-carotene, and carotenoids. However an increasing need to shift attention from individual components to whole foods is being recognized. In fact, it seems reasonable to assume that the beneficial effects may depend on the interaction of potentially relevant substances in whole foods rather than on single supplements. A clear need for this concept arose from the results of several intervention studies where supplementation with pure compounds was associated with no benefit or adverse effects.[1,2]

Over the last few years the question has been raised whether tomato consumption might have protective and anticarcinogenic properties. Lycopene, the carotenoid pigment responsible for the red color, is the most distinctive compound present in

0-8493-0038-X/97/$0.00+$.50

tomatoes and it has been recognized as the most effective antioxidant among the carotenoids. That is why we have more information about lycopene than the tomato itself and why data referring to lycopene also often refers to tomatoes and vice versa.

Even though more research is needed to understand the role and potential mechanism of action of foods like tomatoes, some data are already available. This brief review summarizes our present knowledge and future prospects.

4.2 CHEMICAL COMPOSITION OF TOMATO PRODUCTS

Tomato (*Solanum lycopersicum*) is a vegetable crop of the family Solanaceae. It has had a rapid development with large-scale cultivation, and an increasing number of different varieties have been produced. Nowadays, not only are raw tomatoes consumed all over the world, but so are processed tomatoes (tomato juice, paste, puree, ketchup, sauce, salsa, etc.).

Tomato fruit contains about 5 to 10% dry matter and 1% is skin and seeds. About 50% of the dry matter consists of reducing sugars (mainly glucose and fructose), while the remaining part is alcohol-insoluble solids, organic acids, minerals, pigments, vitamins, and lipids.[3] The range of composition of ripe tomatoes is shown in Table 4.1. Some data are also available on the carotenoid content of different tomato products.[4-8]

What is special about the composition of tomato and tomato products with respect to other fruits and vegetables is their high content of lycopene, the acyclic carotenoid containing 11 conjugated double bonds (Figure 4.1). There is a small amount of lycopene in just a few other foods (watermelon, pink guava, pink grapefruit, papaya) but tomatoes and tomato products are the major sources in the diet. Tomatoes contain low amounts of α-, β-, γ-, ξ-carotene and lutein and also neurosporene, phytoene, and phytofluene. The lycopene content can vary greatly depending on the variety of the tomatoes considered and obviously on the type of processing undergone. Table 4.2 shows the range of lycopene content for several tomato products.[9]

In fresh tomatoes lycopene is present in the all-trans geometrical configuration, and isomerization has been suggested to derive from thermal treatment in food processing. However, it has recently been shown that lycopene is stable in the tomato matrix and that, if isomerization occurs, it is due to sample handling.[10] On the other hand, as will be subsequently discussed, it has been reported that cis isomers are bioavailable and have been detected both in plasma[11-13] and tissues.[13]

When reporting data on carotenoids composition, and especially on lycopene, it is important to carefully consider the reliability of the analytical method used. There is a great between-laboratory variation in the determination of lycopene content and this is why conflicting data are reported in the literature. Since epidemiologists and clinical investigators use databases to estimate food intake, the data becomes of utmost importance.

Apart from lycopene, tomato is also a source of vitamin C, providing a significant contribution to dietary intake.[14] Raw tomato contains more vitamin C than processed tomato, and there is a higher loss of the vitamin during the production of tomato

TABLE 4.1
Composition of Raw Tomato[4–8]

Constituent	Range of Concentration
	g/100 g
Water	93.1–94.2
Protein	0.7–1.0
Fat	0.2–0.3
Carbohydrate	3.1–3.5
	mg/100 g
Vitamin C	16.0–24.2
Vitamin E	0.80–1.22
Lycopene	0.90–9.30
β-Carotene	0.30–0.52
Lutein	0.04–0.10
Phytoene	0.49–2.80
γ-Carotene	0.04–1.61
	μg/100 g
Fe	400–600
Zn	100–240
Mn	90–140
Cu	10–90
Se	trace–600
Folates	17–39

TABLE 4.2
Lycopene Contents of Common Tomato-Based Foods

Tomato Products	Lycopene (μg/g weight)
Fresh Tomatoes	8.8—42.0
Cooked Tomatoes	37.0
Tomato Sauce	62.0
Tomato Paste	54.0—1500.0
Tomato Soup (condensed)	79.9
Tomato Powder	1126.3—1264.9
Tomato Juice	50.0—116.0
Pizza Sauce	127.1
Ketchup	99.0—134.4

Source: From Rao, A.V. and Argawal, S., *Nutr. Res.*, 19(2), 305, 1999. With permission.

concentrates than in tomato juice or whole canned tomatoes.[15] It is necessary to underline that the contribution of vitamin C (extensively studied per se), and its possible interaction with the other compounds in tomatoes, has not been sufficiently investigated.

Phenolic compounds are other potential important substances that, although in a lesser amounts, could contribute to the beneficial effects of tomato products. Qualitative and quantitative distribution in tomato products has been reported by different authors.[16-18] It is true that tomato is not a main source of these compounds but neither has it been demonstrated they are not absorbed. Particularly, the few reports in literature on the flavonoid composition of tomatoes are not consistent and univocal, due mainly to methodological problems. We found recently that tomato puree contains a small amount of rutin and that this compound can be absorbed *in vivo;*[19] however, no other data are reported in literature.

There is a need to update our knowledge about tomato composition, taking into account the new and more sensitive analytical resources developed over the last few years.

4.3 BIOAVAILABILITY OF COMPOUNDS IN TOMATOES

When studying the relation between fruit and vegetable intake and the risk of disease, it is important to focus on the bioavailability of the different nutrients from these foods.

At present, there is no validated method for the quantitative assessment of lycopene bioavailability. In general, bioavailability of carotenoids can be studied using several methods[20,21] including (a) oral-fecal balance studies; (b) plasma or chylomicron response studies; and (c) stable isotope and compartmental modeling studies in humans. The stable isotope labeling approach appears to be the best way to study carotenoid bioavailability, however, few data using this method are available. Plasma or chylomicron response studies can be useful in determining the relative efficiency of absorption of carotenoids and are also easier to perform. Most data on lycopene bioavailability have been based on this approach.

Several studies have pointed out that by restricting dietary sources of lycopene there is a progressive decline in plasma lycopene concentrations, and that by adding natural sources of lycopene to the diet plasma concentrations can be restored.[7,22-26] This fact should be carefully considered when interpreting data from epidemiological studies, as just a single blood sample may not be representative of the habitual dietary pattern of the subjects studied. This could also be the reason for the low correlation found between plasma concentrations (from one blood sample) and dietary intake evaluated by several days of food regimentation or by dietary history methods.[27,28] Furthermore, great attention must be paid to lycopene bioavailability which, like that of the other carotenoids, is influenced by several physiological and dietary factors.[21,29] The absorption of lycopene is thought to be quite a slow process involving passive diffusion through the intestinal membrane. Lycopene is fat soluble and follows the same four-step absorptive pathway as other dietary lipids: digestion of the food matrix, formation of lipid-mixed micelles, uptake into the intestinal mucosal cells, and transport into the general circulation via the lymph system. A crucial step of the absorptive mechanism is the transfer of the carotenoid from the emulsion particles to mixed bile salt micelles: carotenoid absorption is minimal

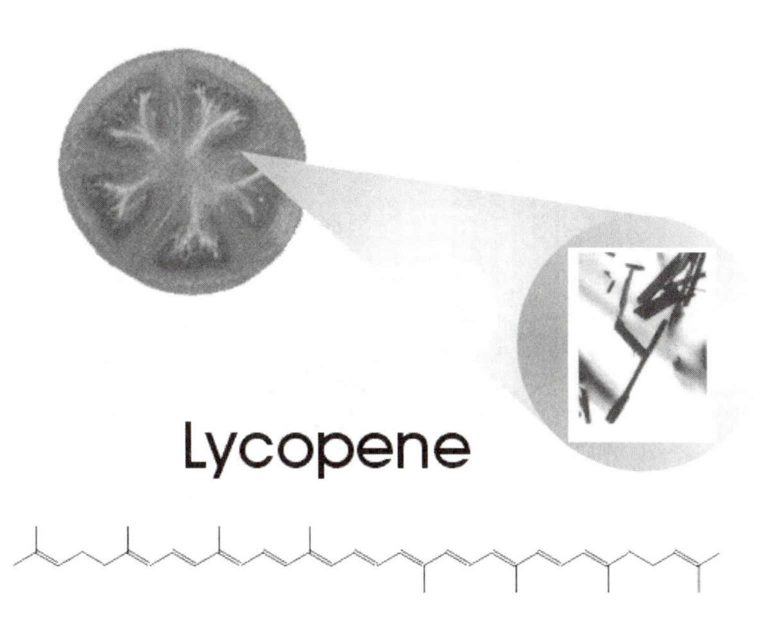

FIGURE 4.1 Lycopene crystals and lycopene structure in tomato.

when intraluminal bile salts are below the concentration required for aggregation into micelles. The rate of incorporation into chylomicrons is another important factor, as carotenoids are transported into the plasma by lipoproteins. These events explain the role of the presence of fat in the lumen: a sufficient amount of fat is necessary for solubilization of lycopene and for stimulation of chylomicron synthesis. Nonabsorbable lipids, such as sucrose polyesters used nowadays as fat substitutes, may behave as a hydrophobic trap in the intestinal lumen and reduce lycopene absorption.[30] It has been estimated that the intake of 18 g/day olestra for 16 weeks effects a reduction in serum lycopene concentration of about 30%,[30] but still unknown is the role of fat substitutes in carotenoid absorption under conditions of usual consumption.

Before absorption, lycopene must be released from the food matrix, as it is not free in food but in the form of crystalline aggregates in specific plant cell structures (Figure 4.1). Aggregation changes the physical properties of lycopene as well as aiding in its solubilization, thereby affecting its bioavailability. Consequently, physically altering food by cooking, blending, and finely chopping it can improve the release of lycopene from the food matrix.

Stahl and Sies[31] were the first researchers to investigate the absorption of lycopene from a food source. They found a significant increase in serum lycopene concentration after the intake of tomato juice boiled for 1 h in the presence of corn oil, but not after the intake of the same amount of unprocessed tomato juice. Later, differences in lycopene bioavailability were also observed between raw tomato and

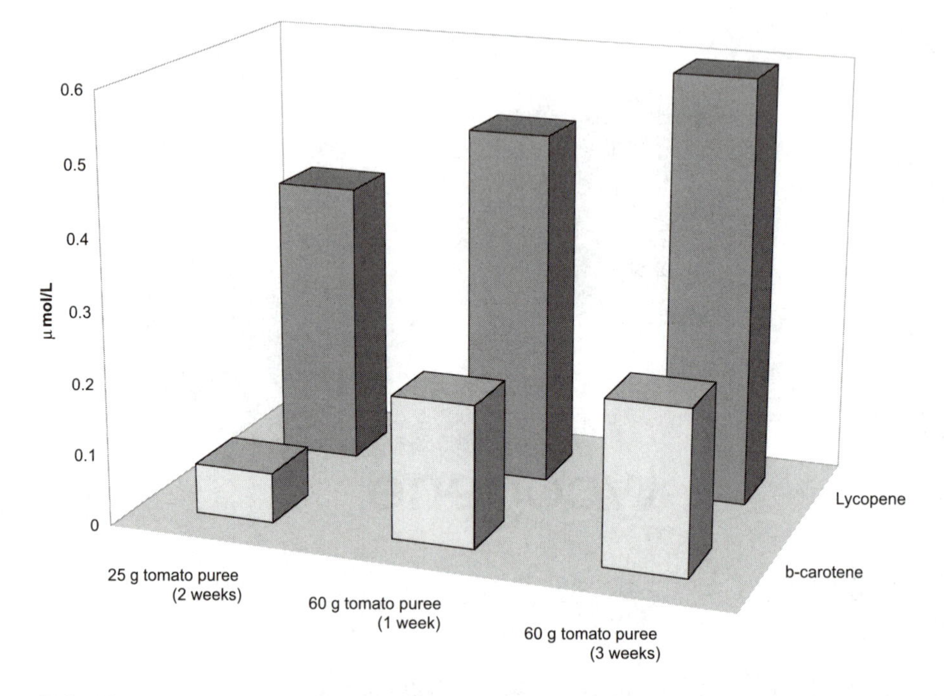

FIGURE 4.2 Increase of lycopene and β-carotene concentrations (μmol/l) in human plasma after the intake of 60 g or 25 g tomato puree for different intervals of time (1, 2, 3 weeks).

processed tomato (homogenized and heated) when studying both plasma[7,26] and chylomicron[32] response to different amounts of the carotenoid; absorption of lycopene was always greater from the processed tomato than the raw tomato. In all these studies, to assure a sufficient amount of fat tomato products were consumed either with oil or with the meal.

From these data we can conclude that the mechanical disruption of the food matrix and heat treatment must be considered important factors influencing lycopene bioavailability as they affect the structure of vegetable tissues and, consequently, the efficiency of extraction of lycopene from the food matrix into the lipophilic phase.

One aspect that at present is not sufficiently clear concerns the quantitative relationship between lycopene intake and lycopene plasma concentration. We have found that 16.5 mg lycopene (provided by 60 g tomato puree) consumed daily for 1 or 3 weeks, elicited an increase in lycopene plasma concentration of about 0.5 and 0.6 μmol/l, respectively,[7,33] while the intake of 7 mg lycopene (provided by 25 g of the same tomato puree) daily for 2 weeks, elicited an increase of 0.4 μmol/l[34] (Figure 4.2). Consequently, it seems that plasma lycopene concentrations do not respond in a dose-dependent manner and that small amounts are enough to improve and maintain plasma levels. Furthermore, in the same studies β-carotene increased significantly during tomato consumption and decreased during the tomato-free diet, showing that despite the small amount consumed (0.6 and 0.3 mg, respectively) β-carotene absorption is an efficient process which does not seem to be affected by the high quantity of lycopene present (Figure 4.2).

Apart from these data on plasma or chylomicron response, at present little is known about the relationship between the intake of foods rich in carotenoids and their concentration in specific cells. We found that the daily consumption of 25 g tomato puree (containing 7 mg lycopene) increased not only the plasma, but also the lymphocyte lycopene concentration.[34]

Several, but limited, reports are also available on lycopene distribution in tissues, however, these data are highly variable. The difference in tissues pattern supports the hypothesis that the specific effects of lycopene are mainly concentrated in the adrenal glands, testes, liver, and prostate (see Clinton[35] for a review).

Another aspect closely related to lycopene bioavailability is the contribution of its structural configuration. Some studies report that lycopene is present in plasma and tissue in several geometrical configurations,[32,36-38] mainly all-*trans*, 9-*cis*, 13-*cis*, and 15-*cis* isomers. Clinton et al.,[39] using a C_{30} HPLC column, were able to separate 12 to 13 geometric lycopene isomers in serum extracts and 15 to 18 in prostate extracts. Altogether, *cis*-isomers account for more than 50% of total lycopene in tissues.[9,39] However, in tomatoes and tomato-based products, all-*trans* lycopene comprises 79–91% of total lycopene.[39] The mechanism by which all-*trans* lycopene is converted to the *cis* isomers in plasma and tissues is still unknown. Isomerization could occur during heat treatment of food or during digestion before absorption. It has been suggested that *cis*-isomers of lycopene have a lower tendency to crystallize or aggregate in foods[40] and thus are better absorbed than all-*trans* isomers.[31,32] Probably this is due to the enhanced solubility of *cis*-lycopene in bile acid micelles and its preferential incorporation into chylomicrons, as supported by Boileau et al.[41] who studied the absorption of lycopene isomers both *in vitro* (with bile acid micelles containing crystalline lycopene) and *in vivo* (using mesenteric lymph duct cannulated ferrets). However, the physiological role of all these isomers in biological tissues is still unknown.

4.4 EXPERIMENTAL EVIDENCE OF TOMATO'S EFFECTS

Intervention trials on a large scale are fundamental to understand the action of foods or particular substances on human health; however, they are often very expensive, difficult to carry out, and time consuming. Furthermore, it is necessary that consistent experimental evidence supports the use of a substance in intervention studies on human beings.

In the case of tomato, some studies exist showing that its consumption may exert a protective effect on specific targets in a short time. Consequently, over the last few years the number of investigations using relevant *in vitro* and *in vivo* models has been increasing. However, the experimental data on tomato and tomato products are limited, more if lycopene is considered.

In order to simplify the analysis of studies reported in the literature we have divided them into *in vitro* studies, cell culture studies, animal studies, and human studies.

4.4.1 *In Vitro* Studies

It is generally accepted that the beneficial effect of tomato and tomato products go beyond the accomplishment of what is called the "antioxidant capacity." Obviously, the potential antioxidant properties of tomato depend on the contribution of all the compounds present, even if lycopene is recognized as being the most powerful.

Many *in vitro* studies demonstrated that lycopene has the best singlet oxygen quenching properties[42] and radical scavenging activity[43] among the carotenoids. This action occurs mainly via physical interaction.

Weisburger[44] reported that lycopene can block the conversion of food mutagens in fried or cooked foods in reactive mutagenic products, suggesting that the small amounts of these mutagens in the Mediterranean diet could not be activated by the contemporaneous presence of antioxidants from fruit and vegetables, tomato included.

Lavelli et al.[45] demonstrated that tomato extracts can act as radical scavengers against reactive oxygen species and lipid peroxidation in *in vitro* models. The model systems used simulated the key reactions involved in the pathogenesis of several chronic diseases. Wang et al.[46] showed the radical scavenging activity of water and acetone extracts of tomato; the methanol/water fraction of tomato had an inhibitory effect on the peroxidation of microsomes containing cytochrome P450s isoenzymes, which have an important role in nonenzymic microsomal lipid peroxidation.[47] In another study the methanol/water fraction was able to inhibit the copper-catalyzed oxidation of LDL.[18] Pellegrini et al.[48] recently developed a method that can analyze the antioxidant activity of both the lipophilic and aqueous methanolic extracts of tomatoes; with this method, the aqueous methanolic extract, rich in flavonoids and phenolics, seems to contribute significantly toward the antioxidant capacity — three times more than the lipophilic extract.

Despite this convincing evidence, data coming from the *in vitro* studies cannot be simply shifted *in vivo*, as the real contribution of such compounds is strictly subordinate to the relative bioavailability and absorption *in vivo*.

4.4.2 Cell Culture Studies

Cell culture studies have been addressed as a potential model for the evaluation of the activity of antioxidant substances.[49] Animals cannot be considered good models for studying the mechanistic effects of dietary components, as there are differences between humans and animals in the absorption and distribution in tissues of many compounds. For this reason, cell models have been developed; they are less invasive and could help in providing a few tentative explanations as to the healthy properties of these substances. For tomato, however, data are still insufficient and are limited mainly to the action of lycopene. One important problem with the study of lycopene in cell culture is that this high lipophilic compound is difficult to supplement in a bioavailable form. The supplementation of carotenoids is generally made by the use of beadlets (mainly for β-carotene), liposomes, and several organic solvents (e.g., tetrahydrofuran).

Most cell culture studies have concentrated on the antitumorigenic activity using cancer cells derived from both animal and human tumors (Table 4.3); however, it would also be advisable to have data on primary cells that could be good markers of the *in vivo* response in physiological conditions.

Lycopene is a good inhibitor of proliferation of several types of cancer cells in culture. This is a characteristic common with a lot of other antioxidant compounds (other carotenoids, flavonoids, etc). However, it is not clearly understood how they act and the relation with the dosage used. Generally the concentrations reached in cell culture studies are much higher than those achievable *in vivo* by food consumption and it is likely that such high doses could be toxic for cells. However some interesting results have been reported that have stimulated research on lycopene action.

Levy et al.[50] found that lycopene was much more effective than α-carotene and β-carotene in inhibiting human endometrial (Ishikawa) mammary (MCF-7) and lung (NCI-H226) cancer cells in culture. This higher activity of lycopene seems not to depend on its preferential uptake into cells, however, the inhibitory mechanism is still under study. The authors suggested that lycopene could act by inhibiting the IGF-induced growth of cancer cells. Differently from cancer cells, human fibroblasts were less sensitive to lycopene.

Countryman et al.[51] showed that lycopene also was effective in inhibiting the proliferation of the HL-60 human promyelocitic leukemia cells and increasing cell differentiation. The same effect was shown by Bankson et al.[52] and Amir et al,[53] who furthermore demonstrated that the inhibition of the HL-60 cell growth by lycopene, as well as by β-carotene, was associated with a slowing of cell cycle progression at the G_0/G_1 phase and induction of cell differentiation. Interestingly, lycopene showed a synergistic effect with 1,25-dihydroxyvitamin D_3. In this regard, it is interesting to point out that while $1,25(OH)_2D_3$ seemed effective at high and toxic concentrations, lycopene was active at physiological concentrations. When the two were supplemented together they were effective at concentrations close to their physiological levels. This supports the importance of the food matrix, and more generally the whole diet rather than the single substances or ingredients for "therapeutic approaches."

Bertram et al.[54] demonstrated that several carotenoids, lycopene included, were able to inhibit the neoplastic transformation induced by methylcholantrene in a mouse embryo fibroblast cell line. The compounds exerted their activity when added 7 days after treatment with the carcinogen, thus suggesting a role of inhibition of the events occurring post-initiation. Furthermore, carotenoids and retinoids were able to cause a reversible inhibition of cell transformation initiated by carcinogens. This activity was correlated with the ability of the different carotenoids to upregulate gap junction communication by increasing the gene expression of connexin 43,[55,56] a component of the gap junction structure. Loss of gap junctional communication may be important for malignant transformation, and its restoration may reverse the malignant process.

Other reports have supported the chemopreventive action of lycopene. Tsushima et al.[57] found that the carotenoid was able to inhibit 12-O-tetradecanoylphorbol-13-acetate-induced Epstein-Barr virus activation in Raji limphoblastoid cells. Kim[58]

TABLE 4.3
Evidence of Lycopene/Tomato Action from Cell Culture Studies

Model	Supplementation	Effect	Ref.
C3H/10T1/2 mouse embryo fibroblast cell line	Lycopene and other carotenoids	Dose-dependent inhibition of malignant transformation	54
C3H/10T1/2 mouse embryo fibroblast cell line	Lycopene and other carotenoids	Increase of connexin43 gene expression involved in gap junction communication	55, 56
HL-60 human leukemia cell line	Lycopene (10 μmol/l) and other carotenoids	Inhibition of tumor cell growth	51
HL-60 human leukemia cell line	Lycopene and other carotenoids	Increase in cell differentiation	52
Raji lymphoblastoid cells (carrying Epstein-Barr virus genome)	Lycopene and other carotenoids	Inhibition of virus activation	57
Endometrial (Ishikawa), mammary (MCF-7), lung (NCI-H226) human cancer cell lines and normal fibroblast	Lycopene and other carotenoids	Inhibition of tumor cell growth but not of normal fibroblast	50
Rat hepatocytes	Lycopene and other carotenoids	Increased protection from CCL_4, decrease of lipid peroxidation	58
Mouse hepatocytes	Lycopene and other carotenoids	Increased protection from microcystin-LR-inducing liver tumor	59
Colo205 human colon cancer cells	Lycopene, other carotenoids, and vitamins	No effect on NAD(P)H: quinone reductase/ glutathione-*S*-transferase	60
HL-60 human leukemia cell line	Lycopene and 1,25-dihydroxyvitamin D_3	Inhibition of cell cycle progression in the G_0/G_1 phase, synergistic effect with vitamin D	53
J774A.1 macrophahage cell line	Lycopene and β-carotene	Reduction of cholesterol synthesis	61
Human aortic endothelial cells (EaHy-1)	Incubation with lycopene-enriched LDL	No effect on LDL lipid peroxidation	62
Lymphocyte from human blood	Cells coated with lycopene + sensitizer of singlet oxyen	Protections from photodynamic reaction	63
Lymphocyte from human blood	Cells coated with lycopene + NO_2 radical generator	Protection from nitrogen dioxide radical	64
HT29 colon carcinoma cell line	Lycopene supplementation + xanthine/xanthine oxidase	Protection from oxidative DNA damage	65

found that lycopene suppressed lipid peroxidation and increased survival of rat hepatocytes exposed to CCl_4, and Matushima-Nishiwaki et al.[59] found lycopene to be effective in protecting against microcystin-LR-induced liver tumors in mouse hepatocytes. They suggested that lycopene may inhibit tumor promotion by suppressing the hyperphosphorylation of cellular proteins.

On the contrary, Wang and Higuchi,[60] after supplementation of Colo205 human colon cancer cells with different vitamins and carotenoids, found no effect of lycopene on the induction of the detoxifying phase II enzymes (NAD(P)H: quinone reductase and glutathione-*S*-transferase), a possible mechanism of dietary anticarcinogenesis.

Cellular models also have been used to demonstrate the antioxidant activity of lycopene as well as other functions. Fuhrman et al.[61] showed that lycopene was able to reduce cholesterol synthesis in a macrophage cell line, providing support for a moderating effect of the carotenoid as a hypocholesterolemic agent. Dugas et al.[62] evaluated the effect of enriching LDL *in vitro* or *in vivo* with lycopene on oxidation by human aortic endothelial cells EaHy-1. After *in vitro* enrichment there was increased oxidation. On the contrary, on LDL isolated from subjects supplemented daily with tomato juice for 3 weeks, no effect was present. This study is important as it points out that different procedures of enrichment can produce controversial results.

Tinkler et al.[63] showed that lycopene is able to protect lymphoid cells against the photodynamic reaction sensitized by rose bengal or meso-tetra(4-sulphonatophenyl)porphine and it effectively protects lymphocyte cells from nitrogen dioxide radical damage.[64]

Lowe et al.[65] established that lycopene and β-carotene also protect the colon carcinoma cell line HT29 against oxidative DNA damage induced by xanthine/xanthine oxidase. The protection was exerted at a concentration lower than 3 μmol/l while higher concentrations registered an increase in the extent of DNA damage (pro-oxidant action). However, as previously discussed, it is important to consider that *in vivo* such concentrations can not be reached; in fact, in human subjects, daily tomato intake increased the plasma lycopene concentration up to about 1 μmol/l, reaching a plateau.[33]

4.4.3 Animal Studies

Animals have been used in experiments whereby they have been injected with or had a diet incorporating tomato extracts or lycopene, in order to evaluate the role of these substances in preventing cancer. The results have often been promising, even if some controversial results have also been reported (Table 4.4).

The first study was conducted in 1959 by Lingen et al.[66] who found an increase in the survival time of bacterially infected mice that underwent intraperitoneal or intravenous injection of lycopene. However, it has only been in the last decade that literature has been published about the increasing evidence that tomato products may protect from cancer.

Lycopene was shown to inhibit the growth and development of brain tumor cells in rats,[67] and of mammary tumor in both SHN virgin mice[68] and in rats treated with

TABLE 4.4
Evidence of Lycopene/Tomato Action from Animal Studies

Model	Intervention	Effect	Ref.
Bacterially infected mice	Intraperitoneal/intravenous injection of lycopene	Increase in survival rate	66
Wistar rates inoculated with brain tumor cells	Lycopene supplementation	Inhibition of growth and development of tumor cells	67
High mammary tumor strain of SHN virgin mice	Lycopene supplementation	Lower development of mammary tumor (decrease in the activity of thymidilate synthetase, lower levels of free fatty acids and prolactin)	68
Sprague-Dawley rats treated with MNU	Lycopene supplementation	Inhibition of formation of aberrant crypt foci	72
Weanling Rats	Lycopene supplementation	No effect on liver drug metabolizing enzymes	79
Sprague-Dawley rats treated with DMBA	Injection of lycopene-enriched tomato oleoresin	Decreased number of tumors and tumor size	69
Fisher rats treated with aflatoxin	Feeding by intubation with tomato paste extract	Decreased number of preneoplastic foci, effect in the early stages of hepatocarcinogenesis	70
S PF Wistar rats treated with DEN	Ingestion of a diet containing lycopene	Decrease in the size of liver preneoplastic foci	71
$B6C3F_1$ Mice treated with DEN, MNU, DMH	Lycopene supplementation	Protection on DEN-, MNU-, DMH-induced lung neoplasia	77
Wistar rats	Ingestion of tomato paste	Inhibition of nitrosamine production	76
F344/nsic rats	Supplementation with a diet containing lycopene-rich tomato juice	Protective on colon carcinogenesis	73
Fisher 344 rats	Ingestion of tomato juice	Inhibitory effect on the development of urinary bladder carcinogenesis	75
Fisher 344 rats treated with azoxymethane	Ingestion of oleoresin containing lycopene	Reduced number and size of aberrant crypt foci. Lower lipid and protein oxidation	74
A/J mice treated with benzo[a]pyrene	Lycopene-enriched oleoresin	No effect on lung tumor multiplicity	78
Wistar rats	Lycopene supplementation	No effect on P450 enzyme activity of extrahepatic tissues	80
Hypercholesterolemic mice	Ingestion of tomato	Protection from lipid peroxidation and decrease in the vaso-relaxing activity in the aorta	81

DMBA (7,12-dimethyl-benz(a)anthracene).[69] Nagasawa et al.[68] suggested that the protective role of lycopene against mammary tumor development could be due to the reduction of thymydilate synthetase activity and pituitary prolactin secretion.

The intubation of rats with a carotenoid-rich extract from tomato paste decreased the preneoplastic foci induced by aflatoxin during the initiation period, suggesting a role of lycopene in the early stages of hepatocarcinogenesis.[70] Astorg et al.[71] also found a decrease in the size of preneoplastic foci in rat livers as well as in the fraction of liver volume occupied after lycopene supplementation, but not after β-carotene, cantaxanthin, and astaxanthin supplementation.

Narisawa et al. wrote in 1996 that lycopene[72] and later in 1998, that tomato juice rich in lycopene[73] showed a protective effect against colon carcinogenesis. Rats receiving tomato juice differently diluted showed a significant reduction of cancer incidence with respect to a control group. The best effect was obtained with the less-diluted tomato juice (17 ppm lycopene) while no results were obtained when lycopene was provided in a water solution. Recently, Jain et al.[74] also reported a trend towards reduced numbers and size of aberrant crypt foci in rats after the addition of oleoresin containing lycopene to the diet. Furthermore, there was a decrease in serum TBARS and an increase in thiols measured as indicators of lipid and protein oxidation. Differently from what reported by He et al.[70] the efficiency of the oleoresin supplementation was better during the promotion stage than during the initiation stage. Similarly, other works suggested a protective effect of tomato juice against urinary bladder carcinoma[75] and of tomato paste against nitrosamine production[76] in rats, while there are some controversial results concerning the effect of lycopene and lycopene-enriched tomato oleoresin on lung neoplasia, as the former provided protection[77] and the latter had no effect[78] on mice.

No effect of lycopene, β-carotene, and lutein was shown on liver drug metabolizing enzymes[79] and on P450 enzyme activities of extrahepatic tissues[80] in rats.

Few animal studies exist that investigate the effect of tomato products on pathologies different from cancer. Recently, Suganuma and Inakuma[81] reported that the dietary ingestion of tomato for 4 months decreased plasma lipid peroxide and the vaso-relaxing activity in the aorta induced by acetylcholine in hypercholesterolemic mice. These results suggest a role of tomato in protecting plasma lipids from oxidation *in vivo*.

4.4.4 Human Studies

Although very few, human studies are very promising and fundamental to confirm the effect of lycopene and tomato consumption on health. The studies considered here include both intervention trials on small groups of subjects and *ex vivo* treatments and evaluations.

An aspect that is receiving great attention is the role of lycopene and tomato on lipid and lipoprotein oxidation, which is highly implicated in atherogenesis and coronary heart disease. In this regard, in order to have a more comprehensive presentation of the results, some *in vitro* supplementation studies will be considered.

In vitro LDL enrichment with lycopene and other carotenoids has been investigated by a few authors with controversial results. Fuhrman et al.[82] were the first to indicate that the supplementation of LDL with 3 μmol/l lycopene or β-carotene reduced their susceptibility to metal ion-dependent oxidation by 65 and 37%, respectively. The inhibitory effect of these carotenoids on LDL oxidation was positively correlated with the vitamin E content, and a synergistic effect was observed when the carotenoids and vitamin E were supplemented together. This was attributed to a different antioxidant action (vitamin E acts as a free radical scavenger by hydrogen atom donation, carotenoids scavenge radicals by their addition to a double bond) or to their action at different sites in the lipoprotein (vitamin E at the surface, carotenoids in the lipid core). These data were confirmed supplementing human LDLs with tomato oleoresin (containing 5% lycopene, 0.1% β-carotene, and 1% vitamin E).

Romanchik et al.,[83] in another *in vitro* study, found that the supplementation of human LDL with lycopene or lutein did not improve LDL protection from copper-mediated oxidative damage. They also studied the relative rates of destruction of individual carotenoids during LDL oxidation and found that lycopene, above all, was destroyed very quickly before the formation of lipid peroxidation products. On the contrary, β-carotene enrichment had a small but significant effect on LDL oxidation and was also able to decrease the rate of destruction of the other carotenoids. These findings are in agreement with what Dugas et al.[62] reported in a cell culture study.

Similar results have been obtained by intervention studies conducted *in vivo*. Argawal and Rao[84] supplemented healthy volunteers for 1 week with tomato juice (about 50 mg/day lycopene), spaghetti sauce (about 39 mg/day lycopene), or tomato oleoresin (about 75 mg/day lycopene) and showed a significant decrease in lipid peroxidation and LDL oxidation (evaluated by TBARS and conjugated dienes) after the supplementation, but observed no change in serum cholesterol levels. The decrease in lipid peroxidation after the consumption of the same tomato products was confirmed in a further study by the same authors,[85] who also found a trend towards lower protein oxidation estimated by measuring the loss of reduced thiol groups. Further research is needed to investigate the possible effect of lycopene and tomato products on the prevention of protein oxidation as no other results are available.

In a study carried out by Steinberg and Chait,[86] smokers received a supplementation for 4 weeks of a tomato-based juice fortified with vitamin C (600 mg), E (400 mg), and β-carotene (30 mg) that reduced lipid peroxidation (breath pentane excretion) and susceptibility of LDL to oxidation mediated by copper. The same effect was not seen when the tomato juice was supplemented alone. In all cases the total peroxyl radical trapping potential of plasma (TRAP), as an index of antioxidant capacity, did not vary. The same results were found by other authors after the daily consumption of tomato products containing 5 mg lycopene[26] and 7 mg lycopene.[87] Thus, it may be possible that TRAP test is not appropriate for studing *in vivo* the effect of the consumption of lipophilic antioxidant-rich foods on plasma antioxidant capacity.

Rao and Argawal[85] found that subjects consuming a lycopene-free diet had higher lipid peroxidation than those on their habitual diet. Furthermore, they found that serum lycopene concentration decreased as a result of oxidative stress deriving from both the ingestion of a meal or a glucose solution and from cigarette smoke. They concluded that lycopene could really act as an antioxidant *in vivo*.

From all these results a beneficial effect of tomato and tomato products on the inhibition of lipid and lipoprotein oxidation may be hypothesized but not definitely proved.

More convincing is the evidence about a possible effect of lycopene and/or tomato consumption on DNA protection from oxidative damage involved in cancer-related genetic changes in humans.

In order to assess whether consumption of vegetables including tomatoes could protect against DNA damage and oxidative damage, Pool-Zobel et al.[88] gave a group of subjects 330 ml tomato juice (40 mg lycopene), or 330 g carrots, or 10 g spinach powder daily for 2 weeks. After the supplementation with tomato, carrots, and spinach, there were decreased levels of endogenous strand breaks in lymphocyte DNA evaluated with the comet assay, while after oxidative treatment with H_2O_2 only the carrot intervention was effective.

On the contrary, we found that the consumption of 60 g tomato puree (about 16.5 mg lycopene) for 3 weeks[33] or 25 g tomato puree (about 7 mg lycopene) for only 2 weeks[34] elicited a significant reduction in DNA damage (evaluated by the comet assay) of lymphocytes challenged *ex vivo* with H_2O_2. Treatment with H_2O_2 exacerbates the DNA damage, consequently under this condition it is possible to study the ability of cells to protect themselves against oxidative stress; the damage sustained was related to the dose of H_2O_2 used.[89] On the contrary, the levels of endogenous DNA damage evaluated in untreated lymphocytes were not related to the tomato intake.[89] We also found an inverse relation between DNA damage and plasma and lymphocyte lycopene concentration, supporting the hypothesis of a real contribution by lycopene on cell protection from oxidative damage, even if we cannot exclude the potential role of the other compounds present in tomato.[34]

A trend towards lower lymphocyte DNA oxidation evaluated by 8-oxodeoxyguanosine was also reported by Rao and Argawal[25] after daily consumption for one week of two types of spaghetti sauces, a tomato juice, and a lycopene-rich oleoresin from tomato in the form of capsules.

Few studies exist suggesting a role of lycopene in protecting other antioxidant compounds in the diet and preventing tissue damage *in vivo*. Ribaya-Mercado et al.[90] hypothesized that lycopene may protect other carotenoids and antioxidant substances. In a human study they observed up to 46% reduction in *skin* lycopene after a single exposure to a dose of simulated solar light. This seems to suggest a role of this carotenoid is mitigating oxidative damage in tissues. At this regard Clinton et al.[13] and Rao et al.[91] hypothesized a role for lycopene in prostate tissue, however, more research is needed to clarify this action.

4.5 EPIDEMIOLOGICAL EVIDENCE OF THE RELATIONSHIP BETWEEN TOMATO CONSUMPTION AND HEALTH

For a better understanding of the potential salutary effect of tomato it is essential to consider the results of the epidemiological studies in the last decades. Most of the studies are focused on the relation between food consumption and cancer prevention, however, some evidence also exists about other diseases.

4.5.1 Cancer

Numerous studies have shown that a high consumption of vegetables and fruit is protective against cancers at many sites.[92-95] Dietary recommendations to increase the intake of vegetables and fruit have been made by several organizations, including the National Research Council of the National Academy of Sciences, the American Cancer Society, and the Italian Cancer Institute. However, evidence does not exist concerning which component accounts for this benefit. Furthermore, as previously reported, tomatoes are not only widely consumed raw, but are also used in many processed foods (e.g., tomato sauce, tomato puree, tomato soup, ketchup), consequently they are not exclusively identified with fruit or vegetable consumption.

Over the past few years many researchers have reported the anticarcinogenic properties of tomato, quoting some epidemiological study in which a protective effect is shown.[96,97] Franceschi et al.[96] highlighted the importance of studying the association between cancer and individual vegetables and fruits and also considered that the translation of foods into nutrients is incomplete. Analyzing data from a series of Italian case-control studies, they found a consistent pattern of protection from a high intake of raw tomatoes in cancer of the digestive tract, especially for gastrointestinal neoplasms. Giovannucci et al.[97] reported the results of a prospective cohort study designed to examine the relationship between the intake of various carotenoids, retinol, fruits and vegetables and the risk of prostate cancer. Of 46 vegetables and fruits or related products, only four — tomato sauce (p for trend = .001), strawberries (p for trend = .005), raw tomato (p for trend = .03), and pizza (p for trend = .05) — were significantly associated with lower prostate cancer risk. Three of the four are good sources of lycopene. The other major contributor of lycopene, tomato juice, was not related to the risk. The authors ascribed this fact to the low bioavailability of lycopene from tomato juice, as well as to the poor reporting of the consumption of this item. Among all carotenoids analyzed (β-carotene, α-carotene, lutein, β-cryptoxanthin, and lycopene) only lycopene intake was related to lower risk. More recently, Key et al.,[98] investigating the relationship between dietary factors and the risk for prostate cancer in a case-control study in England, did not confirm the reduction in risk associated with lycopene intake. However, they found a significant reduction in risk associated with baked beans consumption, which could be a good source of lycopene from the tomato sauce.

La Vecchia[99] studied the relationship between tomato intake and the risk of digestive tract cancers (oral cavity, pharynx, esophagus, stomach, colon, and rectum) using data from a series of case-control studies conducted in Italy between 1983 and 1992. The Italian studies can be considered particularly important since, notwithstanding the appreciable rises in intestinal cancer mortality observed in Italy, Spain, Portugal, and Greece,[100] rates are still lower in Italy, Spain, and mostly in Greece. Similarly, oral, esophageal, and stomach cancer rates are comparatively low in southern Italy and Greece.[101] This could be partially attributed to the impact of the Mediterranean diet, where tomato is an important component. The study evidenced a consistent pattern of protection for all sites.

Another large, Italian multicenter study of colorectal cancer[102] confirmed that tomato was protective against this kind of cancer. In these Italian studies the beneficial effect of tomato was comparable or in some cases greater than that given by other fruits and vegetables. The authors attributed this to the fact that tomato is one of the most widely consumed items of the Mediterranean diet. Similarly, Tzonou et al.,[103] in a case-control study in Greece, found that cooked tomato and to a lesser extent raw tomato intake was inversely associated with the risk of prostate cancer.

At present there are few informative reviews that examine the epidemiological evidence regarding tomato and tomato product intake with the risk of cancers at various body sites.[104,105] The problem facing these authors was to try to prove, given the current state of knowledge, that there is evidence that such intake could be beneficial to specific cancer sites, or whether the observed associations are casual. The authors analyzed literature using precise criteria of selection, such as strength of association, consistency of results by study design, method of exposure assessment (questionnaire or biomarkers), and the potential for residual or uncontrolled confounding. Giovannucci[104] reported that of the 72 studies analyzed, 35 found a statistically significant inverse association between tomato or lycopene consumption or blood lycopene concentration and risk of cancer, 22 reported an inverse but not significant association. The remaining 15 studies were inconclusive or indicated a slight direct association (never significant). Evidence was strongest for cancers of the lung, stomach, and prostate, and was suggestive for cancers of the cervix, breast, oral cavity, pancreas, colorectum, and esophagus. The author concluded that the benefits of tomato and tomato products cannot be attributable to lycopene, because a direct benefit of lycopene has not been proven, and consequently he supports the current dietary recommendations to increase the intake of fruit and vegetables, including tomato and tomato products, to reduce cancer risk.

In a report by the European-funded Concerted Action (FAIR CT 97-3233) "Role and Control of Antioxidants in the Tomato Processing Industry" Gerber et al.[105] reviewed the relationship between tomatoes and their constituents (carotenoids, vitamin C, and vitamin E) and diseases. For cancers, they used as a basis the data reported in three books[95,106,107] published in three different countries, updated with studies published since 1996. Their conclusions of the role of tomato and tomato products in preventing cancers were more cautious; the protective effect of tomatoes (without considering whether they are raw, cooked, or processed) seem conclusive for cancers of the upper aero-digestive tract, plus lung and stomach. Also in this review lycopene was not associated to these cancer sites, and the contribution of other compounds present in tomatoes, such as β-carotene and vitamin C, has been advocated. There is evidence of a possible beneficial effect of cooked tomatoes against prostate cancer; in this case a role for lycopene has been suggested since processing tomatoes enhances release of lycopene. For many other cancers the results seem insufficient to draw a conclusion.

4.5.2 Cardiovascular Diseases

The relationship between vegetables and fruit intake and cardiovascular disease risk has been recently reviewed by Ness and Powles[108] and Law and Morris,[109] however, few studies have investigated the role of tomato and tomato products in the prevention of cardiovascular diseases. Consequently, it seems possible to state that fruit and vegetables are protective against CVD, but no conclusion can be drawn for tomato. Conversely, as previously reported, some data from *in vitro* and human studies seem to support the effect of tomato and lycopene in the protection from LDL oxidation involved in CVD.

4.5.3 Lens Opacities and Age-Related Macular Degenerative Disease

Opacification of the ocular lens or cataract is one of the major causes of blindness throughout the world. It is a multifactorial disease process that may be promoted by oxidative damage. Cataract, as well as macular degeneration, is associated with ageing and can cause a great deal of disability and lower the quality of life of elderly people. It has been postulated that carotenoids and vitamin E may deter cataract formation because of their capacity to reduce oxidative damage to lens tissues by scavenging free radicals. Whether tomato may protect against cataract has not yet been clarified. An Italian case-control study[110] showed a significantly decreased risk in people with high tomato intake. These data have not been confirmed by other North America studies.[111-113] So it is more than likely that other foods commonly consumed in the Mediterranean area could contribute towards protecting the eyes from cataract (certainly spinach, which is rich in lutein).

4.6 CONCLUSION AND SUGGESTIONS FOR FURTHER INVESTIGATION

An aspect of nutrition, nowadays shared by all scientists, is that vegetables and fruit intake must be increased to improve protection from diseases. However, each class of vegetable and fruit, and sometimes, each single product, contains different compounds that should all be present in the diet.

Considering all the evidence previously discussed, tomato is a "healthy" food and consequently, people, especially those whose dietary habits differ from the Mediterranean one, should consume more of this food.

Usually, dietary recommendations are made in order to help in the prevention of diseases, and consuming such healthy foods should become a habit rather than a "fashion". This is true for tomato consumption. But how much tomato should we eat? This is an interesting question. A specific recommendation does not exist, however from the knowledge accumulated until now, we can speculate that it is better to eat a small amount daily rather than a large amount at one time. Processed tomatoes together with a little oil is preferred, in order to improve absorption. At the same time, a high intake of tomato does not seem to have any adverse effect, as the absorption of carotenoids, and lycopene particularly, is limited so that no pro-oxidant effects are possible. We think it is important to improve the diet by the consumption of healthy foods rather than the intake of supplements. In fact, in the case of lycopene, until now there is no research clarifying the possible adverse effects of pure supplementation which, in any case, will never really substitute for the tomato product. This is also true for tomato extracts that are simple surrogates.

Finally, despite what is now known about the positive effect of tomato products on health promotion, there is still not enough data to completely explain their role and mode of action. Further studies are required in different research areas in order to:

- Improve analytical methodology to update tomato composition and identify specific components that could contribute to the protective effect
- Improve knowledge on the interaction between compounds in tomato
- Define technological processes able to improve bioavailability
- Study in depth the mechanisms of action of lycopene and the other compounds in tomato, trying to elucidate further potential mechanisms other than antioxidant properties in the prevention of disease (e.g., gene expression)
- Identify new and reliable markers to use for rapid screening of tomato action
- Increase the number of intervention studies to support the importance of tomato consumption

Furthermore, the role of the various organizations interested in improving the health of the general public, is no less important. Campaigns should concentrate on dietary advice in such a way that people will realize just how important it is to increase tomato consumption.

ACKNOWLEDGMENTS

We are very grateful to Dr. Sue Southon for having introduced us to the "world" of tomato. We would also like to thank Dr. Mariette Gerber, whose invaluable work has helped stimulate research so much, and Dr. Pascal Grolier for the contribution and materials supplied. AMITOM and all the members of the European Concerted Action “Role and Control of Antioxidants in the Tomato Processing Industry” are also gratefully acknowledged.

REFERENCES

1. Hennekens, C.H., Buring, J.E., Manson, J.E., Stampfer, M., Rosner, B., Cook, N.R., Belanger, C., LaMotte, B.S., Gaziano, J.M., Ridker, P.M., Willett, W., and Peto, R., Lack of effect of long-term supplementation with beta-carotene on the incidence of malignant neoplasms and cardiovascular disease, *N. Engl. J. Med.,* 334, 1145, 1996.
2. Omenn, G.S., Goodman, G.E., Thornquist, M.D., Balmes, J., Cullen, M.R., Glass, A., Keogh, J.P., Meyskens, F.L., Valanis, B., Williams, J.H., Barnhart, S., and Hammar S., Effects of a combination of beta carotene and vitamin A on lung cancer and cardiovascular disease, *N. Engl. J. Med.,* 334, 1150, 1996.
3. Thakur, B.R., Singh, R.K., and Nelson, P.E., Quality attributes of processed tomato products: a review, *Food Rev. Int.,* 12(3), 375, 1996.
4. Mangels, A.R., Holden, J.M., Beecher, G.R., Forman, M.R., and Lanza, E., Carotenoid contents of fruits and vegetables: an evaluation of analytical data, *J. Am. Diet. Assoc.,* 93, 284, 1993.

5. Scott, K.J. and Hart, D.J., Development and evaluation of an HPLC method for the analysis of carotenoids in foods and the measurement of carotenoid content of vegetables and fruits commonly consumed in the U.K., *Food Chem.*, 54, 101, 1995.
6. Olmedilla, B., Granado, F., Blanco, I., and Gil-Martinez, E., Carotenoid content in fruit and vegetables and its relevance to human health: some of the factors involved, *Recent Res. Dev. Agric. Food Chem.*, 2, 57, 1998.
7. Porrini, M., Riso, P., and Testolin, G., Absorption of lycopene from single or daily portion of raw and processed tomato, *Br. J. Nutr.*, 80, 353, 1998.
8. Grolier, P., Bartholin, G., Caris-Veyrat, C., Dadomo, M., Dumas, Y., Meddens, F., Sandei, L., and Schuch, W., Antioxidants in the tomato fruit, European-funded Concerted Action (FAIR CT 97-3233): Role and control of antioxidants in the tomato processing industry, Annual Scientific Report, 1999.
9. Rao, A.V. and Argawal, S., Role of lycopene as antioxidant carotenoid in the prevention of chronic diseases: a review, *Nutr. Res.*, 19(2), 305, 1999.
10. Nguyen, M.L. and Schwartz, S.J., Lycopene stability during food processing, *Proc. Soc. Exp. Biol. Med.*, 218, 101, 1998.
11. Khachik, F., Beecher, G.R., Goli, N.B., Lusby, W.R., and Smith J.C., Separation and identification of carotenoids and their oxidation products in the extracts of human plasma, *Anal. Chem.*, 64, 2111, 1992.
12. Stahl, W., Sundquist, A.R., Hanusch, M., Schwarz, W., and Sies, H., Separation of β-carotene and lycopene geometrical isomers in biological samples, *Clin. Chem.*, 39(5), 810, 1993.
13. Clinton, S.K., Emenhiser, C., Schwartz, Bostwick, D.G., Williams, A.W., Moore, B.J., and Erdman, J.W., *Cis-trans* lycopene isomers, carotenoids, and retinol in the human prostate, *Cancer Epidemiol. Biomark. Prev.*, 5, 823, 1996.
14. Davies, J.N. and Hobson, G.E., The costituents of tomato fruit. The influence of environment, nutrition, and genotype, *Crit. Rev. Food Sci. Nutr.*, 15, 205, 1981.
15. Gould, W.A., *Tomato Production, Processing and Technology*, CTI Publications, Baltimore, MD, 1992.
16. Hertog, M.G.L., Hollman, P.C.H., and Katan, M.B., Content of potentially anticarcinogenic flavonoids of 28 vegetables and 9 fruit commonly consumed in The Netherlands, *J. Agric. Food Chem.*, 40, 2379, 1992.
17. Crozier, A., Lean, M.E., McDonald, M.S., and Black, C., Quantitative analysis of the flavonoid content of commercial tomatoes, onions, lettuce, and celery, *J. Agric. Food Chem.*, 45, 590, 1997.
18. Vinson, J.A., Hao, Y., Su, X., and Zubik, L., Phenol antioxidant quantity and quality in foods: vegetables, *J. Agric. Food Chem.*, 46, 3630, 1998.
19. Mauri, P.L., Iemoli, L., Gardana, C., Riso, P., Simonetti, P., Porrini, M., and Pietta, P.G., Liquid chromatography/electrospray ionization mass spectrometric characterization of flavonol glycosides in tomato extracts and human plasma, *Rapid Commun. Mass Spectrom.*, 13, 924, 1999.
20. Bowen, P.E., Mobarhan, S., and Smith, J.C., Absorption of carotenoids in humans, *Methods Enzymol.*, 214, 3, 1993.
21. Parker, R.S., Bioavailability of carotenoids, *Eur. J. Clin. Nutr.*, 51(Suppl.1), S86, 1997.
22. Micozzi, M., Brown, E.D., Edwards, B.K., Bieri, J.G., Taylor, P.R., Khachick, F., Beecher, G.R., and Smith, J.C., Plasma carotenoid response to chronic intake of selected food and β-carotene supplements in men, *Am. J. Clin. Nutr.*, 55, 1120, 1992.
23. Rock, C.L., Swendseid, M.E., Jacob, R.A., and McKee, R.W., Plasma carotenoid levels in human subjects fed a low carotenoid diet, *J. Nutr.*, 122, 96, 1992.

24. Yeum, K.J., Booth, S.L., and Sadowski J.A., Human plasma carotenoid response to the ingestion of controlled diets high in fruits and vegetables, *Am. J. Clin. Nutr.,* 64, 594, 1996.
25. Rao, A.V. and Argawal, S., Bioavailability and in vivo antioxidant properties of lycopene from tomato products and their possible role in the prevention of cancer, *Nutr. Cancer*, 31(3), 199, 1998.
26. Böhm, V. and Bitsch, R., Intestinal absorption of lycopene from different matrices and interactions to other carotenoids, the lipid status, and the antioxidant capacity of human plasma, *Eur. J. Nutr.*, 38, 118, 1999.
27. Ascherio, A., Stampfer, M.J., Colditz, G.A., Rimm, E.B., Litin, L., and Willet, W.C., Correlations of vitamin A and E intakes with the plasma concentrations of carotenoids and tocopherols among American men and women, *J. Nutr.,* 122, 1792, 1992.
28. Scott, K.J., Thurnam, D.I., Hart, D.J., Bingham, G.H., and Day, K., The correlation between the intake of lutein, lycopene and β-carotene from vegetables and fruits, and blood plasma concentrations in a group of women aged 50-65 years in the U.K., *Br. J. Nutr.,* 75, 409, 1996.
29. Furr, H.C. and Clark, R.M., Intestinal absorption and tissue distribution of carotenoids, *J. Nutr. Biochem.,* 8, 364, 1997.
30. Koonsvitsky, B.P., Berry, D.A., Jones, M.B., Lin, P.Y.T., Cooper, D.A., Jones, D.Y., and Jackson, J.E., Olestra affects serum concentrations of α-tocopherol and carotenoids but not vitamin D or vitamin K status in free-living subjects, *J. Nutr.,* 127, 1636S, 1997.
31. Stahl, W. and Sies, H., Uptake of lycopene and its geometrical isomers is greater from heat-processed than from unprocessed tomato juice, *J. Nutr.,* 122, 2161, 1992.
32. Gärtner, C., Stahl, W., and Sies, H., Lycopene is more bioavailable from tomato paste than from fresh tomatoes, *Am. J. Clin. Nutr.,* 66, 116, 1997.
33. Riso, P., Pinder, A., Santangelo, A., and Porrini, M., Does tomato consumption effectively increase the resistance of lymphocyte DNA to oxidative damage?, *Am. J. Clin. Nutr.*, 69, 712, 1999.
34. Porrini, M. and Riso, P., Lymphocyte lycopene concentration and DNA protection from oxidative damage is increased in women after a short period of tomato consumption, *J. Nutr.*, 130(2), 000, 2000
35. Clinton, S.K., Lycopene: chemistry, biology, and implications for human health and disease, *Nutr. Rev.*, 56(2), 35, 1998.
36. Krinsky, N.I., Russett, M.D., Handelman, G.J., and Snodderly, D.M., Structural and geometrical isomers of carotenoids in human plasma, *J. Nutr.,* 120, 1654, 1990.
37. Schmitz, H.H., Poor, C.L., Wellman, R.B., and Erdman, J.W., Jr., Concentrations of selected carotenoids and vitamin A in human liver, kidney and lung tissue, *J. Nutr.,* 121, 1613, 1991.
38. Stahl, W., Schwarz, W., Sundquist, A.R., and Sies, H., *cis-trans* isomers of lycopene and β-carotene in human serum and tissues, *Arch. Biochem. Biophys.,* 294, 173, 1992.
39. Clinton, S.K., Emenhiser, C., Schwartz, S.J., Bostwick, D.G., Williams, A.W., Moore, B.J., and Erdman, J.W., *Cis-trans* lycopene isomers, carotenoids, and retinol in the human prostate, *Cancer Epidemiol., Biomark. Prev.*, 5, 823, 1996.
40. Britton, G., Structure and properties of carotenoids in relation to function, *FASEB J.,* 9, 1551, 1995.
41. Boileau, A.C., Merchen, N.R., Wasson, K., Atkinson, C.A., and Erdman, J.W., *Cis*-lycopene is more bioavailable than *trans*-lycopene in vitro and in vivo in lymph-cannulated ferrets, *J. Nutr.*, 129, 1176, 1999.

42. Di Mascio, P., Kaiser, S., and Sies, H., Lycopene as the most efficient biological carotenoid singlet oxygen quencher, *Arch. Biochem. Biophys.*, 274(2), 532, 1989.
43. Miller, N.J., Sampson, J., Candeias, L.P., Bramley, P.M., and Rice-Evans, C.A., Antioxidant activities of carotenes and xantophylls, *FEBS Lett.*, 384, 240, 1996.
44. Weisburger, J.H., Evaluation of the evidence on the role of tomato products in disease prevention, *Proc. Soc. Exp. Biol. Med.*, 218, 140, 1998.
45. Lavelli, V., Hippeli, S., Peri, C., and Elstner, E.F., Evaluation of radical scavenging activity of fresh and air-dried tomatoes by three model reactions, *J. Agric. Food Chem.*, 47, 3826, 1999.
46. Wang, H., Cao, G., and Prior, R.L., Total antioxidant capacity of fruit, *J. Agric. Food Chem.*, 44, 701, 1996.
47. Plumb, G.W., Chambers, S.J., Lambert, N., Wanigatunga, S., and Williamson, G., Influence of fruit and vegetable extracts on lipid peroxidation in microsomes containing specific cytochrome P 450 S, *Food Chem.*, 60, 161, 1997.
48. Pellegrini, N., Re, R., Yang, M., and Rice-Evans, C., Screening of dietary carotenoids and carotenoid-rich fruit extracts for antioxidant activities applying 2,2'-azinobis(3-ethylenebenzothiazoline-6-sulphonic acid radical cation decolorization assay, *Methods Enzymol.*, 299, 379, 1999.
49. Krinsky, N.I., Cellular aspect of carotenoid actions, in *Handbook of Antioxidant*, Cadenas, E. and Packer, L., Eds., Marcel Dekker, New York, 1996, chap. 11.
50. Levy, J., Bosin, E., Feldman, B., Giat, Y., Miinster, A., Danilenko, M., and Sharony, Y., Lycopene is a more potent inhibitor of human cancer cell proliferation than either alpha-carotene or beta-carotene, *Nutr. Cancer*, 24, 257, 1995.
51. Countryman, C., Bankson, D., Collins, S., Mar, B., and Lin, W., Lycopene inhibits the growth of the HL-60 promyelocytic leukemia cell line (abstract), *Clin. Chem.*, 37, 1056, 1991.
52. Bankson, D.D., Countryman, C., and Collins, S., Potentiation of the retinoic acid-induced differentiation of HL-60 cells by lycopene, (abstract), *Am. J. Clin. Nutr.*, 53(Suppl.), 13, 1991.
53. Amir, H., Karas, M., Giat, J., Danilenko, M., Levy, R., Yermiahu, T., Levy, J., and Sharoni, Y., Lycopene and 1,25-dihydroxyvitamin D_3 cooperate in the inhibition of cell cycle progression and induction of differentiation in HL-60 leukemic cells, *Nutr. Cancer*, 33(1), 105, 1999.
54. Bertram, J.S., Pung, A., Churly, M., Kappock, T.J., Wilkins, S.R., and Cooney, R.V., Diverse carotenoids protect against chemically induced neoplastic transformation, *Carcinogenesis*, 12, 671, 1991.
55. Zhang, L.-X., Cooney, R.V., and Bertram, J.S., Carotenoids enhance gap junctional communication and inhibit lipid peroxidation in C3H/10T1/2 cells: relationship to their cancer chemopreventive action, *Carcinogenesis*, 12, 2109, 1991.
56. Zhang, L.-X., Cooney, R.V., and Bertram, J.S., Carotenoids up-regulate connexin43 gene expression independent of their provitamin A or antioxidant properties, *Cancer Res.*, 52, 5707, 1992.
57. Tsushima, M., Maoka, T., Katsuyama, M., Kozuka, M., Matsuno, T., Tokuda, H., Nishino, H., and Iwashima, A., Inhibitory effects of natural carotenoids on Epstein-Barr virus activation activity of a tumor promotor in Raji cells. A screening study for anti tumor promotors, *Biol. Pharm. Bull.*, 18, 227, 1995.
58. Kim, H., Carotenoids protect cultured rat hepatocytes from injury caused by carbon tetrachloride, *Int. J. Biochem. Cell Biol.*, 27, 1303, 1995.

59. Matsushima-Nishiwaki, R., Shidoji, Y., Nishiwaki, S., Yamada, T., Moriwaki, H., and Muto, Y., Suppression by carotenoids of microcystin-induced morphological changes in mouse hepatocytes, *Lipids,* 30, 1029, 1995.
60. Wang, W. and Higuchi, C.M., Induction of NAD(P)H: Quinone reductase by vitamins A, E, and C in Colo205 colon cancer cells, *Cancer Lett.,* 98, 63, 1995.
61. Fuhrman, B., Elis, A., and Aviram, M., Hypocholesterolemic effect of lycopene and β-carotene is related to suppression of cholesterol synthesis and augmentation of LDL receptor activity in macrophage, *Biochem. Biophys. Res. Commun.,* 233, 658, 1997.
62. Dugas, T.R., Morel, D.W., and Harrison, E.H., Dietary supplementation with beta-carotene, but not with lycopene, inhibits endothelial cell-mediated oxidation of low-density lipoprotein, *Free Rad. Biol. Med.,* 26(9-10), 1238, 1999.
63. Tinkler, J.H., Bohm, F., Schalch, W., and Truscott, T.G., Dietary carotenoids protect human cells from damage, *J. Photochem. Photobiol.,* 26, 283, 1994.
64. Bohm, F., Tinkler, J.H., and Truscott, T.G., Carotenoids protect against cell membrane damage by nitrogen dioxide radical, *Nat. Med.,* 1, 98, 1995.
65. Lowe, G.M., Booth, L.A., Young, A.J., and Bilton, R., Lycopene and β-carotene protect against oxidative damage in HT29 cells at low concentrations but rapidly lose this capacity at higher doses, *Free Rad. Res.,* 30, 141, 1999.
66. Lingen, C., Ernster, L., and Lindenberg, O., The promoting effects of lycopene on the non-specific resistance of animals, *Exp. Cell Res.,* 16, 384, 1959.
67. Wang, C.J., Chou, M.Y., and Lin, J.K., Inhibition of growth and development of the transplantable C-6 glioma cells inoculated in rats by retinoids and carotenoids, *Cancer Lett.,* 48, 135, 1989.
68. Nagasawa, H., Mitamura, T., Sakamoto, S., and Yamamoto, K., Effects of lycopene on spontaneous mammary tumour development in SHN virgin mice, *Anticancer Res.,* 15, 1173, 1995.
69. Sharony, Y., Giron, E., Rise, M., and Levy, J., Effects of lycopene enriched tomato oleoresin on 7,12-dimethylbenz[a]anthracene-induced rat mammary tumors, *Cancer Detect. Prev.,* 21, 118, 1997.
70. He, Y., Root, M.M., Parker, R.S., and Campbell, T.C., Effects of carotenoid-rich food extracts on the development of preneoplastic lesions in rat liver and on *in vivo* and *in vitro* antioxidant status, *Nutr. Cancer,* 27(3), 238, 1997.
71. Astorg, P., Gradelet, S., Berges, R., and Suschetet, M., Dietary lycopene decreases the initiation of liver preneoplastic foci by diethylnitrosamine in the rat, *Nutr. Cancer,* 29, 60, 1997.
72. Narisawa, T., Fukaura, Y., Hasebe, M., Ito, M., Aizawa, R., Murakoshi, M., Uemura, S., Khachik, F., and Nishino, H., Inhibitory effects of natural carotenoids, α-carotene, β-carotene, lycopene and lutein, on colonic aberrant crypt foci formation in rats, *Cancer Lett.,* 107, 137, 1996.
73. Narisawa, T., Fukaura, Y., Hasebe, M., Seiko, N., Oshima, S., Sakamoto, H., Inakuma, T., Ishiguro, Y., Takayasu, J., and Nishino, H., Prevention of N-Methylnitrosourea-induced colon carcinogenesis in F344 rats by lycopene and tomato juice rich in lycopene, *Jpn. J. Cancer Res.,* 89, 1003, 1998.
74. Jain, C.K., Argawal, S., and Rao, V., The effect of dietary lycopene on bioavailability, tissue distribution, in vivo antioxidant properties and colonic preneoplasia in rats, *Nutr. Res.,* 19 (9), 1383, 1999.

75. Okajima, E., Tsutsumi, M., Ozono, S., Akai, H., Denda, A., Nishino, H., Oshima, S., Sakamoto, H., and Konishi Y., Inhibitory effect of tomato juice on rat urinary bladder carcinogenesis after N-butyl-N-(4hydroxybutyl)nitrosamine initiation, *Jpn. J. Cancer Res.,* 89, 22, 1998.
76. Atanasova-Goranova, V.K., Dimova, P.I., and Pericharova, G.T., Effect of food products on endogenous generation of N-nitrosamines in rats, *Brit. J. Nutr.,* 78(2), 335, 1997.
77. Kim, D.J., Takasuka, N., Kim, J.M., Sekine, K., Ota, T., Asamoto, M., Murakoshi, M., Nishino, H., Nir, Z., and Tsuda, H., Chemoprevention by lycopene of mouse lung neoplasia after combined initiation treatment with DEN, MNU, and DMH, *Cancer Lett.,* 120, 15, 1997.
78. Hecht, S.S., Kenney, P.M., Wang, M., Trushin, N., Argawal, S., Rao, A.V., and Upadhyaya, P., Evaluation of butylated hydroxyanisole, myo-inositol, curcumin, esculerin, resveratrol and lycopene as inhibitors of benzo[a]pyrene plus 4-(methylnitrosamino)-1-(3-pyridyl)-1-butanone-induced lung tumorigenesis in A/J mice, *Cancer Lett.,* 137(2), 123, 1999.
79. Gradelet, S., Astorg, P., Leclerc, J., Chevalier, J., Vernevaut, M.F., and Siess, M.H., Effects of canthaxanthin, astaxanthin, lycopene and lutein on liver xenobiotic metabolizing enzymes in the rat, *Xenobiotica*, 26, 49, 1996.
80. Jewell, C. and O'Brien, N.M., Effect of dietary supplementation with carotenoids on xenobiotic metabolizing enzymes in the liver, lung, kidney and small intestine of the rat, *Br. J. Nutr.,* 81, 235, 1999.
81. Suganuma, H. and Inakuma, T., Protective effect of dietary tomato against endothelial dysfunction in hypercholesterolemic mice, *Biosci. Biotech. Biochem.,* 63(1), 78, 1999.
82. Fuhrman, B., Elis, A., and Aviram, M., Hypocholesterolemic effect of lycopene and beta-carotene is related to suppression of cholesterol synthesis and augmentation of LDL receptor activity in macrophages, *Biochem. Biophys. Res. Commun.,* 233(3), 658, 1997.
83. Romanchik, J.E., Harrison, E.H., and Morel, D.W., Addition of lutein, lycopene, or β-carotene to LDL or serum in vitro: effects on carotenoid distribution, LDL composition and LDL oxidation, *J. Nutr. Biochem.,* 8, 681, 1997.
84. Argawal, S. and Rao, A.V., Tomato lycopene and low density lipoprotein oxidation: a human dietary intervention study, *Lipids,* 33, 981, 1998.
85. Rao, A.V. and Argawal, S., Effect of diet and smoking on serum lycopene and lipid peroxidation, *Nutr. Res.,* 18(4), 713, 1998.
86. Steinberg, F.M. and Chait, A., Antioxidant vitamin supplementation and lipid peroxidation in smokers, *Am. J. Clin. Nutr.,* 68, 319, 1998.
87. Pellegrini, N., Riso, P., and Porrini, M., Tomato consumption does not affect total antioxidant capacity of plasma, *Nutrition*, 16, 268-271, 2000.
88. Pool-Zobel, B.L., Bub, A., Muller, H., Wollowski, I., and Rechkemmer, G., Consumption of vegetables reduces genetic damage in humans: first results of a human intervention trial with carotenoid-rich foods, *Carcinogenesis,* 18(9), 1847, 1997.
89. Riso, P., Santangelo, A., and Porrini, M., The Comet assay for the evaluation of cell resistance to oxidative stress, *Nutr. Res.,* 19(3), 325, 1999.
90. Ribaya-Mercado, J.D., Garmyn, M., Gilchrest, B.A., and Russel, R.M., Skin lycopene is destroyed preferentially over β-carotene during ultraviolet irradiation in humans, *J. Nutr.,* 125, 1854, 1995.
91. Rao, A.V., Fleshner, N., and Argawal, S., Serum and tissue lycopene and biomarkers of oxidation in prostate cancer patients: a case-control study, *Nutr. Cancer,* 33(2), 159, 1999.

92. Negri, E., La Vecchia, C., Franceschi, S., D'Avanzo, B., and Parazzini, F., Vegetable and fruit consumption and cancer risk, *Int. J. Cancer,* 48, 350, 1991.
93. Block, G., Patterson, B., and Subar, A., Fruit, vegetables, and cancer prevention: a review of the epidemiological evidence, *Nutr. Cancer,* 18, 1, 1992.
94. Potter, J.D. and Steinmetz, K., Vegetables, fruit and phytoestrogens as preventive agents, in Stewart, B.W., McGregor, D., Kleihues, P., Eds., Principles of Chemioprevention, IARC Sci. Pub. No. 139, International Agency for Research on Cancer, Lyon, 1996.
95. World Cancer Research Fund, Food, Nutrition, and the Prevention of Cancer: A Global Perspective, American Institute for Cancer Research, Washington, D.C., 1997.
96. Franceschi, S., Bidoli, E., La Vecchia, C., Talamini, R., D'Avanzo, B., and Negri, E., Tomatoes and risk of digestive-tract cancers, *Int. J. Cancer,* 59, 181, 1994.
97. Giovannucci, E., Ascherio, A., Rimm, E.B., Stampfer, M.J., Colditz, G.A., and Willet, W.C., Intake of carotenoids and retinol in relation to risk of prostate cancer, *J. Natl. Cancer Inst.,* 87(23), 1767, 1995.
98. Key, T.J.A., Silcocks, P.B., Davey, G.K., Appleby, P.N., and Bishop, D.T., A case-control study of diet and prostate cancer, *Br. J. Cancer,* 76, 678, 1997.
99. La Vecchia, C., Mediterranean epidemiological evidence on tomatoes and the prevention of digestive-tract cancers, *Proc. Soc. Exp. Biol. Med.,* 218, 125, 1998.
100. La Vecchia, C., Lucchini, F., Negri, E., and Levi, F., Patterns and trends in mortality from selected cancers in Mediterranean countries, in *Epidemiology of Diet and Cancer,* Hill, M.J., Giacosa, A., and Caygill, C.P., Eds., Ellis Horwood, New York, 1994, 169.
101. Levi, F., La Vecchia, C., Lucchini, F., and Negri, E., Cancer mortality in Europe, 1990-92, *Eur. J. Cancer Prev.,* 4, 389, 1995.
102. Franceschi, S., Favero, A., La Vecchia, C., Negri, E., Conti, E., Monsella, M., Giacosa, A., and Decarli, A., The influence of food groups on cancer of the colon and rectum, *Int. J. Cancer,* 72, 56, 1997.
103. Tzonou, A., Signorello, L.B., Lagiou, P., Wuu, J., Trichopoulos, D., and Trichopoulou, A., Diet and cancer of the prostate: a case-control study in Greece, *J. Cancer,* 80, 704, 1999.
104. Giovannucci, E., Tomatoes, tomato-based products, lycopene, and cancer: review of the epidemiologic literature, *J. Natl. Cancer Inst.,* 91(4), 317, 1999.
105. Gerber, M., Amiot, M.J., Offord, E., and Rock, E., Report on the relationship between tomatoes and their constituents (carotenoids, vitamin C and vitamin E), and diseases. European-funded Concerted Action (FAIR CT 97-3233): Role and control of antioxidants in the tomato processing industry, Annual Scientific Report, 1999.
106. CNERNA, Alimentation et cancer. Evaluation des donnees scientifiques, Riboli et al., Eds., Tec Doc, Lavoisier, Paris, 1996.
107. COMA, Nutritional aspects of the development of cancer. Report of the working group on diet and cancer of the Committee on Medical Aspects of Food and Nutrition Policy, Her Majesty's Stationnery Office, London, 1998.
108. Ness, A.R. and Powles, J.W., Fruit and vegetables, and cardiovascular disease: a review, *Int. J. Epidemiol.,* 26, 1, 1997.
109. Law, M.R. and Morris, J.K., By how much does fruit and vegetable consumption reduce the risk of ischaemic heart disease?, *Eur. J. Clin. Nutr.,* 52, 549, 1998.
110. Tavani, A., Negri, E., and La Vecchia, C., Food and nutrient intake and risk of cataract, *Ann. Epidemiol.,* 6, 41, 1996.

111. Mares-Perlman, J.A., Brady, W.E., Klein, B.E.K., Klein, R., Haus, G.J., Palta, M., Ritter, L.L., and Shoff, S.M., Diet and nuclear lens opacities, *Am. J. Epidemiol.,* 141, 322, 1995.
112. Brown, L., Rimm, E.B., Seddon, J.M., Giovannucci, E.L., Chasan-Taber, L., Spiegelman, D., Willet, W.C., and Hankinson, S.E., A prospective study of carotenoid intake and risk of cataract extraction in U.S. men, *Am. J. Clin. Nutr.,* 70, 517, 1999.
113. Lyle, B.J., Mares-Perlman, J.A., Klein, B.E.K., Klein, R., Palta, M., Bowen, P.E., and Greger, J.L., Serum carotenoids and tocopherols and incidence of age-related nuclear cataract, *Am. J. Clin. Nutr.,* 69, 272, 1999.

Section II

Vegetable Extracts and Nutrient Supplementation: Health Promotion

5 Phytomedicines: Creating Safer Choices

Piergiorgio Pietta

CONTENTS

5.1 INTRODUCTION

Plants have been used for medicinal purposes for centuries, and today about 80% of the world population relies primarily on botanical preparations as medicines for their health needs.[1,2] Phytotherapy is common in Europe, where Germany holds the largest share (49%), followed by Italy, France, U.K. (10% each), Spain, Netherland, Belgium (2% each), and the rest of Europe (15%). Overall, the European market is predicted to grow at an annual rate of 4%.[3] In the U.S. about one-third of adults use herbal remedies (only 5% is sold in pharmacies), and the total market is projected to reach $5.9 billion by the year 2000.

Despite this use, most physicians are not aware of the herbal medicines available, as well as understanding their beneficial and adverse effects.[4,5] This may be related to their lack of a phytotherapeutic background. Indeed, phytotherapy is infrequently taught in medical schools, scarcely prescribed, and therefore erroneously regarded as unconventional medicine. This assumption is not appropriate, since there are no conventional or unconventional or alternative medicines, only scientifically proved evidence-based medicine. This is the critical point. Mainstream medicine argues that phytomedicines are not based on controlled studies, i.e., subjected to properly

0-8493-0038-X/97/$0.00+$.50

designed clinical trials to establish their efficacy and safety, as is done for synthetic drugs. This is not surprising, since many herbal medicines were introduced before the advent of randomized clinical trials. This is also the case for some current drugs: aspirin, warfarin, heparin, and chloroquine are examples.

Herbal remedies are amenable to the **same testing as is used for standard medicines**. However, it has to be remembered that in the case of herbal medicines these studies are not profitable. There is little motivation for companies to perform highly expensive trials for a product that cannot be patented (no cost recovery). Companies prefer to convert the bioactive natural compound into a modified synthetic analogue that permits it to obtain intellectual property rights. Consequently, only a few phytomedicines have been examined to the same level of scientific scrutiny (chemical, pharmacological, and clinical) that is required for synthetic drugs. Nevertheless, several promising herbs rooted in traditional medicine have been examined for their chemistry, and many studies aimed to provide **basic** assessment of efficacy and safety (in terms of experimental pharmacology and clinical trial data) are currently performed (Commission E, ESCOP, WHO Monographs).

A particular feature of phytomedicines is their complex composition, i.e., the "phytocomplex" which includes a variety of phytochemicals with different biological activities. Some of these phytochemicals are responsible for specific effects, while other components play an additive role. Differently from synthetic drugs that act as "single bullets" against distinct targets, phytomedicines provide a wider array of effects, and the healing properties are frequently guaranteed only by the phytocomplex.

Herbs and herbal remedies may offer an alternative or a support to synthetic drugs in preventing or treating **mild/moderate** states of illnesses, including hyperlipidemia, impaired microcirculation, high blood pressure,[6] and depression.[7] Herbal medicines may also provide benefit to people suffering from common cold, moderate digestive or hepatic disorders, and common dermatologic conditions, and may enhance the immune system or protect it against chronic diseases correlated with oxidative stress, i.e., the persistent imbalance between prooxidants and antioxidants.[8,9] All these conditions may be treated successfully with phytomedicines, **provided** they are of adequate quality and properly used. Indeed, the quality control of herbs and their standardized (i.e., with known potency) preparations is essential to guarantee efficacy, safety, and therapeutic reproducibility.

Another important determinant of efficacy and safety is proper usage. Like other medicinal products, herbal remedies may reduce adverse reactions depending on the dosage, the age, specific physiologic circumstances like pregnancy, concomitant diseases, and related therapy with synthetic drugs.

The chapter aims to describe the state of the art, with particular attention to the quality and safe use of herbal medicines.

5.2 QUALITY ASSURANCE

Detailed procedures for the authentication of the herbal source, for identification and quantification of active constituents, and for the absence of possible adulterants and contaminants are available. The first step involves the identity (authentication) of the raw herbal material through macroscopic and microscopic examination of its botanical characteristics and comparison with authentic materials. Near-infrared and X-ray diffraction may be promising alternatives to microscopy for the authentication of powdered herbs. This step is important for ensuring batch-to-batch reproducibility. In some cases, batches of the same herb may differ, since several factors may influence the quality of the herbs, including climate, altitude, soil characteristics, time and mode of harvesting, storage, and processing.

The content of the active principles can vary during the growing cycle, and the optimum time for harvesting should be selected. Inappropriate storage may cause microbial contamination and/or loss of active components; inappropriate drying may destroy thermolabile constituents. In addition, the herbal raw materials may be adulterated with the same plant material that is poor in active constituents, with other plants, and even with synthetic drugs. Possible contaminants of herbs include pesticides, heavy metals, pathogenic organisms, and radionuclides.

The next step may involve simple identity tests, e.g., color formation or precipitation with specific reagents. Usually, chromatographic procedures are preferred to establish the identity of a herbal ingredient. To this purpose, thin-layer chromatography (TLC) still represents a valuable procedure. The technique provides a "fingerprint" (chromatogram showing particular spots with proper visualization, e.g., UV exposure, or spraying with specific reagents) for the extract. TLC is normally rapid and reproducible, and it does not require expensive instrumentation. Unfortunately, TLC suffers from a relative lack of resolution and sensitivity that limits its use to a preliminary qualitative evaluation of an herbal extract. By contrast, high performance liquid chromatography (HPLC) permits separation of the components of complex herbal mixtures wth high resolution and sensitivity.[10] Coupling of HPLC with a diode array detector provides an "on-line" UV spectrum for each of the constituents, and quantification is easily achieved from calibration curves obtained with known concentrations of reference compounds. The HPLC chromatograms can be stored in a computer-assisted library and used for comparison with those of samples under investigation, thereby allowing the identification of an herbal extract with great accuracy. A further analytical improvement is obtained by mass spectrometry (MS).[11] This technique measures mass-to-charge ratios of ions generated by ionization of the analyte molecule under vacuum, and provides information about the molecular mass and the structure of the analytes. The herbal extract can be analyzed by direct infusion into the mass spectrometer or after separation by HPLC or by gas chromatography. The latter is mandatory for volatile components, like essential oils present in different herbs, and also may be the method of choice for some constituents amenable to be converted into volatile derivatives. Complex natural matrices can be satisfactorily analyzed by capillary electrophoresis (CE),[12] which can be regarded as a technique complementary to HPLC, since it allows separations not achievable by HPLC.

Reference standards are usually available to assure the accuracy and the robustness of the analytical methods. When not available, reference compounds need to be isolated from the native matrix, and their identity and purity have to be checked by chemical and physical methods.

In regard to possible contaminants and adulterants, specific well-validated procedures are available to detect heavy metals, pesticides, aflatoxins, pathogenic microorganisms, radionuclides, and synthetic drugs. In particular, toxic metals like lead, zinc, mercury, arsenic, and aluminum have been found as contaminants in Ayurvedic and Chinese preparations.[13] In addition, it has been reported that these preparations may also contain as adulterants some synthetic drugs, including aspirin, paracetamol, diazepam, corticosteroids, caffeine, diclofenac, thiazide diuretics, ephedrine, phenylbutazone ....[14]

By using all these techniques, it is possible to properly evaluate the identity of an herbal extract, to measure the content of its bioactive components, and to exclude the presence of contaminants/adulterants. This results in a "standardized" ingredient with a consistent level of active principles, that can be used to prepare phytomedicines with the same known, guaranteed, and reproducible level of activity, efficacy and safety as is the case for synthetic drugs.

5.3 SAFE USE OF PHYTOMEDICINES

Herbs generally have a safe consumption history. However, while some herbs have been proved to be effective and safe, others are toxic and must be avoided. Indeed, the common assumption that "because they are natural they should be harmless" is misleading. Herbs and their products are mixtures of different compounds, some of which could be harmful. Overall, according to a recent survey of 400 users of herbal remedies,[15] 8% had experienced adverse effects, and most of these were due either to falsification of the herbal ingredient or to contaminants or to added synthetic drugs. However, this estimate may suffer from the limit that botanical products (except for derivatives represented by single-molecule active principles like paclixatel, camptotheticin, tiocolchicoside, colchicin, and others that are regulated as ethical drugs) are often supplied as dietary supplements, even if most of them do not provide any integration of nutrients. Echinacea, saw palmetto, Saint John's wort, aged garlic extract, and ginkgo are examples. This implies that consumers, healthcare professionals, manufacturers, or distributors are not aware of the need to report any adverse event associated with these products to the health authority. Herbal remedies cannot be dismissed as dietary supplements, since they have important biological activities.[16] Consequently, they should be categorized as phytopharmaceuticals and require drug surveillance to ascertain possible adverse effects, as occurs in countries where phytomedicines are properly regulated.

Several medicinal plants have been proved to be free of serious adverse effects when used appropriately. However, only a limited number of phytomedicines conform to the same efficacy and safety criteria established for synthetic drugs. These are listed in Table 5.1, and are among the top selling botanical remedies. Side effects reported for these phytomedicines are summarized in Table 5.2. Other potential side effects[17] associated with a number of medicinal plants are described as follows.

5.3.1 Allergic Reactions

A list of herbs that may cause allergic reactions is given in Table 5.3.

TABLE 5.1
Examples of Phytomedicines Whose Safety and Efficacy Conform to the Same Testing Standards as Used for Synthetic Drugs

Phytomedicine	Chemical Group	Uses
Cascara/Senna	Anthraquinones	Constipation
Chamomile	Chamazulene, bisabolol, flavones	Inflammatory disorders of GI with spasticity
Garlic	*S*-allyl-cysteine Alliin/alliinase	Support in patients with high serum lipid levels, prevention of age-related diseases, adjunct in treatment of hypertension
Ginkgo biloba	Ginkgoflavonols, ginkgolides, bilobalide	Synthomatic treatment of cerebral vascular insufficiency and peripheral vascular disease
Hawthorn	C-glycosylflavonoids Proanthocyanidins	Mild heart failure (early stages)
Horse chestnut	Aescin	Lower extremity venous disease
Kava	Methysticin	States of nervous anxiety, tension, and restlessness
Milk thistle	Silybinin	Dyspeptic complaints, toxic liver disease
Peppermint	Menthol	Symptomatic treatment of irritable bowel
Saw palmetto	Fatty acids, β-sitosterol glucoside	Benign prostatic hyperplasia
St. John's wort	Hypericin analogues Hyperforin analogues	Mild and moderate depression

5.3.2 Gastrointestinal/Renal Irritants

Herbs containing **anthraquinones, capsaicinoids,**[23] and **saponins** are generally regarded as irritants to the gastrointestinal mucosa. Irritant properties have been observed particularly for herbs containing saponins, like senega (*Polygala senega*), horse chestnut (*Aesculus hippocastanum*), cowslip (*Primula veris*), sarsaparilla (*Smilax officinalis*), and blue cohosh (*Caulophyllum thalictroides*). High doses of these herbs may cause diarrhea and vomiting. Even small doses may produce gastrointestinal irritation in sensitive subjects.

Volatile oils consist mainly of terpenes (hydrocarbons and alcohols), and many of them induce irritation of the urinary tract if ingested. Irritant volatile oils are contained in juniper (*Juniperus communis*), sage (*Salvia officinalis*), eucalyptus (*Eucalyptus globulus*), tea tree (*Melaleuca alternifolia*) oil, buchu (*Barosma betulina*), and yarrow (*Achillea millefolium*). These herbs are contraindicated in subjects

TABLE 5.2
Potential Side Effects of Evidence-Based Phytomedicines

Herb	Class[b]	Side Effects
Cascara/senna (*Rhamnus p./Cassia senna*)	2[b]	Long-term abuse results in electrolyte imbalance
Chamomile (*Matricaria chamomilla*)	1	Allergic reactions in sensitive individuals
Garlic (*Allium sativum*)	2[c]	Gastrointestinal disturbances in sensitive individuals
Ginkgo biloba	2[d]	Occasional headaches and gastrointestinal upset
Horse chestnut (*Aesculus hippocastanum*)	2[b]	Gastrointestinal disturbances
Kava (*Piper methysticum*)	2[b]	Gastrointestinal disturbances, allergic skin reactions
Milk thistle (*Silybum marianum*)	1	Occasional mild laxative effects
Peppermint (*Mentha piperita*)	1	Contraindicated by biliary tract obstruction and cholecystitis
Saw palmetto (*Serenoa repens*)	1[a]	Gastric complaints (rarely)
St. John's wort (*Hypericum perforatum*)	2[d]	Not to be taken with synthetic antidepressants, induces photosensitivity

[a] Safe under regular physician supervision.
[b] According to the American Herbal Products Association,[18] herbs can be sorted in different classes:
Class 1: Herbs that can be safely consumed when used appropriately.
Class 2: Herbs with specific use restrictions, unless otherwise directed by an expert health professional: (2a) For external use only; (2b) Not to be used during pregnancy; (2c) Not to be used while nursing; (2d) Specific restrictions, including not for long-term use/do not exceed recommended dosage/avoid intense sun exposure.
Class 3: Herbs with high risk of serious adverse effects.
Many herbs of Class 1 are suitable for self medication, while those of the other classes should be used under the supervision of an expert health-care professional.

with existing renal disease, and the internal use of their oils must be restricted to expert health-care professionals.

All the herbs and related phytomedicines containing anthraquinones, capsaicinoids, saponins, and irritant volatile oils should be avoided during pregnancy and lactation.[24]

5.3.3 Endocrine/Hormonal Effects

Some commonly used herbs with estrogenic effects are listed in Table 5.4. Licorice has an additional mineralocorticoid effect.

TABLE 5.3
Herbs with Allergenic Potential

Herbs	Class	Components
Angelica (*Angelica* spp.)	2d (Avoid prolonged sun exposure)	Furanocoumarins[a]
Arnica	2d (external use)	Sesquiterpene lactones[b]
Celery (*Apium graveolens*)	2d (avoid in renal disorders)	Furanocoumarins
Feverfew (*Thanacetum parthenium*)	2b	Sesquiterpene lactones
Melaleuca oil	Not classified	Terpenes
Poplar bud (Propolis)	Not classified	Prenylcaffeate[c]
St. John's wort	2d (avoid sun exposure)	Naphthodianthrones
Yarrow (*Achillea millefolium*)	2b	Sesquiterpene lactones

[a] Furanocoumarins may provoke photosensitive allergic reactions.[19]
[b] Sesquiterpene lactones that contain an alpha-methylene butyrolactone ring are known to be allergenic compounds[20,21] and are constituents of several herbs of the *Asteraceae*.
[c] The presence of this caffeoyl ester may induce skin allergic reactions.[22]

TABLE 5.4
Herbs with Estrogenic Effects

Herbs	Class	Components
Fucus	2d (short-term use, may induce hyperthyroidism[25])	Iodine
Chaste tree (*Vitex agnus-castus*)	2b, 2d (interference with endocrine therapies[26])	Flavonoids/iridoids
Black cohosh (*Cimicifuga racemosa*)	2b	Triterpenes
Licorice (*Glycyrrhiza glabra*)	2b, 2c, 2d (contraindicated in hypertension and diabetes; mid-term use)	Triterpenoids
Ginseng	2d (contraindicated in hypertension and pregnancy; mid-term use)	Saponins

5.3.4 Anticoagulant Effects

Due to the presence of components with anti-aggregating properties, the herbs listed in Table 5.5 display an anticoagulant effect. Interestingly, the enhancing effect of aspirin on anticoagulant drugs has not been observed for salicin-containing herbs like willow (*Salix alba*), meadowsweet (*Filipendula ulmaria*), white and black birch (*Betula* spp.), wintergreen (*Gaultheria* procumbens), and balsam poplar (*Populus nigra*).[27]

TABLE 5.5
Herbs with Anticoagulant Effects

Herbs	Class	Components
Garlic	2c	Sulfur compounds[a]
Ginkgo	2d (occasional headache and mild gastric upset)	Ginkgolide B (PAF inhibitor)
Fenugreek (*Trigonella foenum-graecum*)	2b	Coumarins[b]
Angelica	2d (phototoxicity)	Coumarins and furocoumarins
Feverfew	2b	Sesquiterpene lactones (inhibits platelet aggregation)
Ginger (*Zingiber officinalis*)	2d (contraindicated during pregnancy and lactation)	Gingerol derivatives (inhibits platelet aggregation)

[a] Fresh garlic may induce heartburn and thin blood if more than five cloves a day are ingested. This is an unusual dietary consumption, but it is nearly the dose recommended for health effects (Commission E). To overcome this limit, extract of aged garlic with a standardized content of a stable and bioavailable sulfur compound (*S*-allyl-cysteine) is available.
[b] Coumarins are blood-thinning agents, and may potentiate existing anticoagulant therapies. Besides angelica and fenugreek, coumarins are also present in alfalfa, chamomile, horseradish, meadowsweet, passionflower, melilot, and horse chestnut. In view of this, excessive use of these herbs should be avoided.[24]

5.4 HERBS ASSOCIATED WITH TOXIC REACTIONS

The herbs listed in Table 5.6 are characterized by the presence of components that have been described to cause serious adverse reactions, and their use is not advised.

5.5 HIGHLY TOXIC MEDICINAL PLANTS

A number of potent medicinal plants **are not considered a part of herbal medicine.**[29,30] These plant are characterized by the presence of specific alkaloids and steroid cardiac glycosides. For instance, *Atropa belladonna* (belladonna), *Hyoscyamus niger* (henbane), and *Datura stramonium* (stramonium or jimson weed) contain atropine and its racemate hyoscyamine, that are tropane alkaloids with great potential toxicity. Both atropine and hyoscyamine are anticholinergic (they block the muscarinic activity of acetylcholine in the parasympathetic nervous system) and provide antispasmodic (excess motor activity of the gastrointestinal tract and spasm of urinary tracts) as well as antisecretory (gastric and nasal secretions) and mydriatic effects. These herbs must be used cautiously. Similar caution is needed for *Catharanthus roseus* (vinca), which contains the indole alkaloids vinblastine and vincristine (effective antineoplastic co-agents), or *Ephedra* spp. (ephedra or ma huang) for the presence of ephedrine, a potent sympathomimetic that relaxes bronchial muscles, produces in the heart a positive inotropic effect, and promotes vasoconstriction.

TABLE 5.6
Herbs with Toxic Constituents

Herbs (Class)	Components
Comfrey(2a), Coltsfoot(2b), Liferoot(3) (*Senecio*)	Pyrrolizidine alkaloids[a] (liver damage)
Borage (2a)	Sparteine (oxytocic)
Broom (3)(*Cytisus scoparius*)	Sparteine, lectins[b] (abortifacient)
Calamus (2b) (*Acorus calamus*)	β-Asarone
Sassafras (2d)	Safrole[c] (genotoxic-chromosomal aberrations)
Pennyroyal (2b) (*Mentha pulegium*)	Pulegone (liver damage, abortifacient)
Chaparral (2d) (contraindicated in kidney and liver diseases) (*Larrea tridentata*)	Nordihydroguaiaretic acid (liver damage)
Mistletoe (2d) (berries are highly poisonous; contraindicated during pregnancy and lactation) (*Viscum album*)	Lectins (hemagglutinating and mitogenic activity), viscotoxins (toxic constituents)
	Lectins (hemagglutinating activity)
	Lectins and saponins (toxic agents)
Poke (3) (*Phytolacca americana*)	
Juniper (2b), sage (2d), tansy(2b)	Thujone[d] (abortifacient)

[a] Some specific pyrrolizidine alkaloids have been demonstrated to be associated with liver disease, and to be mutagenic and carcinogenic. *Symphytum* spp. (comfrey), *Tussilago farfara* (coltsfoot), and *Borago officinalis* (borage) are examples of herbs containing toxic unsaturated pyrrolizidine alkaloids.[28]

[b] Lectins are glycoproteins with highly diversified chemical structures and biological activities. Some have carbohydrate-binding properties (phytohemagglutinins, i.e., able to agglutinate red blood cells), while others exert immune-enhancing and mitogenic effects. A number of lectins are toxic. This is not the case for lectins found in common legumes (kidney beans, green beans, soybeans, and lentils) which are freed of the slight potential toxicity during food processing. By contrast, lectins present in mistletoe, poke weed, and in castor bean seeds are highly toxic. In view of this, these herbs must "be used only under the supervision of an expert qualified in their appropriate use".[18]

[c] Safrole, and the other allylbenzenes estragole and beta-asarone, though not directly toxic, are converted in the liver into reactive epoxides. These intermediates, if not deactivated, may promote genetic and cellular damage.[29] Therefore, herbs containing these allylbenzenes (camphor, sassafras, nutmeg or *Myristica fragrans*, calamus, Canadian snakeroot or *Asarum canadense*) should be avoided, or at least consumed in minor amounts as flavors.

[d] Thujone, a bicyclic monoterpene (related to camphor) present in the volatile fraction of some plants, is neurotoxic. High-dose or long-term ingestion of these plants can cause serious adverse effects.[27]

By contrast, *Hydrastis canadensis* (goldenseal), *Mahonia aquifolium* (Oregon grape), *Coptis sinensis* (Chinese gold thread), *Berberis vulgaris* (common barberry), *Chelidonium majus* (greater celandine), and *Sanguinaria canadensis* (bloodroot) contain the quaternary alkaloid berberine, which is only moderately toxic. These herbs are considered safe for external use (skin inflammation and dental hygiene); their internal use should be limited and avoided during pregnancy and lactation.

Medicinal plants containing steroid glycosides able to increase the force of systolic contraction (positive inotropic action), such as digitoxin and digoxin present in *Digitalis* spp. (foxglove), may be associated with hazardous intoxication. Due to their narrow therapeutic range, these cardioactive herbs should be handled with exceptional care.

5.6 POSSIBLE INTERACTIONS OF PHYTOMEDICINES WITH DRUGS

When referring to the ESCOP Monographs[31] of the medicinal use of plant drugs, very few interactions with other medicaments are reported. Nevertheless, interactions between phytomedicines and synthetic drugs are possible,[32-34] and some of them have been studied.

Long-term abuse of stimulant laxatives (cascara, senna, frangula) results in hypokalemia, that enhances the action of cardiac glycosides. Thus, stimulant laxatives may interfere with cardiac glycoside therapy. For the same reason, concomitant use of stimulant laxatives with diuretics and mineralocorticoids (both inducing hypokalemia) is not advised.

Saint John's wort should not be used with other known photosensitizers, such as piroxicam or tetracycline hydrochloride. Furthermore, taking Saint John's wort with synthetic antidepressants, like tricyclic antidepressants or selective serotonin reuptake inhibitors (fluoxetine), is not advised.

Valerian should not be used with barbiturates, as it prolongs the barbiturate-induced sleep. Similarly, concomitant use of kava (*Piper methysticum*) with sedative benzodiazepines is not recommended.

Due to their immunostimulating properties, echinacea (*Echinacea* spp.), astragalus (*Astragalus membranaceous*), and licorice (*Glycyrrhiza* spp.) should be avoided when immunosuppressive drugs (corticosteroids) are given.

Phytomedicines with an aquaretic effect, including goldenrod (*Solidago virgaurea*), elder (*Sambucus nigra*), and yarrow (*Achillea millefolium*) may decrease the effects of antihypertensive diuretic drugs, as sodium is retained.

Ginseng (*Panax ginseng*), feverfew (*Thanacetum parthenium*), garlic (*Allium sativum*), ginger (*Zingiber officinalis*), and ginkgo (*Ginkgo biloba*) may potentiate anticoagulant therapy, as they contain blood-thinning agents.

Volatile oils rich in camphor and thujone (*Salvia officinalis* or sage, *Thanacetum vulgare* or tansy) or gamma-linolenic acid-rich oils (*Oenothera perennis* or evening primrose, *Borago officinalis* or borage, *Ribes nigrum* or blackcurrant seeds) are reported to increase the risk of seizure. Thus, their concomitant use with phenobarbital, phenytoin, and other drugs known to lower the seizure threshold (e.g., tricyclic antidepressants and phenothiazines) should be avoided.

Horseradish (*Radicula armoracia*), like other members of the Brassicaceae, may depress thyroid function, and should not be used with thyroid replacement drugs (thyroxine). These drugs also interfere with kelp (*Fucus* vesiculosus, that provides iodine), resulting in hyperthyroidism.

The use of phytomedicines with hypoglycemic properties, like fenugreek (*Trigonella foenum-graecum*), garlic (*Allium sativum*), ginger (*Zingiber officinalis*), ginseng (*Panax ginseng*), gymnema (*Gymnema sylvestris*), nettle (*Urtica dioica*), or with hyperglycemic activity like licorice (*Glycyrrhiza* spp.), devil's claw (*Harpagophytum procumbens*), and hydrocotyle (*Centella asiatica*) may interfere with diabetes therapy, and should be carefully monitored.

Finally, the effect of MAOIs may be potentiated by different herbal medicines, including Californian poppy (*Eschschtzia californica*), ginkgo (*Ginkgo biloba*), ginseng (*Panax ginseng*), licorice (*Glycyrrhiza* spp.), and Saint John's wort (*Hypericum perforatum*).

5.7 CONCLUSIONS

An increasing number of phytomedicines has been proved to conform with evidence-based criteria required for modern drugs, and they can be integrated into mainstream medicine for the treatment of some mild/moderate and chronic diseases. Other herbal products need further evaluation prior to being considered part of the therapeutic armamentarium, while specific herbs must be avoided because of their toxicity.

Accurate quality control and proper use under supervision of expert health-care professionals are mandatory to guarantee efficacy and safety, and to reduce the risk of interactions with other medicaments.

ACKNOWLEDGMENTS

Supported by a grant from the National Council of Research, Italy.

REFERENCES

1. Winslow, L.C. and Kroll, D.J., Herbs as medicines, *Arch. Int. Med.*, 158, 2192, 1998.
2. Winston, J.C., Health-promoting properties of common herbs, *Am. J. Clin. Nutr.*, 70, 4915, 1999.
3. Johnston, B.A., One-third of nation's adults use herbal remedies, *Herbalgram*, 40, 49, 1997.
4. Jonas, W.B., Alternative medicine — Learning from the past, examining the present, advancing to the future, *J. Am. Med. Assoc.*, 280, 1616, 1998.
5. O'Hara, M., Kiefer, D., Farrell, K., and Kemper, K., A review of 12 commonly used medicinal herbs, *Arch. Fam. Med.*, 7, 523, 1998.
6. Mashour, N.H., Lin, G.I., and Frishman, W.H., Herbal medicine for the treatment of cardiovascular disease, *Arch. Int. Med.*, 158, 2225, 1998.
7. Upton, R., Ed., St John's Wort Monograph, *American Herbal Pharmacopoeia*, 1997.
8. Brown, D.J. and Dattner, A.M., Phytotherapeutic approaches to common dermatologic conditions, *Arch. Dermatol.*, 134, 1401, 1998.
9. Pietta, P.G. and Pietta, A., *Fitomedicine e Nutrienti*, Ricchiuto Editore, Verona, 1998.
10. Pietta, P.G., in *Flavonoids in Health and Disease*, Packer, L. and Rice-Evans, C.A., Eds., Marcel Dekker, New York, 1998, chap. 3.

11. Mauri, P.L. and Pietta, P.G., Electrospray characterization of selected medicinal plant extracts, *J. Pharm. Biomed. Anal.*, in press.
12. Pietta, P.G., in *Handbook of Capillary Electrophoresis Applications*, Shintoni, H. and Polonsky, J., Eds., Blackie Academic, London, chap. 3.
13. Debbie, S., House, I., Stoyko, K., and Murray, V., Should herbal medicines be licensed?, *Br. Med. J.*, 311, 451, 1995.
14. Ko, R.J., Adulterants in Asian patent medicines, *N. Engl. J .Med.*, 339, 847, 1998.
15. Abbot, N.C., *Nature*, 1996, 381.
16. Marwick, C., Growing use of medicinal botanicals forces assessment by drug regulators, *J. Am. Med. Assoc.*, 273, 607, 1995.
17. De Smet, P.A.G.M., *Adverse Reactions of Herbal Drugs*, Vol. 3, Springer-Verlag, New York, 1997.
18. McGuffin, M., Hobbs, C., Upton, R., and Goldberg, A., Eds., *Botanical Safety Book*, CRC Press, Boca Raton, FL, 1997.
19. Berkley, S.F., Dermatitis associated with high natural concentrations of furanocoumarins in celery, *Am. Int. Med.*, 105, 351, 1986.
20. Hausen, B.M., Identification of allergenes of Arnica montana, *Contact Dermatitis*, 4, 308, 1978.
21. Mitchell, J.C. and Dupnis, G., Allergenic contact dermatitis from sesquiterpenoids of the Compositae family, *Br. J. Dermatol.*, 84, 139, 1971.
22. Wollenweber, E., Asakawa, Y., Schillo, D., Lehman, U., and Weigel, H., A novel caffeic acid derivative and other constituents of Populus bud excretion and propolis, *Z. Naturforsch.*, 42C, 1030, 1987.
23. Locock, R.A., Capsicum, *Can. Pharm. J.*, 118, 517, 1985.
24. Newall, C.A., Anderson, L.A., and Phillipson, D., *Herbal Medicines — A Guide for Health-Care Professionals*, Pharmaceutical Press, London, 1996.
25. Shilo, S. and Hirsch, H.J., Iodine-induced hyperthyroidism in a patient with a normal thyroid gland, *Postgrad. Med. J.*, 62, 661, 1986.
26. Roeder, D., Therapie von Zyklusstoerungen mit *Vitex agnus-castus*, *Z. Phytther.*, 15, 155, 1994.
27. Wichtl, M. and Bisset, N.G., Eds., *Herbal Drugs and Phytopharmaceuticals*, Medpharm GmbH Scientific, Stuttgart, 1994.
28. Bruneton, J., *Pharmacognosy, Phytochemistry, Medicinal Plants*, Hatton, C.K., translator, Lavoisier Publishers, Paris, 1995.
29. Luo, G. and Guenther, T.M., Metabolism of allylbenzene-2',3'-oxide and estragole-2',3'-oxide in the isolated perfused rat liver, *J. Pharmacol. Exp. Ther.*, 272, 588, 1995.
30. Robbers, J.E., Speedie, M.K., and Tyler, V.E., *Pharmacognosy and Pharmacobiotechnology*, Williams & Wilkins, Baltimore, 1996.
31. ESCOP, *Monographs on the Medicinal Use of Plant Drugs*, Exeter, U.K., 1997
32. Ernst, E., Harmless herbs? A review of recent literature, *Am. J. Med.*, 104, 170, 1998.
33. Miller, L.G., Herbal medicinals — Selected clinical considerations focusing on known or potential drug-herb interactions, *Arch. Int. Med.*, 158, 2200, 1998.
34. De Smet, P.A.G.M. and D'Arcy, P.F., Drug interactions with herbal and other non-orthodox remedies, in *Mechanisms of Drug Interactions*, D'Arcy, P.F., Ed., Springer-Verlag, Berlin, 1996.

6 Fruit and Vegetable Micronutrients in Diseases of the Eye

Herbert T. Greenway and Steven G. Pratt

CONTENTS

6.1 INTRODUCTION

Cataracts and macular degeneration constitute the most common causes of visual impairment in the U.S. Indeed, the leading cause of blindness in people older than 65 years is age-related macular degeneration (AMD).[1] It has been estimated that 13 million people in the U.S. have evidence of AMD and that the disease causes visual impairment in 1.2 million. At present, there are no effective treatments for most patients with the disease. Cataracts affect more than 15% of people older than 43 years and increase in prevalence among older people so that more than 50% of people older than 75 years are estimated to have evidence of cataracts.[2,3]

Recent studies have found strong evidence that consumption of specific fruits and vegetables can play an important role in reducing the incidence of cataracts and AMD.[4] This chapter will summarize the role of these compounds in these eye diseases.

6.2 EFFECTS OF FRUIT AND VEGETABLE CONSUMPTION ON THE INCIDENCE OF AMD

Population studies have provided evidence that consumption of specific fruits and vegetables can reduce the incidence of AMD. Goldberg et al.[5] analyzed data from the National Health and Nutrition Examination Survey (NHANES I) and found an

0-8493-0038-X/97/$0.00+$.50

association between dietary antioxidant intake and protection from AMD. They found that people who consumed fruits and vegetables that were rich sources of vitamin A at least once per day had a significant protection from AMD compared to those who consumed such foods less than once per week.[5] This study did not establish vitamin A as the important factor. Indeed, recent studies suggest that specific carotenoids, found in many of the same foods, may be responsible.

Investigators from the Eye Disease Case-Control Study used a case-control experimental design to examine how consumption of specific foods affected the incidence of AMD.[6] They employed a multivariate model that related the incidence of AMD to consumption of broccoli, cabbage-related vegetables, carrots, spinach or collard greens, sweet potatoes, and winter squash. In their analysis, consumption of spinach was associated with robust protection from AMD; subjects in the highest quintile for consumption of spinach had an 86% lower odds of advanced AMD.

In an earlier report,[7] the same investigators divided patients into three groups on the basis of their plasma levels of various micronutrients. They found that high levels of plasma carotenoids were associated with the lowest incidence of AMD. They also analyzed specific carotenoids and found that the patients with the highest levels of lutein/zeaxanthin in their plasma had an odds ratio for AMD of 0.3 (95% CI 0.2–0.6; $p = .0001$). Certain other carotenoids, such as β-carotene, α-carotene, and cryptoxanthan were also associated with a reduced odds of AMD. However, lycopene, the major carotenoid in tomatoes, was not associated with a reduced odds of AMD.

Not all studies have found an association between serum carotenoids and protection from AMD. For example, a case-control study that used the population from the Beaver Dam Eye Study found no such association for lutein or zeaxanthin, but it did find a weak protective effect of serum lycopene.[8] However, this study included many fewer subjects than did the Eye Disease Case-Control Study. In agreement with the Eye Disease Case-Control Study, a prospective cohort study, the Baltimore Longitudinal Study of Aging, found an association between blood levels of antioxidants and protection from AMD.[9]

Randomized, prospective trials have yet to demonstrate that the incidence of AMD can be reduced by consumption of specific fruits and vegetables or dietary supplements. However, strong evidence exists that leafy green vegetables and fruits containing the carotenoids lutein and zeaxanthin may play an important role in protection from AMD.

6.3 BIOLOGICAL ROLE OF CAROTENOIDS

The term macula lutea refers to a pigmented region of the retina that includes the fovea, which is the region responsible for highest visual acuity and which contains the highest density of cone photoreceptors.

The human macular pigment is composed primarily of a mixture of the two carotenoids, lutein and zeaxanthin.[10-13] Toward the periphery of the retina, the concentration of zeaxanthin declines rapidly whereas the concentration of lutein declines gradually.[13-15] Similar results have been reported in nonhuman primates.[16] This spatial inhomogeneity has been proposed to be consistent with the role of the macular pigment in reducing chromatic aberration.[17] Interestingly, lutein and zeaxanthin are the two dominant carotenoids in the retina. Indeed, only traces of β-carotene or other carotenoids have been detected in human retinas and these may have come from blood contamination of the samples.[15]

Lutein and zeaxanthin are closely related carotenoids and lutein may be converted to zeaxanthin in the retina.[18] The remainder of retinal zeaxanthin most likely comes from dietary sources.[19] The two carotenoids are also related to β-carotene, but there is no evidence for interconversion between β-carotene and lutein or zeaxanthin, although the various carotenoids may interact.[20] Neither lutein nor zeaxanthin can be synthesized by the human body.

The macular pigment filters blue light, which is particularly damaging to photoreceptors and to the retinal pigment epithelium.[21,22] Snodderly et al.[10] performed experiments concluding that most of the macular pigment is positioned between the incoming light and the photoreceptor outer segments. Hence, it is positioned where it would be an effective optical filter. The filtering of blue light has been proposed as one of the primary functions of the macular pigment. This hypothesis is supported by the finding that lutein and zeaxanthin absorb blue light.[23,24]

Another mechanism by which these nutrients may protect the retina is by limiting the oxidant stress to the tissue that results from metabolism and light.[21,25,26] It has been shown that one of the ways light damages the retina is by generating free radicals that lead to peroxidation of membrane lipids.[27,28] Preclinical studies have found that animals given a diet rich in antioxidant vitamins (A, C, and E) developed less retinal degeneration than animals given a diet low in antioxidants.[29-31] Furthermore, carotenoids have long been known as powerful antioxidants[26,32] and lutein and zeaxanthin have been proposed to serve this role in protecting the macula. Khachik et al.[25] found oxidation products of lutein in the human retina and proposed that the presence of such metabolites indicates an antioxidant role of lutein in this tissue.

Another component to the proposed antioxidant role of macular carotenoids is the role of lipofuscin, a group of autofluorescent lipid and protein aggregates that accumulate in cells of the retina, particularly the retinal pigment epithelium (RPE).[33] Lipofuscin produces reactive oxygen species when exposed to blue light.[34] This effect may cause death of RPE cells.[35]

Although the pathophysiology of AMD is not well understood, the integrity of the macular pigment is believed to protect this region of the retina from degeneration.[24] For example, it has been found that people older than 60 years who have a low macular pigment density also have reduced visual sensitivity. In contrast, people of the same age but who have a high macular pigment density have visual sensitivity similar to younger people.[36,37] Loss of visual sensitivity can be a precursor to many retinal diseases and may be an early sign of AMD.[37]

Other studies examining the protective role of the macular pigment have found that its density is correlated with other risk factors for AMD. For example, some studies have concluded that people with light-colored irises are at higher risk for AMD.[23] Furthermore, Hammond et al.[38] have reported that people with light-colored irises are more likely to have a low macular pigment density. Interestingly, sunlight exposure is a risk factor for AMD and sunlight exposure reduces levels of carotenoids in plasma.[39]

A similar association has been found between smoking (a risk factor for AMD[40-44]) and macular pigment density. Early as well as more recent studies found that smoking reduced plasma levels of carotenoids.[45,46] An additional study found that macular pigment density was reduced in smokers in a dose-dependent manner,[47] supporting a link between plasma carotenoids and their accumulation in the macula.[45] Another risk factor for AMD is excessive alcohol consumption.[48,49] As with smoking, excessive alcohol consumption is associated with reduced plasma levels of antioxidant vitamins and carotenoids.[45,50]

Several areas of basic research have underscored the importance to eye health of fruits and vegetables rich in carotenoids. A recent study has shown that increasing dietary intake of fruits and vegetables high in these nutrients leads to a large increase in the concentration of lutein in plasma.[51] Indeed, these authors proposed that measurements of plasma carotenoids could be used as measurements of fruit and vegetable intake. Animal studies have also found that plasma levels of specific carotenoids are directly related to dietary intake of these nutrients.[52]

Further along the biological route, plasma levels of lutein and zeaxanthin are believed to affect the density of the macular pigment. As discussed, low density of the macular pigment is associated with loss of visual sensitivity.[36,37] In a recent study,[53] subjects were given a diet rich in fruits and vegetables that are known to be good sources of the carotenoids lutein and zeaxanthin. Control subjects were given an otherwise similar diet but that was low in fruits and vegetables that contained these carotenoids. Most of the subjects consuming lutein and zeaxanthin experienced an increase in their plasma levels of these nutrients and in the density of their macular pigment over the 15 weeks of the trial. The control group experienced no such changes. Additional evidence that consumption of such fruits and vegetables leads to thickening of the macular pigment comes from animal studies in which macular carotenoids were measured more directly. These studies have shown that the concentrations of lutein and zeaxanthin in the macula are strongly influenced by dietary intake of these nutrients.[54]

Although randomized trials have yet to be conducted, Landrum et al.[55] have shown that a lutein supplement given to two subjects led to a measurable increase in the optical density of the macular pigment in both subjects (21 and 39% increases). Interestingly, the plasma concentrations rose rapidly at the beginning of the supplementation period, but the macular pigment density began to rise only after 20 to 40 days. Likewise, when the subjects stopped taking the supplement, the plasma concentration declined rapidly but the macular pigment density remained elevated for a prolonged period. These findings led the investigators to speculate that the turnover rate of the carotenoids in the macula is relatively slow and may represent an average of carotenoid consumption over a long period. A recent pilot study has also concluded that visual function is improved in patients with AMD who increase their consumption of dark-green leafy vegetables.[56]

Thus, basic research studies have generated biologically plausible mechanisms whereby carotenoids and antioxidant vitamins could protect the retina from light-induced degeneration.

6.4 EFFECTS OF FRUIT AND VEGETABLE CONSUMPTION ON THE INCIDENCE OF CATARACTS

Cataracts are opacifications of the lens of the eye. The incidence of cataracts increases sharply with age. As with AMD, there are no prospective, randomized trials of dietary components or supplements that have demonstrated a protective effect against development of cataracts. However, population-based and case-control studies have provided evidence that specific vitamins and dietary components may reduce the risk of cataracts.

The strongest evidence currently available comes from two prospective, cohort studies, which have recently reported that the risk of cataract extraction is reduced in women and men who consume diets rich in specific carotenoids. The Nurses' Health Study[57] followed 50,461 women between the ages of 45 and 71 years for up to 12 years. They obtained information on diet by repeatedly administering a questionnaire designed to assess the frequency of consumption of specific foods. From these data, the consumption of specific nutrients was estimated and correlated with the risk of cataract extraction during the follow-up period. The studies examined the risk of cataract associated with intakes of foods containing several carotenoids, retinol, and vitamin A. In a multivariate analysis, only the carotenoids lutein and zeaxanthin were associated with a significant reduction in the odds of cataract extraction ($p < .04$). When specific foods were examined, intake of spinach was consistently associated with reduced risk of cataract extraction. They reported that participants who consumed cooked spinach at lease twice per week had a 30 to 38% lower risk of cataract extraction compared to those who consumed it less that once per month. In general, raw spinach had a similar effect. The conclusions from this study were robust when the data were adjusted for intakes of other nutrients and for other markers of a healthy life style.

A similar prospective, cohort study was performed in men participating in the Health Professionals Follow-up Study.[58] This study followed 51,529 male health professionals for up to 8 years. Dietary intake of specific foods was assessed with periodic food-frequency questionnaires. The risk of cataract extraction was significantly lower among men with the highest consumption of fruits and vegetables rich in lutein and zeaxanthin in a multivariate analysis ($p < .03$). When the investigators examined specific foods, intake of spinach and broccoli were associated with a reduced risk of cataract extraction.

Interestingly, Hammond et al.[59] have found a correlation between macular pigment density and clarity of the lens. As discussed, macular pigment density is determined largely by the presence of lutein and zeaxanthin. Thus, increased levels of these nutrients may be associated with maintenance of lens clarity.

Reduced risk of cataracts has also been associated with intake of specific vitamins, in particular vitamins A, C, and E. In a recent population-based study conducted as part of the Beaver Dam Eye Study,[60] tocopherols (forms of vitamin E) and carotenoids were assessed for their association with cataracts. High serum levels of both alpha-tocopherol and gamma-tocopherol were associated with a significantly lower risk of nuclear cataracts 5 years after baseline assessment. Interestingly, participants with higher levels of serum lutein had a lower incidence of nuclear cataracts, although the effect was not statistically significant. These results with tocopherols are in agreement with previous studies, notably the Baltimore Longitudinal Study on Aging[61] and the Lens Opacities Case-Control Study,[62] but not with three other studies.[63-65] Differences in study design and diet assessment are likely to explain the different results. Another recent study, the Longitudinal Study of Cataract,[66] found that regular users of vitamin E supplements and people with high serum concentrations of vitamin E had about 50% fewer cases of cataracts.

The role of vitamin C has been assessed in several epidemiologic studies, and several have reported lower incidence of cataracts in individuals with high blood levels or high intakes of vitamin C.[67-71] In a cohort derived from the Nurses' Health Study, use of vitamin C supplements for 10 years or longer was associated with 77 to 83% lower risk of lens opacity.[72] However, women who used vitamin C supplements for shorter periods did not derive such a benefit.

6.5 OTHER MICRONUTRIENTS IN DISEASES OF THE EYE

Several other micronutrients have been implicated as potentially useful for treatment or prevention of eye diseases. Although there are some data from humans, many of these nutrients have been studied only in animal models and have yet to be studied by epidemiologic or clinical methods in humans.

Deficiency of zinc has been shown to be associated with an increase in the risk of AMD in humans.[73] Zinc is a cofactor for Cu-Zn superoxide dismutase and induces the synthesis of metallothionein.[74,75] It is found in relatively high concentrations in the eye.[76] In animal models, zinc deficiency increases oxidative stress in the retina.[77] Although one study has shown a benefit of zinc supplements in patients with AMD,[78] other studies indicate that excessive zinc supplements (more than 15 mg/day) may have adverse effects on blood lipids.[79,80] There is also evidence that excessive consumption of zinc can cause depression of the immune system and possibly play a role in Alzheimers disease.[81-87] In general, consumption of more than 15 mg/day of zinc should be avoided.[85-87]

Polyphenolic phytonutrients comprise a large group of molecules derived from a variety of plant sources. Many of these compounds are powerful antioxidants and are associated with a variety of potential beneficial effects. For example, polyphenolic phytonutrients may be protective against atherosclerosis and cardiovascular disease and some may have anti-inflammatory or antithrombotic properties.[88-92] Furthermore, there is an accumulating body of evidence that polyphenolic phytonutrients exert beneficial effects synergistically with carotenoids, vitamins C and E, and endogenous antioxidants.[93-98] A few of these compounds have been investigated for their effects on the eyes.

TABLE 6.1
Foods Rich in Micronutrients Important for Eye Health

Nutrient	Foods
Vitamin E	Kale
	Spinach
	Sunflower seeds
	Almonds
	Hazelnuts
	Peanuts
	Wheat germ
	Soybeans
	Avocados
	Sardines
	Oils (sunflower, corn, soybean, canola, wheat germ, almond)
Vitamin C	Citrus fruit
	Kiwi fruit
	Cantaloupe
	Papaya
	Broccoli
	Black currants
	Orange juice
	Strawberries
	Peppers (red, yellow, green)
Lutein	Spinach
	Kale
	Collard greens
	Mustard greens
	Swiss chard
	Watercress
Zeaxanthin	Peaches
	Citrus fruit
	Yellow corn
	Orange bell peppers
	Egg yolk

TABLE 6.1 (cont.)

Polyphenolic phytonutrients	Raspberries
	Blackberries
	Blueberries
	Strawberries
	Boysenberries
	Raisins
	Prunes
	Onions
	Apples
	Red wine
	Green tea
	Dark grape juice
	Soybeans
	Chickpeas
	Flax seed
	Spinach
Zinc	Shellfish
	Sunflower seeds
	Pumpkin seeds
	Wheat germ
	Sirloin (lean)
	Beans
	Brewers yeast
	Sardines
	Veal

Genistein, an isoflavone from soybeans, is an inhibitor of tyrosine kinase, which mediates the cellular effects of many growth factors. Genistein has been shown to inhibit proliferation of vascular endothelial cells. A recent study showed that injection of genistein into the vitreous of rabbits reduced neovascularization of the choriocapillaris, which is a common occurrence in many forms of retinopathy.[99]

Pycnogenol is a standardized extract from the pine tree *Pinus maritima*. It contains a mixture of flavonoids. This extract has been reported to have beneficial cardiovascular effects, such as vasorelaxation and inhibition of angiotensin converting enzyme, and to have strong free-radical scavenging activity.[100] There is currently much interest in the possibility that such compounds may be useful in treating neurogenerative disorders, including those involving the retina.

Finally, an extract from *Ginkgo biloba* has shown promise in reducing light-induced damage to the retina of experimental animals. The extract, Egb 761, is a standardized extract containing largely flavonoid glycosides and terpenoids. A recent study has demonstrated that administration of the extract to rats by gavage can reduce light-induced retinal damage.[101]

6.6 CONCLUSION

Consumption of fruits and vegetables, particularly those high in carotenoids, antioxidant vitamins, and polyphenolic phytonutrients, is likely to dramatically reduce the risk of age-related macular degeneration and cataracts. The best way to increase consumption of these nutrients is to consume foods that contain them in high concentrations (see Table 6.1). In situations where it is impractical to obtain sufficient nutrients from dietary sources, a well-balanced supplement containing vitamins, minerals, antioxidants, and phytonutrients may be a reasonable alternative. In the case of lutein and zeaxanthin, there is no evidence that they are associated with any adverse side effects. Other practical approaches to prevention of eye disease are also warranted. Such approaches include avoiding cigarette smoke, moderating alcohol consumption, avoiding excessive sunlight exposure, wearing a hat in the sun, and wearing sunglasses that block light wavelengths up to 450 nm.

REFERENCES

1. Retinal and Choroidal Diseases Panel, National Advisory Eye Council, Vision Research — a National Plan: 1983-1987, U.S. Department of Health and Human Services, Bethesda, MD, 1984.
2. Klein, B.E., Klein, R., and Linton, K.L., Prevalence of age-related lens opacities in a population, The Beaver Dam Eye Study. *Ophthalmology,* 95, 546, 1992.
3. Sperduto, R.D. and Hiller, R., The prevalence of nuclear, cortical, and posterior subcapsular lens opacities in a general population sample. *Ophthalmology,* 91, 815, 1984.
4. Pratt, S., Dietary prevention of age-related macular degeneration. *J. Am. Optom. Assoc.*, 70, 39, 1999.
5. Goldberg, J., Flowerdew, G., Smith, E., Brody, J.A., and Tso, M.O., Factors associated with age-related macular degeneration. An analysis of data from the first National Health and Nutrition Examination Survey. *Am. J. Epidemiol.,* 128, 700, 1988.
6. Seddon, J.M., Ajani, U.A., Sperduto, R.D., et al., Dietary carotenoids, vitamins A, C, and E, and advanced age-related macular degeneration. Eye Disease Case-Control Study Group. *J. Am. Med. Assoc.,* 272, 1413, 1994.
7. Antioxidant status and neovascular age-related macular degeneration, Eye Disease Case-Control Study Group. *Arch. Ophthalmol.,* 111, 104, 1993.
8. Mares-Perlman, J.A., Brady, W.E., Klein, R., et al., Serum antioxidants and age-related macular degeneration in a population-based case-control study. *Arch. Ophthalmol.,* 113, 1518, 1995.
9. West, S., Vitale, S., Hallfrisch, J., et al., Are antioxidants or supplements protective for age-related macular degeneration? *Arch. Ophthalmol.,* 112, 222, 1994.
10. Snodderly, D.M., Auran, J.D., and Delori, F.C., The macular pigment. II. Spatial distribution in primate retinas. *Invest. Ophthalmol. Vis. Sci.,* 25, 674, 1984.
11. Snodderly, D.M., Brown, P.K., Delori, F.C., and Auran, J.D., The macular pigment. I. Absorbance spectra, localization, and discrimination from other yellow pigments in primate retinas. *Invest. Ophthalmol. Vis. Sci.,* 25, 660, 1984.
12. Bone, R.A., Landrum, J.T., and Tarsis, S.L., Preliminary identification of the human macular pigment. *Vision Res.,* 25, 1531, 1985.

13. Bone, R.A., Landrum, J.T., Fernandez, L., and Tarsis, S.L., Analysis of the macular pigment by HPLC: retinal distribution and age study. *Invest. Ophthalmol. Vis. Sci.*, 29, 843, 1988.
14. Bone, R.A., Landrum, J.T., Friedes, L.M., et al., Distribution of lutein and zeaxanthin stereoisomers in the human retina. *Exp. Eye Res.*, 64, 211, 1997.
15. Handelman, G.J., Dratz, E.A., Reay, C.C., and van Kuijk, J.G., Carotenoids in the human macula and whole retina. *Invest. Ophthalmol. Vis. Sci.*, 29, 850, 1988.
16. Snodderly, D.M., Handelman, G.J., and Adler, A.J., Distribution of individual macular pigment carotenoids in central retina of macaque and squirrel monkeys. *Invest. Ophthalmol. Vis. Sci.*, 32, 268, 1991.
17. Beatty, S., Boulton, M., Henson, D., Koh, H.H., and Murray, I.J., Macular pigment and age related macular degeneration. *Br. J. Ophthalmol.*, 83, 867, 1999.
18. Bone, R.A., Landrum, J.T., Hime, G.W., Cains, A., and Zamor, J., Stereochemistry of the human macular carotenoids. *Invest. Ophthalmol. Vis. Sci.*, 34, 2033, 1993.
19. Schalch, W., Dayhaw-Barker, P., and Barker, F.M., II., The Carotenoids of the Human Retina in *Nutritional and Environmental Influences on the Eye*, Taylor, A., Ed., CRC Press, Boca Ratron, FL, 1999.
20. van den Berg, H., Carotenoid interactions. *Nutr. Rev.*, 57, 1, 1999.
21. Ham, W.T., Jr., Ocular hazards of light sources: review of current knowledge. *J. Occup. Med.*, 25, 101, 1983.
22. Ham, W.T., Jr., Mueller, H.A., Ruffolo, J.J., Jr., et al., Basic mechanisms underlying the production of photochemical lesions in the mammalian retina. *Curr. Eye Res.*, 3, 165, 1984.
23. Snodderly, D.M., Evidence for protection against age-related macular degeneration by carotenoids and antioxidant vitamins. *Am. J. Clin. Nutr.*, 62, 1448S, 1995.
24. Nussbaum, J.J., Pruett, R.C., and Delori, F.C., Historic perspectives. Macular yellow pigment, the first 200 years. *Retina,* 1, 296, 1981.
25. Khachik, F., Bernstein, P.S., and Garland, D.L., Identification of lutein and zeaxanthin oxidation products in human and monkey retinas. *Invest. Ophthalmol. Vis. Sci.*, 38, 1802, 1997.
26. Schalch, W., Carotenoids in the retina--a review of their possible role in preventing or limiting damage caused by light and oxygen. *Exs.*, 62, 280, 1992.
27. Noell, W.K., Possible mechanisms of photoreceptor damage by light in mammalian eyes. *Vision Res.*, 20, 1163, 1980.
28. Wiegand, R.D., Giusto, N.M., Rapp, L.M., and Anderson, R.E., Evidence for rod outer segment lipid peroxidation following constant illumination of the rat retina. *Invest. Ophthalmol. Vis. Sci.*, 24, 1433, 1983.
29. Hayes, K.C., Retinal degeneration in monkeys induced by deficiencies of vitamin E or A. *Invest. Ophthalmol.*, 13, 499, 1974.
30. Katz, M.L., Parker, K.R., Handelman, G.J., Bramel, T.L., and Dratz, E.A., Effects of antioxidant nutrient deficiency on the retina and retinal pigment epithelium of albino rats: a light and electron microscopic study. *Exp. Eye Res.*, 34, 339, 1982.
31. Organisciak, D.T., Wang, H.M., Li, Z.Y., and Tso, M.O., The protective effect of ascorbate in retinal light damage of rats. *Invest. Ophthalmol. Vis. Sci.*, 26, 1580, 1985.
32. Zhang, L.X., Cooney, R.V., and Bertram, J.S., Carotenoids enhance gap junctional communication and inhibit lipid peroxidation in C3H/10T1/2 cells: relationship to their cancer chemopreventive action. *Carcinogenesis,* 12, 2109, 1991.
33. Winkler, B.S., Boulton, M.E., Gottsch, J.D., and Sternberg, P., Oxidative damage and age-related macular degeneration. *Mol. Vis.*, 5, 32, 1999.

34. Rozanowska, M., Jarvis-Evans, J., Korytowski, W., Boulton, M.E., Burke, J.M., and Sarna, T., Blue light-induced reactivity of retinal age pigment. In vitro generation of oxygen-reactive species. *J. Biol. Chem.*, 270, 18825, 1995.
35. Brunk, U.T., Wihlmark, U., Wrigstad, A., Roberg, K., and Nilsson, S.E., Accumulation of lipofuscin within retinal pigment epithelial cells results in enhanced sensitivity to photo-oxidation. *Gerontology,* 41(Suppl. 2), 201, 1995.
36. Haegerstrom-Portnoy, G., Short-wavelength-sensitive cone sensitivity loss with aging: a protective role for macular pigment? *J. Opt. Soc. Am.,* [A] 5, 2140, 1988.
37. Hammond, B.R., Wooten, B.R., and Snodderly, D.M., Preservation of visual sensitivity of older subjects: association with macular pigment density. *Invest. Ophthalmol. Vis. Sci.,* 39, 397, 1998.
38. Hammond, B.R., Jr., Fuld, K., and Snodderly, D.M., Iris color and macular pigment optical density. *Exp. Eye Res.,* 62, 293, 1996.
39. White, W.S., Kim, C.I., Kalkwarf, H.J., Bustos, P., and Roe, D.A., Ultraviolet light-induced reductions in plasma carotenoid levels, *Am. J. Clin. Nutr.,* 47, 879, 1988.
40. The Eye Disease Case-Control Study Group, Risk factors for neovascular age-related macular degeneration, *Arch. Ophthalmol.,* 110, 1701, 1992.
41. Vingerling, J.R., Hofman, A., Grobbee, D.E., and de Jong, P.T., Age-related macular degeneration and smoking. The Rotterdam Study. *Arch. Ophthalmol.,* 114, 1193, 1996.
42. Smith, W., Mitchell, P., and Leeder, S.R., Smoking and age-related maculopathy, The Blue Mountains Eye Study. *Arch. Ophthalmol.,* 114, 1518, 1996.
43. Seddon, J.M., Willett, W.C., Speizer, F.E., and Hankinson, S.E., A prospective study of cigarette smoking and age-related macular degeneration in women. *J. Am. Med. Assoc.,* 276, 1141, 1996.
44. Christen, W.G., Glynn, R.J., Manson, J.E., Ajani, U.A., and Buring, J.E., A prospective study of cigarette smoking and risk of age-related macular degeneration in men. *J. Am. Med. Assoc.,* 276, 1147, 1996.
45. Stryker, W.S., Kaplan, L.A., Stein, E.A., Stampfer, M.J., Sober, A., and Willett, W.C., The relation of diet, cigarette smoking, and alcohol consumption to plasma beta-carotene and alpha-tocopherol levels. *Am. J. Epidemiol.,* 127, 283, 1988.
46. Handelman, G.J., Packer, L., and Cross, C.E., Destruction of tocopherols, carotenoids, and retinol in human plasma by cigarette smoke. *Am. J. Clin. Nutr.,* 63, 559, 1996.
47. Hammond, B.R., Jr., Wooten, B.R., and Snodderly, D.M., Cigarette smoking and retinal carotenoids: implications for age-related macular degeneration. *Vision. Res.,* 36, 3003, 1996.
48. Ritter, L.L., Klein, R., Klein, B.E., Mares-Perlman, J.A., and Jensen, S.C., Alcohol use and age-related maculopathy in the Beaver Dam Eye Study. *Am. J. Ophthalmol.,* 120, 190, 1995.
49. Moss, S.E., Klein, R., Klein, B.E., Jensen, S.C., and Meuer, S.M., Alcohol consumption and the 5-year incidence of age-related maculopathy: the Beaver Dam eye study. *Ophthalmology,* 105, 789, 1998.
50. Forman, M.R., Beecher, G.R., Lanza, E., et al. Effect of alcohol consumption on plasma carotenoid concentrations in premenopausal women: a controlled dietary study. *Am. J. Clin. Nutr.,* 62, 131, 1995.
51. Martini, M.C., Campbell, D.R., Gross, M.D., Grandits, G.A., Potter, J.D., and Slavin, J.L., Plasma carotenoids as biomarkers of vegetable intake: the University of Minnesota Cancer Prevention Research Unit Feeding Studies. *Cancer Epidemiol. Biomark. Prev.,* 4, 491, 1995.

52. Snodderly, D.M., Shen, B., Land, R.I., and Krinsky, N.I., Dietary manipulation of plasma carotenoid concentrations of squirrel monkeys (Saimiri sciureus). *J. Nutr.*, 127, 122, 1997.
53. Hammond, B.R., Jr., Johnson, E.J., Russell, R.M., et al., Dietary modification of human macular pigment density. *Invest. Ophthalmol. Vis. Sci.*, 38, 1795, 1997.
54. Malinow, M.R., Feeney-Burns, L., Peterson, L.H., Klein, M.L., and Neuringer, M., Diet-related macular anomalies in monkeys. *Invest. Ophthalmol. Vis. Sci.*, 19, 857, 1980.
55. Landrum, J.T., Bone, R.A., Joa, H., Kilburn, M.D., Moore, L.L., and Sprague, K.E., A one year study of the macular pigment: the effect of 140 days of a lutein supplement. *Exp. Eye Res.*, 65, 57, 1997.
56. Richer, S., ARMD--pilot (case series) environmental intervention data. *J. Am. Optom. Assoc.*, 70, 24, 1999.
57. Chasan-Taber, L., Willett, W.C., Seddon, J.M., et al., A prospective study of carotenoid and vitamin A intakes and risk of cataract extraction in U.S. women. *Am. J. Clin. Nutr.*, 70, 509, 1999.
58. Brown, L., Rimm, E.B., Seddon, J.M., et al., A prospective study of carotenoid intake and risk of cataract extraction in U.S. men. *Am. J. Clin. Nutr.*, 70, 517, 1999.
59. Hammond, B.R., Jr., Wooten, B.R., and Snodderly, D.M., Density of the human crystalline lens is related to the macular pigment carotenoids, lutein and zeaxanthin. *Optom. Vis. Sci.*, 74, 499, 1997.
60. Lyle, B.J., Mares-Perlman, J.A., Klein, B.E., et al., Serum carotenoids and tocopherols and incidence of age-related nuclear cataract. *Am. J. Clin. Nutr.*, 69, 272, 1999.
61. Vitale, S., West, S., Hallfrisch, J., et al., Plasma antioxidants and risk of cortical and nuclear cataract. *Epidemiology*, 4, 195, 1993.
62. Leske, M.C., Wu, S.Y., Hyman, L., et al., Biochemical factors in the lens opacities. Case-control study, The Lens Opacities Case-Control Study Group. *Arch Ophthalmol.*, 113, 1113, 1995.
63. Rouhiainen, P., Rouhiainen, H., and Salonen, J.T., Association between low plasma vitamin E concentration and progression of early cortical lens opacities. *Am. J. Epidemiol.*, 144, 496, 1996.
64. The Italian-American Cataract Study Group, Risk factors for age-related cortical, nuclear, and posterior subcapsular cataracts. *Am. J. Epidemiol.*, 133, 541, 1991.
65. Mohan, M., Sperduto, R.D., Angra, S.K., et al., India-U.S. case-control study of age-related cataracts, India-U.S. Case-Control Study Group, *Arch. Ophthalmol.*, 107, 670, 1989.
66. Leske, M.C., Chylack, L.T., Jr., He, Q., et al., Antioxidant vitamins and nuclear opacities: the longitudinal study of cataract. *Ophthalmology*, 105, 831, 1998.
67. Jacques, P.F. and Chylack, L.T., Jr., Epidemiologic evidence of a role for the antioxidant vitamins and carotenoids in cataract prevention. *Am. J. Clin. Nutr.*, 53, 352S, 1991.
68. Leske, M.C., Chylack, L.T., Jr., and Wu, S.Y., The Lens Opacities Case-Control Study, Risk factors for cataract. *Arch. Ophthalmol.*, 109, 244, 1991.
69. Hankinson, S.E., Stampfer, M.J., Seddon, J.M., et al., Nutrient intake and cataract extraction in women: a prospective study. *Br. Med. J.*, 305, 335, 1992.
70. Mares-Perlman, J.A., Klein, B.E., Klein, R., and Ritter, L.L., Relation between lens opacities and vitamin and mineral supplement use. *Ophthalmology*, 101, 315, 1994.
71. Robertson, J.M., Donner, A.P., and Trevithick, J.R., Vitamin E intake and risk of cataracts in humans. *Ann. N.Y. Acad. Sci.*, 570, 372, 1989.

72. Jacques, P.F., Taylor, A., Hankinson, S.E., et al., Long-term vitamin C supplement use and prevalence of early age-related lens opacities. *Am. J. Clin. Nutr.,* 66, 911, 1997.
73. Mares-Perlman, J.A., Klein, R., Klein, B.E., et al., Association of zinc and antioxidant nutrients with age-related maculopathy. *Arch. Ophthalmol.,* 114, 991, 1996.
74. Marklund, S.L., Westman, N.G., Lundgren, E., and Roos, G., Copper- and zinc-containing superoxide dismutase, manganese-containing superoxide dismutase, catalase, and glutathione peroxidase in normal and neoplastic human cell lines and normal human tissues. *Cancer Res.,* 42, 1955, 1982.
75. Sato, M. and Bremner, I., Oxygen free radicals and metallothionein. *Free Rad. Biol. Med.,* 14, 325, 1993.
76. Karcioglu, Z.A., Zinc in the eye. *Surv. Ophthalmol.,* 27, 114, 1982.
77. Miceli, M.V., Tate, D.J., Jr., Alcock, N.W., and Newsome, D.A., Zinc deficiency and oxidative stress in the retina of pigmented rats. *Invest. Ophthalmol. Vis. Sci.,* 40, 1238, 1999.
78. Newsome, D.A., Swartz, M., Leone, N.C., Elston, R.C., and Miller, E., Oral zinc in macular degeneration. *Arch. Ophthalmol.,* 106, 192, 1988.
79. Goodwin, J.S., Hunt, W.C., Hooper, P., and Garry, P.J., Relationship between zinc intake, physical activity, and blood levels of high-density lipoprotein cholesterol in a healthy elderly population. *Metabolism,* 34, 519, 1985.
80. Hiller, R., Seigel, D., Sperduto, R.D., et al., Serum zinc and serum lipid profiles in 778 adults. *Ann. Epidemiol.,* 5, 490, 1995.
81. Schlesinger, L., Arevalo, M., Arredondo, S., Lonnerdal, B., and Stekel, A., Zinc supplementation impairs monocyte function. *Acta. Paediatr.,* 82, 734, 1993.
82. Fosmire, G.J., Zinc toxicity. *Am. J. Clin. Nutr.,* 51, 225, 1990.
83. Abdel-Mageed, A.B. and Oehme, F.W., A review of the biochemical roles, toxicity and interactions of zinc, copper and iron. I. Zinc. *Vet. Hum. Toxicol.,* 32, 34, 1990.
84. Chandra, R.K., Excessive intake of zinc impairs immune responses. *J. Am. Med. Assoc.,* 252, 1443, 1984.
85. Hartstein, J., Pace, U., Harttstein, M.E., Tanzi, R.E., and Bush, A.I., Editorial: Zinc and Macular Degeneration. *Ann. Opthalmol.,* 27, 194, 1995.
86. Sandstead, H.H., Requirements and toxicity of essential trace elements, illustrated by zinc and copper. *Am. J. Clin. Nutr.,* 61, 621S, 1995.
87. Pratt, S.G., Protect Your Patients from Vitamin Toxicity. *Rev. Opthalmol.,* 6, 104, 1999.
88. Ueda, T. and Armstrong, D., Preventive effect of natural and synthetic antioxidants on lipid peroxidation in the mammalian eye. *Ophthal. Res.,* 28, 184, 1996.
89. Ursini, F., Tubaro, F., Rong, J., and Sevanian, A., Optimization of nutrition: polyphenols and vascular protection. *Nutr. Rev.,* 57, 241, 1999.
90. Formica, J.V. and Regelson, W., Review of the biology of Quercetin and related bioflavonoids. *Food Chem. Toxicol.,* 33, 1061, 1995.
91. King, A. and Young, G., Characteristics and occurrence of phenolic phytochemicals. *J. Am. Diet. Assoc.,* 99, 213, 1999.
92. Lotito, S.B. and Fraga, C.G., (+)-Catechin prevents human plasma oxidation. *Free Rad. Biol. Med.,* 24, 435, 1998.
93. Packer, L. and Colman, C., *The Antioxidant Miracle*, John Wiley & Sons, New York, 1999.

94. Niki, E., Noguchi, N., Iwatsuki, M., and Kato, Y., Dynamics of Antioxidation by Phenolic Antioxidants: Physiochemical Issues, Packer, L., Traber, M.G., and Xin, W., Eds., Proc. Int. Symp. Natural Antioxidants: Molecular Mechanisms and Health Effects, American Oil Chemists Society, Champaign, IL, 1996.
95. Packer, L., Antioxidant Defenses in Biological Systems: An Overview, Packer, L., Traber, M.G., and Xin, W., Eds., Proc. Int. Symp. Natural Antioxidants: Molecular Mechanisms and Health Effects, American Oil Chemists Society, Champaign, IL, 1996.
96. AOCS Proc. Int. Symp. Natural Antioxidants: Molecular Mechanisms and Health Effects, American Oil Chemists Society, Champaign, IL, 1996.
97. Terao, J., Dietary Flavonoids as Plasma Antioxidants on Lipid Peroxidation: Significance of Metabolic Conversion, in Packer, L., Hiramatsu, M., and Yoshikawa, T., Eds., *Antioxidant Food Supplements in Human Health*, Academic Press, San Diego, CA, 1999, p. 255.
98. Pietta, P. and Simonetti, P., Dietary Flavonoids and Interaction with Physiologic Antioxidants, in Packer, L., Hiramatsu, M., and Yoshikawa, T., Eds., *Antioxidant Food Supplements in Human Health*, Academic Press, San Diego, CA, 1999, p. 283.
99. Majji, A.B., Hayashi, A., Kim, H.C., Grebe, R.R., and de Juan, E., Jr., Inhibition of choriocapillaris regeneration with genistein. *Invest. Ophthalmol. Vis. Sci.,* 40, 1477, 1999.
100. Packer, L., Rimbach, G., and Virgili, F., Antioxidant activity and biologic properties of a procyanidin-rich extract from pine (Pinus maritima) bark, pycnogenol. *Free Rad. Biol. Med.,* 27, 704, 1999.
101. Ranchon, I., Gorrand, J.M., Cluzel, J., Droy-Lefaix, M.T., and Doly, M., Functional protection of photoreceptors from light-induced damage by dimethylthiourea and Ginkgo biloba extract. *Invest. Ophthalmol. Vis. Sci.,* 40, 1191, 1999.

7 Nutrients and Vegetables in Skin Protection

Jeongmin Lee and Ronald R. Watson

CONTENTS

7.1 INTRODUCTION

With the continuing diminution of the protective ozone layer, concern about the harmful effects of overexposure to sunlight has been growing. Epidemiological and experimental studies here demonstrated that the increasing incidence of skin diseases in the last two decades is caused by an increase of exposure to solar UVR.[1] The biologically reactive solar UVR that attacks the skin is UVB (290–320 nm) and UVA (320–400 nm) irradiation. UVB normally penetrates the epiderma. Although UVA is less damaging at a given dose of irradiation, it penetrates much more deeply into the skin.[2]

UV irradiation causes a variety of biological effects on the skin, including erythema (skin redness) due to inflammation, pigmentation, and immunomodulation.[3] Chronic exposure to UVR also leads to acceleration of the skin aging process and increased risk of skin cancer development over time. UV-induced reactive oxygen species (ROS) are believed to have important roles in skin aging and in development of skin diseases. Free radical have also been shown to be involved in UV-induced and ionizing radiation damage to epidermal cells and in the suppression of the immune system by UVR.[4] The epidermis is the first line of defense against free radicals and contains a variety of antioxidants. Recent studies have demonstrated that the level of skin antioxidants was gradually depleted after UV irradiation in a time-dependent manner.[5] Therefore, it is possible to reduce or prevent skin damage

0-8493-0038-X/97/$0.00+$.50

associated with free radicals by using antioxidants. Fruits and vegetables contain a variety of antioxidants and nutrients such as vitamins, that can activate the immune system and restore the immunosuppression status after UVR exposure.[6]

In this review, the defined mechanisms of UVR on skin damage and the preventive effects of antioxidants and nutrients will be discussed.

7.2 MECHANISMS OF UVR-INDUCED SKIN DAMAGE

The mechanisms of UVR-induced skin damage can be broadly categorized into two aspects: (1) DNA damage, and (2) suppressed immune response including inflammation, immune cell dysfunction, and cytokine dysregulation.[7-9] First, UVB is most efficient in producing oxidative DNA damage in a large group of DNA components, notably the DNA bases like cyclobutane and pyrimidine dimers.[10] Those damaged bases are excised by a DNA repair enzyme, formamido-pyrimidine DNA glycosylase (FPG). UVR can induce oxidative DNA base damage in the form of 7,8-dihydro-8-oxoguanine (8-OHdG) or lesions sensitive to the FPG enzyme.[11] Kvam and Tyrrell reported by testing human skin fibroblasts that production of singlet oxygen by UVA is a major factor in the induction of 8-OhdG at the most effective wavelength of 365 nm.[8] In addition, singlet oxygen seems to be involved in production of other types of oxidative DNA damage induced by sunlight: presumably, nonmutagenic DNA strand breaks and protein-DNA cross-links.[11]

The immunosuppressive effects of UVR exposure have been well documented in both human and animal models. Reported effects of UV have included inhibition of antigen presentation in lymphocytes, reduction in CD4+/CD8+ ratios,[12] as well as suppression of delayed-type hypersensitivity (DTH) response.[13] Interestingly, it is suggested that epidermal Langerhans cells (LC) are targets of UVB irradiation. LC are the principal antigen-presenting cells (APC) in normal epidermis.[9] The capacity of LC to act as APC for T-cell responses has been shown for a wide spectrum of antigens, including nominal proteins, virus-derived proteins, tumor antigens, and reactive haptens.

The idea that epidermal LC serve as targets of UVB radiation was first suggested in experiments with C57BL/6 mice, in which exposure of abdominal skin to relatively low doses of UVB (200 $J/m^2/d$ on four consecutive days) resulted in reduction in the density of LC within epidermis of irradiated skin.[14] In other studies, *in vitro* UVB irradiation (single doses of 25–600 J/m^2) was shown to abrogate the ability of human or mouse epidermal cells containing LC to stimulate proliferation of antigen-specific T cells.[15] Furthermore, studies by Streilein et al.[16] suggest that susceptibility to UV-induced immune suppression of T-cell-mediated contact hypersensitivity responses may be a risk factor for the development of skin cancer in humans. The systemic effects of UVR are mediated in part through the production of *cis*-urocanic acid (cis-UCA) and immunosuppressive cytokines such as tumor necrosis factor (TNF-α) and interleukin-10 (IL-10), that suppress DTH responses to protein antigens by downregulating antigen-presenting cell functions and triggering the formation of antigen-specific suppressor T cells.[17,18]

A number of studies have demonstrated that UVB irradiation of cells of monocyte/macrophage lineage, in doses similar to those used to abrogate the presentation of antigen, also impairs their capacity to produce soluble IL-1 (sIL-1).[9] In contrast to sIL-1, UV-induced downregulation of membrane IL-1 that is already present on the cell surface does not occur, suggesting that UVB radiation impairs the synthesis and/or movement of this molecule to the cell surface but does not reduce its expression once it is there.[19]

UVR induces the generation of reactive oxygen species (ROS), which are responsible for the photooxidative damage to nucleic acids, lipids, and proteins and stimulate the release of NF-kB from IkB that is an inhibitory factor.[20, 21] NF-kB is an inducible transcription factor involved in the transcription of genes whose protein production participate in either inflammatory or immune responses. AP-1 is a dimer composed of proteins from the Fos and Jun families. The expression and the activity of c-fos and c-jun are inducible by UVR through a ras pathway.[22] By the nature of the primary response to UVR in the skin, NF-kB and AP-1, two major transcription factors with recognition sites in the promoter region of genes involved in inflammation, immune response, and cellular proliferation, have been suspected to play a key role in the development of skin disease. Recent studies suggest that levels of cellular NF-kB and AP-1 increased with UVB irradiation.[21] In fact, it is well established that keratinocytes respond to UVR by synthesizing and secreting pro-inflammatory cytokines like IL-1α, IL-6, IL-8, or TNF-α whose expression is also induced upon NF-kB activation.[23]

7.3 ROLE OF ANTIOXIDANTS IN SKIN PROTECTION

7.3.1 Vitamin E and Vitamin C

In a study assessing antioxidant depletion in a human skin model, both ubiquinol and ubiquinone decreased to virtually nondetectable concentrations with higher UV-light exposures (4.2 mJ/cm^2, 3 MED).[5] Vitamin E (*d*-α-tocopherol) was the next most susceptible antioxidant to depletion by UV light. This appears to be a response to increased oxidative stress due to free-radical generation initiated by UV irradiation. Although higher levels of UV irradiation (4.2 J/cm^2) were necessary to demonstrate a significant depletion, a linear relatioship between the UV-irradiation dose and vitamin E depletion was found, in which 1.7 pmol vitamin E per square centimeter skin equivalent surface were destroyed per each Joule per square centimeter of solar-simulated UV irradiation. The ubiquinol loss prior to vitamin E suggests that it may spare vitamin E by regenerating it from its oxidized form. Additionally, vitamin E may have absorbed some of the energy from the UV light directly and was thereby oxidized.[24]

Vitamin E provided a protective effect against erythema and mechanoelectrical changes when applied to the skin of rabbits and humans prior to irradiation.[25] However application of vitamin E after UVR treatment gave no protection from phototoxic effects. The observed protective effect of vitamin E was maximal at intermediate vitamin E concentrations and high radiation doses. In another study in rabbits, application of topical vitamin E and BHT before and within two minutes after irradiation greatly inhibited the erythemal response of skin to UVR.[26] Treatment of the skin with antioxidants 5 h after irradiation had almost no effect on the minimal erythemal dose (reddening observed in 20 to 24 h after irradiation).

When *d*-α-tocopherol acetate, a derivative of vitamin E, is administered in the diet, it can decrease tumor incidence in UV-irradiated mice and provide some protection against photocarcinogenesis when supplied in a polyunsaturated fatty acid-rich diet.[27] However, when the synthetic form, *d,l*-α-tocopherol acetate, is applied to the skin, it is unable to prevent UV-induced tumor formation although the reason still remains controversial. Berton et al.[27] demonstrated that when the synthetic form of *d,l*-α-tocopherol acetate in a neutral cream is applied 15 min before UV irradiation, there was a significant reduction in thymine dimer formation in mouse epidermis. However, the degree of effectiveness is less than the natural form of *d*-α-tocopherol acetate.

A combination of topical vitamin C and E significantly protected the skin from UVB damage (sunburn cell formation).[28] Vitamin C was more effective than vitamin E in protecting the skin from UVA-mediated skin damage. This may be explained by the fact that vitamin C is quite resistant to oxidative damage by UVR and high levels of vitamin C are present in the epidermis plasma. Indeed, more than 16.8 J/cm^2 were required to demonstrate a significant decrease in vitamin C.

In another study of the effect of vitamin E on UV-induced skin damage in hairless mice, lipid peroxidation and suppression of incorporation of thymidine into DNA were used to assess the degree of damage.[29] Lipid peroxidation decreased in mice treated with topical vitamin E 1 to 24 h before irradiation, but not in mice fed high dietary vitamin E levels. In both groups of mice, thymidine incorporation into DNA was restored to the levels of nonirradiated mice. The researchers observed that both dietary and topical vitamin E protect the skin against some of the early changes induced by UVR.

Skin lipid peroxidation was also decreased in carotene-supplemented hairless mice before and after UV irradiation.[30] At 24 h after irradiation, indices of lipid peroxidation were lower in mice orally supplemented with palm fruit carotene (mixed natural carotenoids) than in β-carotene-supplemented mice. In a small double-blind study of 12 adult subjects, oral vitamin E supplementation (400 I.U. per day for 6 months) did not significantly protect the skin against UV-induced damage.[31]

7.3.2 β-Carotene

Animal studies have shown that β-carotene reduces UV-induced tumor development, and β-carotene also inhibited UV-induced peroxidation of linolenic acid micelles *in vitro*.[32] *In vitro* studies have shown that canthaxanthin and β-carotene protect peripheral blood monocytes from functional damage due to UV exposure.[33] In the study of the interaction between β-carotene, UV, and immune function in humans, β-carotene supplementation protected young men from photosuppression of DTH response caused by UV exposure.[13] The efficacy of β-carotene supplementation (30 mg/day for 10 days) and comparison with a topical UV sunscreen to protect against harmful effects of UVR was investigated in a double-blind study of 20 female volunteers.[34] Development of redness in selected skin areas exposed to natural sunlight was lower in the β-carotene-supplemented group than in the placebo group.

In the β-carotene-supplemented group, body areas protected with sunscreen showed lower median degrees of skin redness than in the group protected with sunscreen only. The researcher concluded that supplementation with β-carotene before and during natural sunlight exposure, combined with topical sunscreens, is more effective than sunscreen alone. β-carotene supplementation (30 mg/day for 28 days) was also protective against the UV-induced suppression of immune response in a study of adult male subjects.

However, the photoprotective effect of β-carotene is under great controversy. Recently, Garmyn et al. reported that oral β-carotene supplementation (a single 120 mg dose or 90 mg daily for 23 days) is unlikely to modify the severity of sunburn in normal individuals to a clinically meaningful degree.[35] In a recent clinical trial with 24 young adults in our laboratory, long-term supplementation of β-carotene for 24 weeks (30 mg/day for the first 8 weeks; the concentration was then increased in 30-mg increments at 8-week intervals to a final dose of 90 mg/day) showed only a modest effect against UV irradiation.[36] Although the plasma level of β-carotene reached a plateau at 8 weeks, significance in skin protection from UVR occurred at 18 weeks, implicating that β-carotene is required long-term to be uptaken into the epidermal cells and exert photoprotective effects. These data indicated that the duration of supplementation rather than the dose of β-carotene is more important, and the slight change of skin pigmentation due to β-carotene supplementation might exert the additional protective effect against UV irradiation.

7.3.3 *N*-Acetylcysteine

N-acetylcysteine (NAC), a precursor of glutathione (GSH), can protect keratinocytes against UVB by enhancing the removal of UV-induced DNA damage and modulating the apoptotic process.[37] Mice that were topically treated with NAC showed a significant increase in their epidermal GSH level. It has been believed that GSH synthesized from NAC may act as a skin-protective antioxidant by UV irradiation. However, a recent study using the GSH inhibitor suggested that GSH synthesis is not involved in the protection by NAC against UVB immunosuppression, indicating that the antioxidant potential of NAC itself is sufficient for the protective effect, independent of the epidermal GSH level.[38] In another study, NAC did not influence the induction of pyrimidine dimers in DNA or the formation of *cis*-UCA, the two parameters thought to initiate the cascade that ultimately induces UVB immunosuppression, suggesting that NAC probably interferes at a later stage in the induction without affecting the initiating factors.[39] NAC is found to be very effective in scavenging ROS and inhibiting NF-kB activation and c-fos and c-jun expression in UVB-exposed normal keratinocytes *in vitro*.[21] By doing so, NAC can prevent synthesis of the cytokines that ultimately cause the immunosuppression and inflammation. In addition, in human epidermal cell cultures NAC can inhibit the induction of prostaglandin E_2 by UVR, which also plays a role in the suppression of the immune system by UV. However, the concentration needed to achieve the inhibition is in the millimolar range and that could be a limitation to its therapeutic use.

7.3.4 α-Lipoic Acid and Silymarin

The antioxidants, α-lipoic acid and silymarin, have been shown to elevate intracellular GSH levels *in vitro* by increasing *de novo* synthesis[40] and after an oxidative challenge by a mechanism currently unidentified.[41] In hairless mice, a relatively low concentration of α-lipoic acid (250 μM) can efficiently modulate UV-mediated NF-kB activation.[42] This could contribute the mechanism whereby the dihydrolipoic acid/α-lipoic acid couple prevents oxidant-induced skin inflammation.

Silymarin displayed a photoprotective effect when topically applied on mice skin and in humans it protected against UV-induced erythema. Katiyar et al. demonstrated an inhibition of cyclooxygenase (Cox) activity by silymarin.[43] This action can be accounted for by the inhibition of NF-kB activation due to the presence of two kB sites in the promoter region of the human Cox-2 gene encoding the inducible Cox. Consequently, the inhibition of NF-kB activation by silymarin causes both the blockage of prostaglandin synthesis via the Cox-2 pathway and the suppression of the pro-inflammatory cytokines and adhesion molecule gene expression, resulting in reduction of skin redness (erythema).

7.3.5 Flavonoids

Fruit and vegetable components have modulating effects on the immune system.[6,44] Antioxidants and vitamins are critical components of fruits and vegetables that can activate the immune system and restore the immunosuppressive status due to UVR exposure.

Fruits and vegetables contain many other types of bioactive compounds, such as the flavonoids. Flavonoids belong to a group of polyphenolic antioxidants that display remarkable *in vitro* and *in vivo* antioxidant activity that is a basis for their various biological properties. Flavonoids, consisting of flavonols, flavones, flavonones, catechins, and anthocyanidins, have been shown to affect the immune system, both by suppressing or by enhancing its activity.[45] Flavonoids protect against UV-induced suppression of the contact hypersensitivity.[46] This is found after topical administration of polyphenol extracts of garlic and green tea and after oral administration of quercetin, a flavonoid with a high number of hydroxyl groups. One explanation might be that flavonoids have an anti-inflammatory activity via the arachidonic acid pathway. In addition, it has been reported that flavonoids may act as a sunscreen and prevent DNA damage of dermal cells or cells of the immune system, or prevent the subsequent initiation of conversion of *trans*- to *cis*-UCA, and/or prevent production of IL-1β and TNF-α by keratinocytes, leading to the altered migration pattern and functional activity of LC cells after UV irradiation.[46, 47] However, the photoprotective mechanisms of flavonoids are still controversial.

7.4 CONCLUSIONS

In summary, nutrients and antioxidants, including the components from fruits and vegetables, provide a protective effect against UV-induced immunosuppression and

DNA damage in the epidermal cells. Usually, regardless of the methods applied (topical or oral treatment), duration of treatment turned out to be more critical than doses of treatment. Many nutrients and antioxidants may share a common feature in protection of UV-induced skin damage although the exact mechanisms remain unclear.

ACKNOWLEDGMENT

Research stimulating this review was supported by grants from Cognis and Wallace Genetics Foundation, Inc.

REFERENCES

1. Beissert, S. and Granstein, R.D., UV-induced cutaneous photobiology, *Rev. Biochem. Mol. Biol.*, 31, 381, 1996.
2. van Beijersbergen, H., de Vries, V., van Broeke, D., and Junginger, H., RRR-Tocopherols and their acetates as a possible scavenger of free radicals produced in the skin upon UVA-exposure — an *in vivo* screening method, *Fat Sci. Technol.*, 94, 24, 1992.
3. Taylor, C.R., Stern, R.S., Leyden, J.J., and Hilchrest, B.A., Photoaging/ photodamage and photoprotection, *J. Am. Acad. Dermatol.*, 22, 1, 1990.
4. Fuchs, J., Huflejt, M., Rothfuss, L., Wilson, D., Carcamo, G., and Packer, L., Impairment of enzymatic and nonenzymatic antioxidants in skin by UVB irradiation, *J. Invest. Dermatol.*, 93, 769, 1989.
5. Podda, M., Traber, M.G., Weber, C., Yan, L.J., and Packer, L., UV-irradiation depletes antioxidants and causes oxidative damage in a model of human skin, *Free Rad. Biol. Med.*, 24, 55, 1998.
6. Chandra, R.K., Effect of vitamin and trace element supplementation on the immune responses and infection in elderly subjects, *Lancet*, 340, 1124, 1992.
7. Mcvean, M. and Liebler, D.C., Prevention of DNA photodamage by vitamin E compounds and sunscreens: roles of UV absorbance and cellular uptake, *Mol. Carcinogenesis*, 24, 169, 1999.
8. Kvam, E. and Tyrrell, R.M., Induction of oxidative DNA base damage in human skin cells by UV and near visible radiation, *Carcinogenesis*, 18, 2379, 1997.
9. Cruz, P.D., UVB-induced immunosuppression: biologic, cellular, and molecular effects, *Adv. Dermatol.*, 9, 79, 1994.
10. Cadet, J., Anselmino, C., Douki, T., and Voituriez, L., Photochemistry of nucleic acids in cells, *J. Photochem. Photobiol. B. Biol.*, 15, 277, 1992.
11. Kielbassa, C., Roza, L., and Epe, B., Wavelength dependence of oxidative DNA damage induced by UV and visible light, *Carcinogenesis*, 18, 811, 1997.
12. Hersey, P., Hasic, E., Edwards, A., Bradley, M., Haran, G., and McCarthy, W.H., Immunological effects of solarium exposure, *Lancet*, 1, 545, 1983.
13. Herraiz, L.A., Hsieh, W.C., Parker, R.S., Swanson, J.E., Bendich, A., and Roe, D.A., Effect of UV exposure and β-carotene supplementation on delayed-type hypersensitivity response in healthy older men, *J. Am. Coll. Nutr.*, 17, 617, 1998.

14. Cruz, P.D. and Bergstresser, P.R., Antigen processing and presentation by epidermal Langerhans cells. Induction of immunity or unresponsiveness, *Dermatol. Clin.*, 8, 633, 1990.
15. Dittmar, H.C., Weiss, J.M., Termeer, C.C., Denfeld, R.W., Wanner, M.B., Baadsgaard, O., and Simon, J.C., *In vivo* UVA and UVB irradiation differentially perturbs the antigen-presenting function of human epidermal Langerhans cells, *J. Invest. Dermatol.*, 112, 322, 1999.
16. Yoshikawa, K., Rae, V., Bruins-Slot, W., Taylor, J.R., and Streilein, J.W., Vitamin C abrogates the deleterious effects of UVB radiation on cutaneous immunity by a mechanism that does not depend on TNF-alpha, *J. Invest. Dermatol.*, 109, 20, 1997.
17. Ullrich, S.E., Mechanisms involved in the systemic suppression of antigen-presenting cell function by UV irradiation, *J. Immunol.*, 152, 3410, 1994.
18. Noonan, F.P. and Fabo, E.C., Immunosuppression by UVB radiation: initiation by urocanic acid, *Immunol. Today*, 13, 250, 1992.
19. Elmets, C.A., Photocarcinogenesis: mechanisms, models and human health implications, *Photochem. Photobiol.*, 63, 356, 1996.
20. Wei, H., Zhang, X., Zhao, J.F., Wang, Z.Y., Bickers, D., and Lebwohl, M., Scavenging of hydrogen peroxide and inhibition of UV light-induced oxidative DNA damage by aqueous extracts from green and black teas, *Free Rad. Biol. Med.*, 26, 1427, 1999.
21. Saliou, C., Kitazawa, M., McLaughlin, L., Yang, J.P., Lodge, J.K., Okamoto, T., and Packer, L., Antioxidants modulate acute solar UV radiation-induced NF-kB activation in a human ketatinocyte cell line, *Free Rad. Biol. Med.*, 26, 174, 1999.
22. Sun, Y. and Oberley, L.W., Redox regulation of transcriptional activators, *Free Rad. Biol. Med.*, 21, 335, 1996.
23. Ullrich, S.E., The role of epidermal cytokines in the generation of cutaneous immune reactions and UV radiation-induced immune suppression, *Photochem. Photobiol.*, 62, 389, 1995.
24. Kagan, V.E., Witt, E., Goldman, R., Scita, G., and Packer, L., UV light-induced generation of vitamin E radicals and their recycling. A possible photosensitizing effect of vitamin E in skin, *Free Rad. Res. Commun.*, 16, 51, 1992.
25. Potapenko, A., Abijev, G., Pistsov, M., Roshchupkin, D., and Evstigneeva, R., PUVA-induced erythema and changes in mechanoelectrical properties of skin: inhibition by tocopherols, *Arch. Dermatol. Res.*, 276, 12, 1984.
26. Roshchupkin, D., Pistsov, M., and Potapenko, A., Inhibition of UV light-induced erythema by antioxidants, *Arch. Dermatol. Res.*, 266, 91, 1979.
27. Berton, T.R., Conti, C.J., Mitchell, D.L., and Fischer, S.M., The effect of vitamin E acetate on UV-induced mouse skin carcinogenesis, *Mol. Carcinogenesis*, 23, 175, 1998.
28. Darr, D., Dunston, S., Faust, H., and Pinnell, S., Effectiveness of antioxidants (vitamin E and C) with and without sunscreens as topical photoprotectants, *Acta Derm. Venereol.*, 76, 264, 1996.
29. Record, I.R., Dreosti, I.E., Konstantinopoulos, M., and Buckley, R.A., The influence of topical and systemic vitamin E on UV light-induced skin damage in hairless mice, *Nutr. Cancer*, 16, 219, 1991.
30. Someya, K., Totsuka, Y., Murakoshi, M., and Miyazawa, T., The effect of natural carotenoid (palm fruit carotene) intake on skin lipid peroxidation in hairless mice, *J. Nutr. Sci. Vitaminol.*, 40, 303, 1994.
31. Werninghaus, K., Neydani, M., Bhawan, J., and Gilchrest, B.A., Evalution of the photoprotective effect of oral vitamin E supplementation, *Arch. Dermatol.*, 130, 1257, 1994.

32. Bose, B. and Chatterjee, S.N., Effect of UVA irradiation on linoleic acid micelles, *Radiat. Res.*, 133, 340, 1993.
33. Schoen, D.J. and Watson, R.R., Prevention of UV irradiation-induced suppression of monocyte functions by retinoids and carotenoids in vitro, *Photochem. Photobiol.*, 5, 659, 1988.
34. Fuller, C.J., Faulkner, H., Bendich, A., Parker, R.S., and Roe, D.A., Effect of beta-carotene supplementation on photosuppression of DTH in normal young men, *Am. J. Clin. Nutr.*, 56, 684, 1992.
35. Garmyn, M., Ribaya-Mercado, J.D., Russell, R.M., Bhawan, J., and Gilchrest, B.A., Effect of beta-carotene supplementation on the human sunburn reaction, *Exp. Dermatol.*, 4, 104, 1995.
36. Lee, J., Jiang, S., Levine, N., and Watson, R.R., Carotenoid supplementation reduces erythema in human skin after simulated solar radiation exposure, *Pro. Soc. Exp. Biol. Med.*, 223, 170, 2000.
37. Ho, Y.S., Lee, H.M., Mou, T.C., Wang, Y.J., and Liu, J.K., Suppression of nitric oxide-induced apoptosis by NAC through modulation of glutathione, bcl-2, and bax protein levels, *Mol. Carcinogenesis*, 19, 101, 1997.
38. Steenvoorden, D.P.T. and Henegouwen, M.J., Glutathione synthesis is not involved in protection by NAC against UVB-induced systemic immunosuppression in mice, *Photochem. Photobiol.*, 68, 97, 1998.
39. Bush, J.A., Ho, V.C., Mitchell, D.L., and Li, G., Effect of NAC on UVB-induced apoptosis and DNA repair in human and mouse kerainocytes, *Photochem. Photobiol.*, 70, 329, 1999.
40. Han, D., Handelman, G., Marcocci, L., Sen, C.K., and Packer, L., Lipoic acid increases de novo synthesis of cellular glutathione by improving cysteine utilization, *Biofactors*, 6, 321, 1997.
41. Valenzuela, A., Aspillaga, M., Vial, S., and Guerra, R., Selectivity of silymarin on the increase of the glutathione content in different tissues of the rat, *Planta Med.*, 55, 420, 1989.
42. Fuchs, J. and Milbradt, R., Antioxidant inhibition of skin inflammation induced by reactive oxidants: evaluation of the redox couple dihydrolipoate/lipoate, *Skin Pharmacol.*, 7, 278, 1994.
43. Katiyar, S.K., Korman, N.J., Mukhtar, H., and Agarwal, R., Protective effects of silymarin against photocarcinogenesis in a mouse skin model, *J. Natl. Cancer Inst.*, 89, 556, 1997.
44. Steerenber, P.A., Garssen, J., Dortant, P., Hollman, P.C., and Lovern, H.V., Protection of UV-induced suppression of skin contact hypersensitivity: a common feature of flavonoids after oral administration, *Photochem. Photobiol.*, 67, 456, 1998.
45. Middleton, E. and Kandaswami, C., Effects of flavonoids on immune and inflammatory cell functions, *Biochem. Pharmacol.*, 43, 1167, 1992.
46. Steerenber, P.A., Garssen, J., Dortant, P., Goettsch, Y., Sontag, M., and Lovern, H.V., Quercetin prevents UV-induced local immunosuppression but does not affect UV-induced tumor growth in SKH-1 hairless mice, *Photochem. Photobiol.*, 65, 736, 1997.
47. Luger, T.A. and Schwarz, T., Evidence for an epidermal cytokine network, *J. Invest. Dermatol.*, 95, 100s, 1990.

8 Vitamins and Micronutrients in Aging and Photoaging Skin

Hubert T. Greenway and Steven G. Pratt

CONTENTS

8.1 INTRODUCTION

Photoaging skin and skin cancer constitute a major problem in the U.S. as well as many other areas throughout the world. Natural aging of the skin is associated with many intrinsic changes. The addition of significant ultraviolet exposure creates the potential for benign photoaging changes as well as increasing the potential for skin cancers of all types including basal cell carcinoma, squamous cell carcinoma, melanoma, and a variety of others such as eyelid sebaceous carcinoma. While treatments exist for all types of skin cancers as well as surgical and nonsurgical treatments for photoaging changes (sagging, wrinkles, texture, pigmentation, etc.), prevention and the reduction of the incidence of malignant and nonmalignant conditions offer profound benefit for the individual and for society.

0-8493-0038-X/97/$0.00+$.50

Evidence exists that the oral consumption, and in some cases the topical application, of specific fruits and vegetables or their components may play a role in the reduction of the incidence of both malignant and nonmalignant changes in the skin.

8.2 ULTRAVIOLET RADIATION

The ultraviolet radiation from the sun makes up only 6% of the nonionizing radiation (the remainder being infrared and visible). However, it does have the ability to penetrate the epidermis and induce photochemical reactions. Ultraviolet irradiation consists of UVA, UVB, and UVC. The ozone layer effectively absorbs UVC, leaving UVB and UVA to react with the epidermis. UVB is responsible for the redness, peeling, and burning related to sun exposure. UVB also damages cellular DNA and contributes to skin cancer. UVA penetrates deeper and contributes to both carcinogenic and nonmalignant (wrinkling, premature aging) conditions via a photosensitized reaction mediated in part by reactive oxygen species (primarily singlet oxygen). The subsequent free-radical formation damages not only the cellular skin components (proteins, fats, etc.) but also the genetic material(DNA/RNA). The nucleotide building blocks of cellular DNA absorb UV energy and are susceptible to mutagenesis, with a proportion becoming premalignant or malignant. The epidermal cells carry many UV-caused mutations, with the gene p53 having the highest prevalence (50%) of mutations of any human gene.[1] In its normal state the p53 gene protects the epidermal cell from tumor formation.

Immune suppression increases the risk of the development of skin tumors of all types including nonmelanoma skin cancer. The risk is also increased in AIDs patients. Benign photoaging changes are evident when one compares the facial cutaneous changes of sun-nonexposed and sun-exposed skin. This can be most dramaticaly envisioned by comparing the facial skin of a 60-year-old monk who never sees the sun with that of an American southwest Indian who is constantly exposed to ultraviolet irradiation.

Age-related macular degeneration (AMD) as well as cataracts are also related to UV exposure. AMD is the leading cause of blindness in people older than 65 (see Chapter 6: Fruit and Vegetable Micronutrients in Diseases of the Eye). Evidence suggests that nutrition plays a role in prevention and that two carotenoids (lutein and zeaxanthin) found in spinach may offer protection from AMD by absorbing damaging blue light as well as acting as antioxidants.[2] Nutrition may be important in skin cancer, as the Australians noted that an increased consumption of fish and vegetables, including the cruciferous vegetables (broccoli, brussels sprouts, cabbage, and cauliflower), correlated with a decreased incidence of skin cancer.[3]

8.3 VITAMIN C (ASCORBIC ACID)

Scurvy, the deficiency in Vitamin C characterized by skin hemorrhages, bleeding gums, fragile bones, and death, provides insight into our reluctance to recognize the power of nutrition. In 1753, British physician James Lind published his book *A Treatise of the Scurvy* detailing the cure and prevention via oranges and lemons.

Only in 1795, after Lind's death, did the British Navy adopt his work.[4] Vitamin C acts as an antioxidant in the skin by scavenging and quenching free radicals generated by UV radiation.[5] Dunham et al.[6] found reduced UV-induced tumors in mice given increased Vitamin C. Singlet oxygen formation has been found to be suppressed by antioxidant Vitamin C.[7] Wound healing is dependent on Vitamin C and this vitamin is essential for the production and stabilization of collagen. Older individuals may have lower Vitamin C levels[8] which may contribute to less than optimal cutaneous wound healing.[9,10] Supplemental Vitamin C for skin health should not exceed 1000 mg/day (taken in divided doses).

Topical Vitamin C has been studied both in prevention and treatment of photoaging skin. Forearms treated with 19% *L*-ascorbic acid solution showed reduction in redness as measured by the minimal erythema dose when compared to controls.[11] This protective effect may be related to the antioxidant properties of Vitamin C as it does not appear to offer absorption in either the UVA or UVB range. Topical 12% ascorbic acid solution penetrates the stratum corneum outer epidermis in 72 h,[12] with a 10% solution delivering pharmacologic levels. UV exposure was found to markedly decrease skin levels of Vitamin C in porcine skin.[13] In addition to promotion of its protective effects, multiple commercial preparations now promote restoration of skin tone, improvement in fine wrinkles, and a more youthful look as the positive cosmetic effects of topical Vitamin C.

8.4 VITAMIN E

Various studies evaluating the role of Vitamin E (alpha-tocopherol) both in the prevention of skin cancer, including melanoma, as well as evaluating plasma levels have produced conflicting results.[14,15] Thus, evidence supporting Vitamin E supplementation for skin cancer reduction needs further delineation. Interestingly, oral Vitamin E supplementation has been found to improve hyperpigmentation of the face.

Cultured human melanoma cells were evaluated for the inhibitory effect of alpha-tocopheryl ferulate (alpha-TF) on melanization.[16] Results were positive, suggesting that alpha-TF is a candidate for an efficient whitening agent via melanogenesis suppression and antioxidant function scavenging free radicals produced by UV radiation.

Topical Vitamin E is contained in many sunscreen products, either listed directly (i.e., tocopheryl acetate) or included in "other ingredients." Alberts et al. determined that while alpha-tocopheryl acetate was absorbed by the skin, it failed to undergo conversion to its unesterified free form which reduces UVB carcinogenesis.[17] However, improvement in wrinkle depth and length as well as skin roughness was noted following a 4-week application of topical 5 to 8% tocopherol cream to the face.[18]

Other antioxidants such as Vitamin C may be necessary to enhance tocopherol's photoprotective effects by preventing its degradation in the skin. Natural Vitamin E appears to be more bioavailable than synthetic forms when taken orally. Vitamin E seems to function as the major chain-breaking antioxidant in skin and other body tissues thus offering significant photoaging preventative effects. There appears to be a reduced risk of basal cell carcinoma with vitamin supplementation (including Vitamin E).[15]

Vitamin E supplementation orally for the skin should be at least 200 I.U. plus mixed tocopherols. Topical Vitamin E creams or gels in the *d*-alpha-tocopherol form (as opposed to the acetate form) should be applied every morning. The topical use of oil from capsules of Vitamin E may cause skin irritation in some patients.

8.5 VITAMIN A: RETINOL

Retinoids, including both natural and synthetic Vitamin A derivatives, provide a number of effects on the skin including regulation of both differentiation and growth in epithelial cells.[5] While the lower dosage of 10 mg/day of oral isotretinoin vs. placebo by Tangrea et al.[19] over 3 years failed to demonstrate any difference in reduction of new basal cell carcinoma skin cancers, Kraemer et al.[20] demonstrated that 2 mg/kg/day did provide reduction in the incidence of new nonmelanoma (basal cell and squamous cell) skin cancers. At our institution, patients with a history of multiple nonmelanoma skin cancers are routinely considered for prophylactic preventive oral isotretinoin therapy. Lippman et al.[21] found both advanced squamous cell carcinomas (71%) and basal cell carcinomas (51%) responded partially or completely to oral retinoids. Prolonged retinol supplementation in patients with actinic solar keratosis (precancerous lesions) was shown to increase plasma concentrations of multiple micronutrients and skin concentrations of retinol and retinyl palmitate.[22] Oral Vitamin A supplementation for the skin should not exceed 9000 I.U. daily.

Topical retinoids, namely trans-retinoic acid or tretinoin, have been shown by Kligman et al.,[24] Voorhees et al.,[25] and others [23,24] to decrease roughness, improve fine wrinkles, and lighten dark spots (lentigines) when applied to photodamaged skin. Side effects include dryness and irritation in some patients. Various other retinoids such as topical retinol, while weaker than retinoic acic, provide potent retinoid activity with low irritancy.[25]

In our practice, topical retinoid usage is a critical component of our photoaging topical regimen along with moisturizating regimens to combat dryness. Recently tazarotene, a new topical acetylenic retinoid, was shown to significantly reduce the mean minimal erythema dose (MED) for psoriatic skin exposed to UVB.[26]

8.6 CAROTENOIDS

Dietary beta-carotene, alpha-carotene, and cryptoxanthin are converted into Vitamin A. Beta-carotene was thought to reduce UV erythema but this study was not reproducible. Lutein and zeaxanthin, while related to beta-carotene, do not interconvert in the skin. In the eye, human macular pigment is composed of lutein and zeaxanthin which function as antioxidants as well as filtering and absorbing blue light.[27,28] It is possible that lutein and zeaxanthin could have a similar role on the skin. Sun exposure of as little as 1 h can cause a decrease in serum carotinoids.[29] Lee et al. showed that skin erythema after simulated solar radiation could be reduced with oral natural carotenoid supplementation.[30] This is a most important finding as it opens the door for research on natural materials to protect the skin from UV irradiation.

We evaluated sun-damaged skin in patients with nonmelanoma skin cancer and found a sevenfold higher level of carotinoids, but not retinol, in the skin of the nose of one patient (total of six patients studied) with a similar distribution pattern in skin as in plasma but with much lower values than expected in all six cases.[31]

8.7 VITAMIN B

Biotin, niacin, and riboflavin are essential in normal skin functioning. Panthenol (Vitamin B_5) functions as a humectant, attracting moisture to the hair and skin.

8.8 VITAMIN D

Calcipotriene cream for psoriasis contains the same compound as the Vitamin D found in oral vitamin supplements. Vitamin D supplementation does not appear to be necessary in the majority of healthy individuals using sunscreens on a regular basis.[32] Skin covered with a topical sunscreen with an SPF of 8 or greater fails to produce Vitamin D. Intentional sun exposure is not the optimal way to increase Vitamin D levels in the normal healthy individual.

8.9 SELENIUM

This dietary trace element may play a role in decreasing the risk of nonmelanoma skin cancer.[33] As it is often obtained through seafoods along with omega-3 fats and Vitamins A and D,[34] this positive benefit may only partially be related to the selenium. Selenium supplementation should be in the range of 100 to 200 μg daily.

8.10 COENZYME Q10

Coenzyme Q10 (ubiquinone) functions in part as an antioxidant and has been promoted as a topical treatment to reduce the depth of facial wrinkles.[35] Poda and Packer suggest that coenzyeme Q10 is the first antioxidant to be reduced when there is oxidative stress to the skin.[36]

8.11 VITAMIN K

Historically, Vitamin K has been given orally preoperatively to patients undergoing cosmetic procedures, such as facelifts, to minimize bruising. One recent report touted the use of a topical Vitamin K (phytonadione 1%) and Vitamin A (retinol 0.15%) preparation to provide significant improvement (93% of patients) for the appearance of periorbital hyperpigmentation (dark circles under eyes).[37]

8.12 GREEN TEA

Polyphenolic epicatechin and epicatechin derivatives in green tea extracts reportedly inhibit UV irradiation-induced skin cancer in mice. This antioxidant protective property was demonstrated to be effective with either oral administration or topical application.[38] Interestingly, the Canadian Cancer Society is accepting requests for funding research for alternative cancer therapies, including green tea.

8.13 FATTY ACIDS

Essential fatty acid deficiency can manifest with erythema, dryness, and scaling of the skin. Skin changes lag behind plasma changes by several months. Fat may function as an immune suppressant, with foods high in polyunsaturated fatty acids increasing the risk of melanoma and even premalignant solar keratosis.[15] Omega-3 fatty acids, found in fish (albacore tuna, sardines, salmon, cod, and mackerel) may help block tumor growth.[39]

8.14 SUMMARY

Micronutrients, antioxidants, and vitamins assist in developing and maintaining healthy skin. They are important in reducing aging changes and providing a more youthful appearance. Protecting against free radicals which damage skin cells, antioxidants, vitamins, phytonutrients, essential fatty acids, and proper internal and external hydration help maintain a youthful skin. Future research will certainly explore the use of these substances to naturally protect the skin from solar radiation, both in terms of skin cancer prevention and in protecting and treating the benign photoaging effects so many of us seek to avoid or correct.

REFERENCES

1. Brash, D.E., Rudolph, J.A., Simon, J.A., et al., A role for sunlight in skin cancer: UV-induced p53 mutations in squamous cell carcinoma, *Proc. Natl. Acad. Sci. USA,* 88, 10124, 1991.
2. Pratt, S.G., AMD and nutrition, *Rev. Ophthamol.,* 59, 63, 1998.
3. Steinmetz, K.A. and Potter, J.D., Vegetables, fruit, and cancer prevention: a review, *J. Am. Diet. Assoc.,* 96, 1027, 1996.
4. Packer, L. and Coleman, C., *The Antioxidant Miracle,* John Wiley & Sons, New York, 1999, p. 80.
5. Keller, K.L. and Fenske, N.A., Uses of vitamins A, C, and E and related compounds in dermatology, a review, *J. Am. Acad. Dermatol.,* 39, 611, 1998.
6. Dunham, W.B., Zuckerkandl, E., Reynolds, R., et al., Effects of intake of L-ascorbic acid on the incidence of dermal neoplasms induced in mice by ultraviolet light, *Proc. Natl. Acad. Sci. USA,* 79, 7532, 1982.
7. Chou, P.T. and Khan, A.U., L-Ascorbic acid quenching of singlet delta molecular oxygen in aqueous media: generalized antioxidant property of Vitamin C, *J. Phys. Chem.,* 115, 932, 1983.

8. Finglas, P.M., Bailey, A., Walker, A., et al., Vitamin C intake and plasma ascorbic acid concentration in adolescents, *Br. J. Nutr.*, 69, 563, 1993.
9. Fenske, N.A. and Lober, C.W., Structural and functional changes of normal aging skin, *J. Am. Acad. Dermatol.*, 15, 571, 1986.
10. Leibovitz, B.E. and Siegel, B.V., Aspects of free radical reactions in biological systems: aging, *J. Gerontol.*, 35, 45, 1980.
11. Murray, J., Darr, D., Reich, J., et al., Topical vitamin C treatment reduces ultraviolet B radiation-induced erythema in human skin (abstr.), *J. Invest. Derm.*, 96, 586, 1991.
12. Pinnell, S.R. and Murad, S., Vitamin C and collagen metabolism, in *Cutaneous Aging*, Kligman, A.M. and Takase, Y., Eds., University of Tokyo Press, 1988, p. 275.
13. Darr, D., Combs, S., Dunston, S., et al., Topical vitamin C protects porcine skin from ultraviolet radiation-induced damage, *Br. J. Dermatol.*, 127, 247, 1992.
14. Knekt, P., Vitamin E and cancer: epidemiology, *Ann. NY Acad. Sci.*, 669, 269, 1992.
15. Wei, Q., Matanoski, G.M., Farmer, E.R., Strickland, P., et al., Vitamin supplementation and reduced risk of basal cell carcinoma, *J. Clin. Epidemiol.*, 47, 829, 1994.
16. Funasaka, Y., Chakraborty, A.K., Komoto, M., et al., The depigmenting effect of alpha-tocopheryl ferulate on human melanoma cells, *Br. J. Dermatol.*, 141, 20, 1999.
17. Alberts, S.A., Gouldman, R., Xu, M.J., et al., Disposition and metabolism of topically administered alpha-tocopherol acetate: a common ingredient of commercially available sunscreens and cosmetics, *Nutr. Cancer*, 26, 193, 1996.
18. Mayer, P., The effects of vitamin E on the skin, *Cosmet. Toiletries*, 108, 99, 1993.
19. Tangrea, J.A., Edwards, B.K., Taylor, P.R., et al., Long-term therapy with low dose isotretinoin for prevention of basal cell carcinoma: a multicenter trial, *J. Natl. Cancer Inst.*, 84, 328, 1992.
20. Kraemer, K.H., DiGiovanni, J.J., Moshell, A.N., et al., Prevention of skin cancer in xeroderma pigmentosum with the use of oral isotretinoin, *New Engl. J. Med.*, 318, 1633, 1988.
21. Lippman, S.M., Shimm, D.S., and Meyskens, F.L., Nonsurgical treatments for skin cancer: retinoids and alpha-interferon, *J. Dermatol. Surg. Oncol.*, 14, 862, 1988.
22. Peng, Y.M., Peng, Y.S., Lin, Y., et al., Micronutrient concentrations in paired skin and plasma of patients with actinic keratoses: effect of prolonged retinol supplementation, *Cancer Epidemiol.*, 2, 145, 1993.
23. Kligman, L.H., Do, C.H., and Kligman, A.M., Topical retinoic acid enhances the repair of ultraviolet-damaged dermal connective tissue, *Connect. Tissue Res.*, 12, 139, 1984.
24. Weiss, J.S., Ellis, C.N., and Voorhees, J.J., Topical tretinoin improves photoaged skin, *J. Am. Med. Assoc.*, 259, 727, 1988.
25. Duell, E.A., Kang, S., and Voorhees, J.J., Unoccluded retinol penetrates human skin in vivo more effectively than unoccluded retinyl palmitate or retinoic acid, *J. Invest. Dermatol.*, 109, 301, 1997.
26. Hecker, D., Worsley, J., Yueh, G., et al., Interactions between tazarotene and ultraviolet light, *J. Am. Acad. Dermatol.*, 41, 927, 1999.
27. Snodderley, D.M., Evidence for protections against age-related macular degeneration by carotenoids and antioxidant vitamins, *Am. J. Clin. Nutr.*, 62, 1448S, 1995.
28. Nussbaum, J.J., Pruet, R.C., and Delori, F.C., Historic perspectives. Macular yellow pigment: the first 200 years, *Retina*, 1, 296, 1981.
29. White, W.S., Kim, C., Kalkwalf, H.J., et al., Ultraviolet light-induced reductions in plasma carotinoid levels, *Am. J. Clin. Nutr.*, 47, 879, 1988.

30. Lee, J., Jiang, S., Levine, N., and Watson, R.R., Carotinoid supplementation reduces erythema in human skin after stimulated solar radiation exposure, *PSEBM,* 1, 223, 2000.
31. Greenway, H.T., Pratt, S., and Craft, N., Skin tissue levels of carotinoids, vitamin A, and antioxidants in photodamaged skin, *J. Dermatol. Surg. Oncol.*
32. Naylor, N.F., What you should know about vitamin D and melanoma, *Skin Aging,* 7(6), 48, 1999.
33. Kune, G.A., Bannerman, S., Field, B., et al., Diet, alcohol, smoking, serum beta-carotene, and vitamin A in male nonmelanocytic skin cancer patients and controls, *Nutr. Cancer,* 18(3), 237, 1992.
34. Sahl, W.J., Diet and non-melanoma skin cancer, *J. Geriatr. Dermatol.,* 3(2), 49, 1995.
35. Perricone, N., What we know so far about coenzyme Q10, *Skin Aging,* 7(6), 21, 1999.
36. Poda, M. and Packer, L., Ubiquinol, a marker of oxidative stress in the skin, Proc. 9th Int. Symp. Biomed. Clin. Aspects CoQ10, Ancona, Italy, 1996.
37. Elson, M.I. and Nach, S., Treatment of periorbital hyperpigmentation with topical vitamin K/vitamin A, *Cosmetic Dermatol.,* 12(12), 32, 1999.
38. Katiyar, S.K., Elmets, C.A., Agarwal, R., et al., Protection against ultraviolet B radiation-induced local and systemic suppression of contact hypersensitivity and edema responses in C3H/HeN mice by green tea polyphenols, *Photochem. Photobiol.,* 62, 855, 1995.
39. Black, H., Herd, J.A., Goldberg, L.H., et al., Effect of a low fat diet on the incidence of actinic keratosis, *New Engl. J. Med.,* 330(18), 1272, 1994.
40. Fisher, M.A. and Black, H.S., Modification of membrane composition, eicosanoid metabolism and immunoresponsiveness by dietary omega-3 and omega-6 fatty acid sources, modulators of ultraviolet carcinogenesis, *Photochem. Photobiol.,* 54(3), 381, 1991.

9 Soy Foods and Health Promotion

James W. Anderson, Belinda M. Smith, Kimberly A. Moore, and Tammy J. Hanna

CONTENTS

9.1 INTRODUCTION

The health benefits of soybeans have been recognized for millennia. The pre-Christian era Chinese prized this unique legume as a nutrition powerhouse. In addition, they recognized the important health benefits of the soybean.[1] Introduced into the

0-8493-0038-X/97/$0.00+$.50

U.S. in the early nineteenth century, soybeans languished in obscurity until Dr. John Harvey Kellogg introduced soy milk and soy meat substitutes.[1] Long considered to be a second class citizen in terms of protein value, soy protein has recently been upgraded to a first class protein with an amino acid score similar to the gold standard: egg albumin.[2] Soybeans are rich in polyunsaturated fatty acids, specifically the essential fatty acid linoleic acid, low in saturated fatty acids, and moderate in monounsaturated fatty acids; they also provide n-3 fatty acids.[3] Nearly a century ago animal studies indicated that soy protein, compared to animal protein, decreased development of atherosclerosis in animals fed atherogenic diets.[4] The cholesterol-lowering effects of soy proteins were first documented in animals in 1940[5] and in humans by Sirtori and colleagues in 1977.[6]

During the past decade soy foods have vaulted to the top of the list of health-promoting foods. The meta-analysis of soy protein effects on serum lipids, reported in the *New England Journal of Medicine* in 1995, appears to have consolidated scientific opinion regarding the efficacy of soy protein for decreasing serum cholesterol levels.[7] Recently, the U.S. Food and Drug Administration (U.S. FDA) approved a health claim stating that soy protein as part of a diet low in saturated fat and cholesterol may reduce risk for coronary heart disease (CHD).[8] Of rival significance is the emerging evidence that soy isoflavones have potent effects on the second or beta estrogen receptor. While the first or alpha estrogen receptor is concentrated in traditional estrogen-responsive tissues such as breast and uterus, the beta receptor is present in bone, brain, and blood vessels. Furthermore, the binding affinity — effectiveness — of soy isoflavones is much higher for the beta receptor than for the alpha receptor. Thus, soy isoflavones have the potential to mimic the effects of estrogens on bone, brain, and blood vessels.[9] Consequently, soy foods rich in isoflavones may combat osteoporosis and cognitive function loss while preserving normal blood vessel responsiveness.[9]

Clinical studies and basic research with soy foods and their components are emerging at an exponential rate. We will review current evidence related to the health benefits of soy foods and discuss potential safety issues. After reviewing some of the unique nutrition characteristics of soybeans we will discuss the reported health benefits related to these areas: coronary heart disease (CHD), cancer, diabetes and kidney function, menopausal symptoms, osteoporosis, and cognitive dysfunction.

9.2 NUTRITIONAL CHARACTERISTICS OF SOY FOODS

While soybeans have long been a staple of Asian diets, soy foods have only recently become a health food phenomenon. The soybean itself is a nutrient powerhouse. Soy is rich in high-quality protein and a good source of minerals, B vitamins, and fiber. Soybeans are higher in protein than other beans, and the protein quality of most soy foods is equivalent to animal protein sources. Isolated soy protein has a protein quality score equal to milk and egg protein.[2] Soybeans are a richer source of fat than other dry beans. In addition, 58% of this fat is in the form of health-promoting polyunsaturated fatty acids.[10] Soy foods, being low in saturated fat and cholesterol free, are a heart-healthy choice. The complex carbohydrate and fiber in soy contribute to a blunted post-meal blood glucose response, which is beneficial for persons with diabetes.[11] Uncooked soybeans contain 5.4 g total and 2 g soluble fiber per 1/6 cup (31 g).[12] Many soy foods — such as soybeans, soy nuts, green soybeans, soy flour, textured soy protein, and tempeh — are rich in fiber; isolated soy protein, however, does not include the dietary fiber. Soybeans are low in sodium, but are excellent sources of several minerals, including calcium, copper, iron, magnesium, phosphorus, potassium, and zinc.[10] The mineral content and bioavailablilty of soy foods varies according to the processing and phytate content.[11]

Recent research indicates that soy isoflavones, especially genistein and daidzein, have unique biological actions and specific health-promoting effects. Isoflavones belong to a unique class of plant chemicals or phytoestrogens. These biologically active compounds may have either weak pro-estrogenic (agonist) or anti-estrogenic (antagonist) effects and have relevance for hormone-mediated diseases.[3] Various factors, such as the type of glucose side chain present with genistein and daidzein in foods, affect absorption and metabolism of isoflavones. Also, the amount of isoflavones in soy products varies with type of soybean, geographic area of cultivation, and processing.[13] Products which contain most of the bean, such as mature soybeans, roasted soybeans, soy flour, and textured soy protein are excellent sources of isoflavones and provide approximately 5.1 to 5.5 mg total isoflavones per gram of soy protein. Green soybeans (3.3 mg isoflavone per gram protein) and tempeh (3.1 mg isoflavones per gram protein) are intermediate sources of isoflavones. Tofu, isolated soy protein, and some types of soy milk provide approximately 2 mg isoflavones per gram soy protein. Alcohol-extracted products, such as soy protein concentrate, have lower amounts of isoflavones with values of $\leq$0.3 mg isoflavone per gram soy protein. The isoflavone content of many foods has been measured and is available from the USDA food composition tables.[14]

9.2.1 Soy Safety Concerns

Soy has been touted by many as a miracle food. However, there is concern that a soy food-rich diet may not be beneficial for all populations. In particular, there has been concern regarding allergies to soy, soy-based infant formulas, and potential soybean antinutrients.

Soy protein has been ranked 11th in allergenicity, with 0.5% of young children having an allergy to soy. The incidence among older children and adults is extremely rare.[15] Interestingly, those who have an allergy to soy may be able to tolerate some soy foods, but have an adverse reaction to others. Fermented soy foods and those which have been processed at a high temperature are often more tolerable to those with a soy allergy.[16-18]

Controversy has surrounded the use of soy-based formulas in infant feeding.[19] There is concern in the pediatric community that soy formulas, being phytoestrogen rich, may not be optimal for all children, and may be potentially harmful.[20-22] The long-term biological effects of soy formula fed to infants are under investigation and require further exploration.[23] Soybeans, like other legumes, have an array of antinutrients which could have important adverse nutritional and physiological effects. Soybeans, in particular, are relatively rich in potentially antinutritive compounds, including lectins, phytosterols, phytic acid, saponins, protease inhibitors, and a variety of phenolic acids.[24] Phytic acid in soybeans may adversely affect iron, zinc, and to a much lesser extent, calcium bioavailability in those individuals not eating a well-balanced diet. Interestingly, despite the potential antinutrient effects of these soybean components, there are several reported benefits of these compounds in disease prevention.

9.3 CORONARY HEART DISEASE

Coronary heart disease (CHD) is the major cause of death in most developed countries and is rapidly increasing in prevalence in developing countries. In the U.S., for example, CHD claimed 953,110 lives in 1997. More than 2600 Americans die each day of CHD, an average of 1 death every 33 seconds.[25] While many modifiable risk factors, such as cigarette smoking and hypertension, contribute to risk for CHD, lipid abnormalities are the most important factors. Low-density lipoproteins (LDL) have a central role in the atherosclerotic process. LDL penetrate the walls of blood vessels where they are oxidized by free radicals and accumulate as a gruel-like material that blocks the blood vessel lumen; this material can also leak into the blood vessel to cause a thrombosis. High-density lipoproteins (HDL) have a protective effect and act to prevent LDL oxidation and remove cholesterol that accumulates in the blood vessel wall.[26] Soy foods contain protein and isoflavone components that have specific effects on reducing risk for CHD. The isoflavones or soy estrogens contribute an estimated three-fourths of the protective effect while the soy protein may be responsible for the remaining one-quarter of the protection.[7]

Soy protein and its isoflavones exert at least five anti-atherogenic effects. These effects are itemized below and then reviewed in greater detail. Soy foods have favorable effects on all the blood lipid levels; soy protein and its isoflavones are important antioxidants that prevent oxidation of LDL; soy isoflavones have anti-inflammatory effects; soy foods decrease tendency to form blood clots or thromboses; and soy isoflavones have health-promoting effects on blood vessels.

9.3.1 Correction of Blood Lipid Levels

Our critical statistical analysis of 38 careful human clinical trials noted that soy protein intake significantly decreased serum concentrations of total cholesterol, LDL-cholesterol, and triglycerides, while increasing HDL-cholesterol concentrations. Soy protein intake was associated with a 9.3% reduction in serum cholesterol, a 12.9% reduction in serum LDL-cholesterol, and a 10.5% reduction in serum triglycerides. Serum HDL-cholesterol levels increased by 2.4%, a nonsignificant increase. These findings had a strong consistency because 34 of 38 studies reported that soy protein intake decreased serum cholesterol levels.[7]

The mechanisms responsible for this effect are still under investigation but it appears likely that the soy isoflavones account for >70% of the cholesterol-lowering effects. Recent study in humans[27] and prior work in monkeys[28] document that soy protein from which the isoflavones have been extracted does not lower serum cholesterol levels significantly, while isoflavone-rich soy protein isolates have significant effects. These studies also suggest a dose-response with greater hypocholesterolemic effects with larger amounts of isoflavones. The study of Crouse et al.[27] documents that 25 g of soy protein isolate daily exerts a significant hypocholesterolemic effect.

9.3.2 Antioxidant Effects

Many laboratory studies document the strong antioxidant properties of soy isoflavones. In a recent study using rats, we reported that soy isoflavones appear to be incorporated into lipoprotein particles, such as LDL, and protect it from oxidation.[29] Recent work in humans confirms the antioxidant effects of soy isoflavones on LDL from humans fed isoflavone-rich soy protein isolates.[30] This antioxidant effect would get at the heart of the atherosclerosis problem by decreasing LDL accumulation in blood vessel walls.

9.3.3 Anti-Inflammatory Effects

Recent research indicates that inflammation has an important role in development of atherosclerosis in some individuals.[31] Preliminary research indicates that soy isoflavones act to decrease the inflammatory process that may contribute to atherosclerosis.[32]

9.3.4 Anti-Thrombotic Effects

Soy protein with its isoflavones has a number of effects in the blood, which reduce the risk for blood clot formation. Soy protein intake decreases platelet aggregation or "clumping," an early step in blood clot formation.[33] Soy isoflavones also appear to decrease the tendency of the blood to form thromboses, thus further reducing the risk for thrombotic occlusion of the blood vessel.[34]

9.3.5 Blood Vessel Protection

Blood vessels damaged by atherosclerotic plaque tend to develop spasm or "clamping down" when exposed to stress. This further decreases blood flow though the partially occluded vessel and can aggravate angina or brain symptoms. Soy proteins and their isoflavones restore normal reactivity to damaged blood vessels, protecting them from abnormal spasm or inappropriate "clamping down." This has been best demonstrated in monkeys;[35] however, recent clinical studies document that soy isoflavones have this same effect in humans.[36] Soy isoflavones that have much stronger affinity for the beta-estrogen receptor in vascular tissue than for the alpha-receptor in breast tissue, thus appear to act like human estrogens to promote vascular health.[9]

9.3.6 U.S. FDA Health Claim

Because of the conclusive evidence that soy protein decreases serum cholesterol and LDL-cholesterol concentrations, on October 20, 1999 the U.S. Food and Drug

Administration approved a Health Claim.[8] The FDA reviewed more than 50 research studies to support this claim. This health claim states that "Intake of 25 grams of soy protein a day, as part of a diet low in saturated fat and cholesterol, may reduce risk of heart disease." The FDA reviews all petitions for claims very rigorously and has previously approved only 10 health claims. Based on the body of research the FDA concluded that 25 g of soy protein per day provided an adequate intake to reduce risk for CHD. The study of Crouse et al.[27] documented the benefits of 25 g daily. Some of the heart-protective effects of soy protein, such as the antioxidant effects, are provided by 6–10 g of soy protein daily.

9.4 SOY FOODS AND CANCER RISK

One of the most provocative areas of soy research relates to soybean components and risk for developing cancer, especially breast, prostate, and colon cancer. The vast majority of research has focused on the isoflavones since these phytoestrogens have an array of biological functions.[9] In addition to well-documented antioxidant properties,[29] genistein has potent tyrosine kinase inhibitory activity[37] and anti-angiogenesis properties.[38] While soy foods provide an interesting array of phytochemicals — phenolic acids, protease inhibitors, saponins, and other compounds — most of the evidence points to the isoflavones as the most likely protective components of soy foods.[9] The data related to isoflavones and cancer risk emerge from *in vitro* experiments, animal studies, and observational studies in humans. Controlled clinical trials are in progress but none has yet been reported. We will briefly review the *in vitro* animal and human studies.

Fotsis et al.[38] fractionated urine from subjects consuming a plant-based diet and identified chemicals that had effects on *in vitro* cell growth. Genistein, the major soy isoflavone, was the most potent phytochemical identified. Genistein inhibited *in vitro* proliferation of several tumor cells. It also inhibited *in vitro* angiogenesis, the formation of new blood vessels. Formation of new blood vessels is critical for the growth of human cancers and facilitates tumor cell metastases. Other investigators demonstrated that genistein inhibited tumor cell proliferation,[39] breast cell tumor growth,[40] synthesis of estradiol,[41] binding of transcription factors,[42] and rat myoblast proliferation.[43] Barnes[39] summarized the *in vitro* studies and subsequent investigators[40-43] have updated this area. While these *in vitro* studies do not provide persuasive data related to human cancers, it is reassuring that most *in vitro* studies support a favorable role for genistein in prevention of cancer development, proliferation, and metastases.

Most of the available animal data suggest that soy foods or isoflavones have a protective or preventive role for cancer development. Barnes[39] also summarized these data and reported that soy feeding had protective effects for breast, prostate, colon, liver, and skin cancer in most studies. Subsequent investigators have confirmed and extended these observations.[44-47] Of special interest are the studies suggesting that administration of genistein to rats in the perinatal period reduces the development of breast tumors of the offspring.[48] The effect of soy isoflavones on development of prostate cancer in animal models[39,49] is also of great interest because of the epidemiologic data in humans.

Observational studies suggest that populations with generous intakes of soy foods have lower prevalence rates of breast, prostate, uterine, and colon cancers than Western people.[50-52] Anderson and colleagues[9] reviewed the epidemiological data which largely supports the hypothesis that soy food intake is associated with reduced risk for breast cancer. However, all of the studies have limitations in their interpretability and, of course, do not provide cause and effect relationships. The study of Ingram et al.[53] found an inverse relationship between urinary excretion of isoflavones and risk for breast cancer. As Anderson et al.[9] and Hebert et al.[54] summarize, the epidemiological data are stronger for soy foods having a protective role in respect to prostate cancer than for breast cancer. Soy food intake appears to slow enlargement of the prostate in Asian men and reduce the transformation to prostate cancer.[9,55]

Thus, the available data support hypotheses that intake of soy foods has chemoprevention potential for several types of cancers.[56,57] Currently, prospective clinical trials are in progress for primary prevention of breast cancer and prostate cancer and for prevention of progression or recurrence. We will need to await the outcomes of these controlled clinical trials before developing firm recommendations about use of soy foods and isoflavone-rich products for persons at high risk for these cancers or for protection from progression or recurrence of breast or prostate cancers.

9.5 SOY PROTEIN AND PROTECTION FROM RENAL DISEASE

For more than 150 years it has been recognized that dietary protein plays an important role in the prevention and treatment of renal disease. In 1836, Richard Bright first recommended dietary protein restriction as a therapeutic intervention to slow the progression of chronic kidney disease.[58] Recently, both animal and human trials have found that not only protein restriction, but also modifications in the type of protein consumed, have a favorable affect on renal health. Soy protein has been shown to offer benefits in individuals with Type 1 or Type 2 diabetes,[59,60] end-stage renal disease (ESRD),[61-63] and polycystic kidney disease.[64-66]

9.5.1 Soy and Diabetic Nephropathy

Eighteen million Americans have diabetes mellitus. Sadly, nearly one-third of those with diabetes develops renal disease. Diabetic nephropathy is a major contributor to death in those with diabetes, primarily from end-stage renal disease (ESRD) and cardiovascular disease.[67] Normalization of blood glucose, antihypertensive treatment, and restriction of dietary protein are the primary therapeutic interventions implemented in this population. While it may be ideal for many pre-ESRD patients to restrict their dietary protein intake, this recommendation is not practical in Western society where protein intake is usually almost twice the RDA.[68]

Therefore, researchers are excited by the preliminary evidence showing that substitution of soy protein for animal protein in the diet of individuals with either Type 1 or Type 2 diabetes may be effective in the prevention or treatment of early diabetic nephropathy. The recently coined "soy protein hypothesis" states that substitution of soy protein in these diabetic individuals results in less hyperfiltration and glomerular hypertension with resultant protection from diabetic nephropathy.[59] Our research group recently completed two clinical trials to test this hypothesis. The first included subjects with Type 2 diabetes in conjunction with obesity, hypertension, and proteinuria.[59] Soy protein intake, provided as half of daily dietary protein, had no significant effects on protein excretion, but did have a significant impact on reduction in serum cholesterol and triglyceride concentrations. The second trial, a pilot study of young individuals with Type 1 diabetes, showed that substitution of 55 g of soy protein for animal protein in the diet had benefits on renal health.[60] In particular, after eight weeks of dietary intervention, those subjects who were hyperfiltering at baseline (GFR >120 ml/min/1.73m^2) had a reduction in glomerular filtration rate. Also, the urine albumin:creatinine ratios decreased in those subjects with microalbuminuria (albumin 30 to 300 mg/24 h) at baseline. From these preliminary reports it is evident that soy protein has beneficial effects on diabetic nephropathy characterized by proteinuria.

The mechanisms by which soy protein exerts renal protective effects in diabetes have yet to be elucidated. However, from preliminary *in vitro* and *in vivo* evidence we postulate that the unique amino acid composition, isoflavone, lipid-lowering and antioxidant properties, and anti-inflammatory effects of soy are all important contributors.

The amino acids glutamine, proline, alanine, and tryptophane, are renally metabolized and have direct vasodilatory effects on the kidney. Soy protein contains only small amounts of these amino acids.[69] Isoflavones, independent of protein, have favorable effects on renal glomerular biology and hemodynamic function. *In vitro* trials have shown that increased glomerular intercapillary pressure and capillary dilation activates several intracellular pathways including the tyrosine kinase system. Isoflavones, in particular genistein, block many of these pathways, probably via inhibition of kinase activities.[70-75] Abnormal lipid profiles and an increased propensity to high levels of oxidized LDL-cholesterol may contribute to the onset and progression of diabetic nephropathy. Soy protein has both lipid-lowering and antioxidant effects which may counteract these factors.[7,76-78]

Recent research indicates that inflammation has an important role in development of renal disease in some individuals. Preliminary research indicates that soy isoflavones act to decrease the inflammatory process that may contribute to the pathogenesis of renal failure.[32]

9.5.2 Soy and End-Stage Renal Disease

It has been postulated that genistein and daidzein, the isoflavones particularly concentrated in soy foods, may offer benefits in ESRD. Specifically, the isoflavones may antagonize the immuno-inflammatory system.[61-63, 79]

9.5.3 Soy and Polycystic Kidney Disease

Nutrition intervention in patients with PKD has been shown to significantly improve the disease progression. Recently it has been reported from animal models that soy protein reduces renal cyst growth in both rats and mice. This preliminary research offers exciting support for the potential therapeutic benefit that soy may have in human PKD patients.[64-66]

Although only preliminary in nature, research evaluating the effects of soy protein intake on renal health are very encouraging. Regular intake of soy foods may indeed protect the well being of individuals at risk for developing kidney disease. Future research is needed to evaluate the mechanisms by which soy exerts renal protective affects.

9.6 SOY AND WOMEN'S HEALTH

9.6.1 Soy and Menopausal Symptoms

Menopausal symptoms appear to be much more common among North American women than among Japanese women eating a traditional diet including soy products. Epidemiological studies suggest that ~85% of North American women, compared to ~25% of Japanese women, complain of hot flashes.[80] The undesirable symptoms of menopause can be treated with estrogen replacement and some women choose this option. In the U.S. only 24% of postmenopausal women use hormone replacement therapy (HRT) while 47% of postmenopausal women physicians use HRT.[81] For some women with strong family or personal histories of breast cancer HRT is contraindicated, but most women who do not use HRT opt not to follow this path because of concerns about side effects. Many women of the twenty-first century are seeking natural, yet effective, alternatives to the classic HRT.[82]

Incorporating soy foods into a woman's diet may be a healthy alternative to HRT. Extensive research is currently being done in this area. While there is no conclusive evidence to support the role of soy foods as a replacement for HRT, foods rich in soy protein and isoflavones are a positive addition to a menopausal woman's diet. Soy foods contain phytoestrogens or isoflavones that have weak estrogenic effects. This component of soy alleviates some of the menopausal symptoms in some women, particularly hot flashes. There is conflicting research on this topic. One study found that supplementing the diet of postmenopausal women with 60 g of soy protein and 76 mg of isoflavones significantly decreased the number of hot flashes the women experienced.[80] However, another study showed that supplementing the diet of postmenopausal women with soy foods had little or no effect on the number and frequency of hot flashes.[83] Due to the conflicting research on soy supplementation and menopause, there currently are not any specific guidelines to follow in regard to soy isoflavone and soy protein supplementation in postmenopausal women. It may be beneficial for some postmenopausal women to make an effort to include two or three servings of isoflavone-rich soy protein per day in place of animal protein in their diet. The equivalent of two or three servings of soy foods is 14 to 25 g of soy protein per day and 30 to 65 mg of soy isoflavones per serving. At the present time, the research on soy isoflavone supplements in place of soy foods is inconclusive.[84] The majority of studies that have used soy food products, including both soy protein and isoflavones, have had more significant data. The effect of soy isoflavone supplementation on menopausal symptoms requires more research. Currently, soy isoflavone supplements are NOT recommended as a substitute for hormone replacement therapy.

9.6.2 Osteoporosis

In the U.S. an estimated 23 million women have osteoporosis or low bone mass.[85] Osteoporosis is particularly a concern of postmenopausal women because of the significant decrease in estrogen loss that they experience. Low levels of estrogen contribute to bone loss. The characteristics of women that are more susceptible to osteoporosis are small bone structure and/or build, smokers, inactivity, and heredity factors. Fortunately, it may be preventable with a diet that is adequate in calcium and an exercise regimen that utilizes weight-bearing exercise.[86] The addition of soy foods to a woman's diet may also decrease bone loss and help to enhance bone mineral density by increasing calcium retention.[87] A diet that is high in animal protein tends to increase urinary calcium excretion. Soy protein does not have the same negative effect on calcium loss as animal protein.[88] The isoflavone component of soy that offers weak estrogenic effects may also help to prevent bone loss as that of hormone replacement therapy.[89] There is preliminary data revealing that the isoflavone component of soy may help to preserve bone mineral density.[90] Many soy foods are rich in calcium or are fortified to contain calcium. For this reason, soy foods are even more beneficial to counteract bone loss. Although most people meet their daily requirement of calcium from dairy products, soy milk, tempeh, whole soybeans, and textured vegetable protein are all very good sources of bioavailable calcium. A good recommendation is to include two to three servings of calcium-containing soy foods per day.

9.7 SOY AND COGNITIVE FUNCTION

Alzheimer's disease (AD) is estimated to affect 3.75 million people in the U.S.[91] In a 1993 national survey, 19 million Americans reported having a family member with AD and 37 million knew someone with AD.[92] In addition, dementia, or loss of intellectual function, afflicts nearly 10% of persons over the age of 65 and 50% of those individuals over the age of 85.[93] Approximately $67 billion is spent annually on Alzheimer's disease-related costs.[91] As the baby boomer generation ages public interest and demand for the prevention and treatment of AD has peaked. Recently it has been hypothesized that soy isoflavones, as partial estrogen agonists, may modulate cognitive function, particularly in postmenopausal estrogen-deficient women. Unknown at this time is if this modulation is beneficial or impairs cognitive function.

9.7.1 Estrogen and Cognitive Function

Estrogen has been shown in both animal[94] and clinical trials[95] to affect cognitive function. Estrogen is a neuroactive steroid with receptors in the cerebral cortex, hypothalamus, pituitary, and limbic system (amygdala and hippocampus) regions of the human brain.[96] As such, estrogen has been shown to affect neural function, particularly in the maintenance of verbal memory and enhanced capacity for new learning.[97]

A meta-analysis of 10 observational trials found a 29% reduced risk of dementia among those postmenopausal women on estrogen therapy.[98] The four hypothesized mechanisms by which estrogen may affect cognition include:

1. Promotion of cholinergic and serotonergic activity in specific brain regions.
2. Maintenance of neural circuitry.
3. Favorable lipoprotein alterations.
4. Prevention of cerebral ischemia.[98]

Waring and collaborators recently completed a case-controlled study of the effect of estrogen therapy on risk of AD in 222 postmenopausal women who developed AD between 1980 and 1984 in Rochester, Minnesota. The frequency of estrogen use was higher among control subjects than AD patients — both populations having identical ages of menarche and menopause.[99]

Forty-six postmenopausal women, ages 31 to 61 years, participated in a randomized, double-blind, placebo-controlled trial from 1996 to 1998 to investigate the effects of estrogen on brain activation patterns as the women performed verbal and nonverbal working memory tasks. Treatment with 1.25 mg/day of conjugated equine estrogens for 21 days increased activation of the inferior parietal lobule during storage of verbal material. In addition, inferior parietal lobule activation was decreased during the storage of nonverbal material. Right superior frontal gyrus activity was increased during retrieval tasks while on estrogen supplementation. These results suggest that estrogen therapy in postmenopausal women affects organization of memory in the brain.[95]

9.7.2 Soy Isoflavones and Cognitive Function

Genistein and daidzein are structurally similar to estrogen and have the ability to bind to estrogen receptors, thus exerting agonist or antagonist effects. Isoflavones have a unique structural entity, the phenolic ring, which is able to bind estrogen receptors and thus mediate classic genomic actions, plasma membrane integrity, and cell signaling pathways. The binding affinity of genistein is relatively high for ERβ, being approximately one-third of that of 17β-estradiol.[100] The β-estrogen receptor is the major subtype of receptor in the brain, bone, bladder, and vascular epithelia.[101] As such, is it hypothesized that soy isoflavones may exert potentially biologically important activities in these tissues, in particular, the brain.

Two observational human studies[102,103] and multiple animal and *in vitro* models have evaluated the association between soy isoflavone intake and cognitive function. Interestingly, results from the human trials have been inconsistent with those in cynomolgus monkeys[104] and rats.[105,106]

White and colleagues with the Honolulu Heart Program recently caught the eye of researchers around the globe when they reported that regular consumption of tofu in Japanese-American men has an adverse influence on brain aging. This brain aging may manifest as accelerated brain atrophy, cognitive decline, and lowering of the threshold for the clinical manifestations of AD. The authors indicate that the association between tofu consumption and cognitive function follows a dose-response pattern in these men.[102] Similarly, cross-sectional data from the Kame Project of Japanese-American men and women reports that high tofu consumption is associated with lowered cognitive scores. In addition, regular tofu consumption negated the beneficial association between hormone replacement therapy and cognitive function.[103]

Animal and *in vitro* work has actually shown a beneficial contribution of soy isoflavones in the prevention of Alzheimer's and enhanced cognitive function. Pan and colleagues at Wake Forest University School of Medicine recently evaluated the effect of estradiol and soy phytoestrogens on choline acetyltransferase (ChAT) and nerve growth factor mRNAs (NGF mRNAs) as markers of cognitive function.[105] A reduction in activity of ChAT and loss of cholinergic neurons are associated with AD. Estrogen deficiency has been shown to potentiate these reductions and therefore may be partially responsible for the neurodegeneration in AD. The Wake Forest researchers found that soy phytoestrogens, administered at levels equivalent to a woman's dose of 150 mg total isoflavones per day, may function as estrogen agonists in the brain, upregulating ChAT and NGF mRNAs in female ovariectomized young and retired breeder rats.[105]

In a similar study Weber et al.[106] examined the short-term, 29-day, effects of soy phytoestrogens on regulatory behaviors, such as food and water intake and locomotor activity, and brain androgen-metabolizing enzyme activity in Sprague-Dawley rats. The authors evaluated brain aromatase chytochrome P450 and 5α-reductase activity as measures of regulation of neuroendocrine function and locomotor activities. The aromatase enzyme plays a pivotal role in the local formation of estrogen(s) in the hypothalamus and limbic regions of the brain. No significant changes in aromatase activity were found. However, phytoestrogen supplementation did alter 5α-reductase activity in neural tissue, suggesting the potential benefit of soy isoflavones on brain function.[106]

It is evident that there is a lot to learn in the soy and cognitive function arena. This facet of soy research is still in its infancy and one can predict that there will be a plethora of human trials conducted in the coming years to assess this very important relationship.

9.8 CONCLUSIONS

In the past five years the interest in soy foods among consumers has grown exponentially. Nutritional basic and clinical research has expanded dramatically. Soy foods and their isoflavones appear to have clear protective effects related to CHD and probable protective and therapeutic effects related to osteoporosis. The effects on the kidneys are clear and the protective effects are under study. While the greatest interest may relate to chemopreventive effects related to cancer, much more research is required. The effects of soy foods on cognitive function are unclear and also require further research. The use for menopausal symptoms appear promising and postmenopausal women who cannot or choose not to take HRT may be ideal candidates for daily soy food use.

REFERENCES

1. Messina, M., Messina, V., and Setchell, K.D.R., *The Simple Soybean and Your Health*, New York: Avery Publishing, 1994.
2. Young, V.R., Soy protein in relation to human protein and amino acid nutrition, *J. Am. Diet. Assoc.*, 91, 828-835, 1991.
3. Makrides, M., Neumann, M., Simmer, K., Pater, J., and Gibson, R., Are long-chain polyunsaturated fatty acids essential nutrients in infancy?, *Lancet*, 345(8963), 1463-1468, 1995.
4. Ignatowski, A., Influence de la nourriture animale sur l'organisme des lapins, *Arch. Med. Exp. Anat. Pathol.*, 20, 1-20, 1908.
5. Meeker, D.R. and Kesten, H.D., Experimental atherosclerosis and high protein diets, *Proc. Exp. Biol. Med.*, 45, 543-545, 1940.
6. Sirtori, C.R., Agradi, E., Conti, F., Mantero, O., and Gatto, E., Soybean-protein diet in the treatment of type-II hyperlipoproteinaemia, *Lancet*, 1, 275-277, 1977.
7. Anderson, J.W., Johnstone, B.M., and Cook-Newell, M.E., Meta-analysis of the effects of soy protein intake on serum lipids, *NEJM,* 333, 276-282, 1995.
8. Food and Drug Administration, HHS. Food Labeling: Health Claims; Soy Protein and Coronary Heart Disease, Docket No. 98P-0683, 57700-57733. 99. 4160-01-P, Washington, D.C., 1999.
9. Anderson, J.J.B., Anthony, M., Messina, M., and Garner, S.C., Effects of phyto-oestrogens on tissues, *Nutr. Res. Rev.*, 12, 75-116, 1999.
10. Haytowitz, D.B. and Mathews, R.H., Legume and legume products, U.S. Department of Agriculture, Washington, D.C., 1986.
11. Lo, G.S., Goldbert, A.P., Lim, A., Grundhauser, J.J., Anderson, C., and Schonfeld, G., Soy fiber improves lipid and carbohydrate metabolism in primary hyperlipidemic subjects, *Atherosclerosis*, 62, 239, 1986.
12. Anderson, J.W., *Plant Fiber in Foods*, Lexington, KY: HCF Nutrition Foundation, 1990.
13. Wang, H.J. and Murphy, P.A., Isoflavone composition of American and Japanese soybeans in Iowa; effects of variety, crop year, and location, *J. Agric. Food Chem.*, 42, 1674, 1994.
14. Beecher, G.R., Bhagwat, S., Haytowitz, D., Holden, J.M., and Murphy, P.A., USDA Isoflavone Nutrient Database, 1999. Beltsville, MD, Beltsville Human Nutrition Research Center, ARS, USDA and Iowa State University Department of Food Science and Human Nutrition.
15. Foucard, T. and Yman, I.M., A study on severe food reactions in Sweden — is soy protein an underestimated cause of food anaphylaxis, *Allergy*, 54, 261-265, 1999.
16. Sicherer, S.H. and Sampson, H.A., Food hypersensitivity and atopic dermatitis: pathophysiology, epidemiology, diagnosis, and management, *J. Allerg. Clin. Immunol.*, 104, S114-S122, 1999.
17. Monere-Vautrin, D.A., Cow's milk allergy, *Allerg. Immunol.*, 31, 201-210, 1999.
18. Cantani, A. and Lucenti, P., Natural history of soy allergy and/or intolerance in children, and clinical use of soy-protein formulas, *Pediatr. Allerg. Immunol.*, 8, 59-74, 1997.
19. Zoppi, G. and Guandalin, S., The story of soy formula feeding in infants: a road paved with good intentions, *J. Pediatr. Gastroenterol. Nutr.*, 28(5), 541-543, 1999.
20. American Academy of Pediatrics — Committee on Nutrition. Soy protein-based formulas: Recommendations for use in infant feeding, *Pediatrics,* 101, 48-153, 1998.

21. Setchell, K.D.R., Simmer-Nechemias, L., Cai, J., and Helibi, J.E., Exposure of infants to phyto-estrogens from soy-based infant formulas, *Lancet*, 30, 23-27, 1997.
22. Jensen, K., Chemical substances harmful for the endocrine system, 7-23-1998, European Parliament.
23. Maldonado, J., Gil, A., Narbona, E., and Molina, J.A., Special formulas in infant nutrition: a review, *Early Hum. Dev.*, 53, S23-S32, 1998.
24. Liener, I.E., Implications of antinutritional components in soybean foods, *Crit. Rev. Food Sci. Nutr.*, 34(1), 31-67, 1994.
25. American Heart Association. 2000 Heart and Stroke Statistical Update. 1-32. 2000.
26. Gowri, M.S., Van der Westhuyzen, D.R., Bridges, S.R., and Anderson, J.W., Decreased protection by HDL from poorly controlled type 2 diabetic subjects against LDL oxidation may be due to the abnormal composition of HDL, *Arterioscler. Thromb. Vasc. Biol.*, 9, 2226-2233, 1999.
27. Crouse, J.R. III, Morgan, T., Terry, J.G., Ellis, J., Vitolins, M., and Burke, G.L., A randomized trial comparing the effect of casein with that of soy protein containing varying amounts of isoflavones on plasma concentrations of lipids and lipoproteins, *Arch. Intern. Med.*, 159, 2070-2076, 1999.
28. Anthony, M.S., Clarkson, T.B., Bullock, B.C., and Wagner, JD., Soy protein versus soy phytoestrogens in the prevention of diet-induced coronary artery atherosclerosis of male cynomolgus monkeys, *Arterioscler. Thromb. Vasc. Biol.*, 17(11), 2524-2531, 1997.
29. Anderson, J.W., Diwadkar, V.A., and Bridges, S.R., Selective effects of different antioxidants on oxidation of lipoproteins from rats, *PSEBM*, 218, 376-381, 1998.
30. Tikkanen, M.J., Wahala, K., Ojala, S., Vihma, V., and Aldercreutz, H., Effect of soybean phytoestrogen intake on low density lipoprotein oxidation resistance, *Proc. Natl. Acad. Sci.*, 95, 3106-3110, 1998.
31. Ross, R., Atherosclerosis is an inflammatory disease, *Am. Heart J.*, 138, S419-S420, 1999.
32. Sadowska-Krowicka, H., Mannick, E.E., Oliver, P.D., Sandoval, M., Zhang, X.J., Eloby-Childess, S., Clark, D.A., and Miller, M.J.S., Genistein and gut inflammation: role of nitric oxide, *Proc. Soc. Exp. Biol. Med.*, 217, 351-357, 1998.
33. Gooderham, J.M., Adlercreutz, H., Ojala, S., Wahala, K., and Holub, B.J., A soy protein isolate rich in genistein and daidzein and its effects on plasma isoflavone concentrations, platelet aggregation, blood lipids and fatty acid composition of plasma phospholipid in normal men, *J. Nutr.*, 126, 2000-2006, 1996.
34. Wilcox, J.N. and Blumenthal, B.F., Thrombotic mechanism in atherosclerosis: potential impact of soy proteins, *J. Nutr.*, 125, 631S-638S, 1995.
35. Honore, E.K., Williams, J.K., Anthony, M.S., and Clarkson, T.B., Soy isoflavones enhance coronary vascular reactivity in atherosclerotic female macaques, *Fertil. Steril.*, 67 1(148), 154, 1997.
36. Nestel, P.J., Pomeroy, S., Kay, S., Komesaroff, P., Behrsing, J., Cameron, J.D., and West, L., Isoflavones from red clover improve systemic arterial compliance but not plasma lipids in menopausal women, *J. Clin. Endocrinol. Metab.*, 84(3), 895-898, 1999.
37. Akiyama, S.K. and Yamada, K.M., Biosynthesis and acquisition of biological activity in fibronectin receptor, *J. Biol. Chem.*, 262, 17536-17542, 1987.
38. Fotsis, T., Pepper, M., Adlercreutz, H., Hase, T., Montesano, R., and Schweigerer, L., Genistein, a dietary ingested isoflavonoid, inhibits cell proliferation and in vitro angiogenesis, *J. Nutr.*, 125, 790S-797S, 1995.

39. Barnes, S., Effect of genistein on in vitro and in vivo models of cancers, *J. Nutr.*, 125, 777S-783S, 1995.
40. Li, Y., Bhuiyan, M., and Sarkar, F.H., Induction of apoptosis and inhibition of c-erbB-2 in MDA-MB-435 cells by genistein, *Int. J. Oncol.*, 15, 525-533, 1999.
41. Makela, S., Poutanen, M., Lehtimaki, J., Kostian, M.L., Santti, R., and Vihko, R., Estrogen-specific 17-beta-hydroxysteroid oxidoreductase type 1 (E.C. 1.1.1.62) as a possible target for the action of phytoestrogens, *Proc. Soc. Exp. Biol. Med.*, 208, 51-59, 1995.
42. Zhou, Y. and Lee, A.S., Mechanism for the suppression of the mammalian stress response by genistein, an anticancer phytoestrogen from soy, *J. Natl. Cancer Inst.*, 90, 381-388, 1998.
43. Ji, S., Willis, G.M., Frank, R., Cornelius, S.G., and Spurlock, M.E., Soybean isoflavones, genistein and genistin, inhibit rat myoblast proliferation, fusion and myotube protein synthesis, *J. Nutr.,* 129, 1291-1297, 1999.
44. Hawrylewicz, E.J., Zapata, J.J., and Blair, W.H., Soy and experimental cancer: animal studies, *J. Nutr.*, 125, 698S-708S, 1995.
45. Davies, M.J., Bowey, E.A., Adelercreutz, H., Rowland, I.R., and Rumsby, P.C., Effects of soy or rye supplementation of high-fat diets on colon tumour development in azoxymethane-treated rats, *Carcinogenesis*, 20(6), 927-931, 1999.
46. Li, D., Yee, J.A., McGuire, M.H., Murphy, P.A., and Yan, L., Soybean isoflavones reduce experimental metastasis in mice, *J. Nutr.*, 129, 1075-1078, 1999.
47. Appelt, L.C. and Reicks, M.M., Soy induces phase II enzymes but does not inhibit dimethylbenz[a]anthracene-induced carcinogenesis in female rats, *J. Nutr.*, 129, 1820-1826, 1999.
48. Lamartiniere, C.A., Moore, J.B., Brown, N.M., Thompson, R., Hardin, M.J., and Barnes, S., Genistein suppresses mammary cancer in rats, *Carcinogenesis*, 16, 2833-2840, 1995.
49. Pollard, M., Prevention of prostate-related cancers in lobund-wistar rats, *Prostate*, 39, 305-309, 1999.
50. Steinmetz, K.A. and Potter, J.D., Vegetables, fruit and cancer prevention: a review, *J. Am. Diet. Assoc.*, 96, 1027-1039, 1996.
51. Messina, M.J., Persky, V., Setchell, K.D.R., and Barnes, S., Soy intake and cancer risk: a review of the in vitro and in vivo data, *Nutr. Cancer*, 21, 113-131, 1994.
52. Goodman, M.T., Wilkens, L.R., Hankin, J.H., Lyu, L., Wu, A.H., and Kolonel, L.N., Association of soy and fiber consumption with the risk of endometrial cancer, *Am. J. Epidemiol.*, 146, 294-306, 1997.
53. Ingram, D., Sanders, K., Koybab, M., and Lopez, D., Case-control study of phyto-oestrogens and breast cancer, *Lancet*, 350, 990-994, 1997.
54. Hebert, J.R., Hurley, T.G., Olendzki, B.C., Teas, J., Ma, Y., and Hampl, J.S., Nutritional and socioeconomic factors in relation to prostate cancer mortality: a cross-national study, *J. Natl. Cancer Inst.*, 90, 1637-1647, 1998.
55. Strom, S.S., Yamamura, Y., Duphorne, C.M., Spitz, M.R., Babaian, R.J., Pillow, P.C., and Hursting, S.D., Phytoestrogen intake and prostate cancer: a case-control study using a new database, *Nutr. Cancer*, 33(1), 20-25, 1999.
56. Steele, V.E., Pereira, M.A., Sigman, C.C., and Kelloff, G.J., Cancer chemoprevention agent development strategies for genistein, *J. Nutr.*, 125, 713S-716S, 1995.
57. Kennedy, A.R., The evidence for soybean products as cancer preventive agents, *J. Nutr.*, 125, 733S-743S, 1995.

58. Chan, A.Y.M., Cheng, M.L.L., Keil, L.C., and Myers, B.D., Functional response of healthy and diseased glomeruli to a large, protein-rich meal, *J. Clin. Invest.*, 81, 245-254, 1988.
59. Anderson, J.W., Blake, J.E., Turner, J., and Smith, B.M., Effects of soy protein on renal function and proteinuria in patients with type 2 diabetes, *Am. J. Clin. Nutr.*, 68(Suppl.), 1347S-1353S, 1998.
60. Hanna, T.J., Fanti, P., and Anderson, J.W., Soy protein decreases workload of kidneys in type 1 diabetics at risk for diabetic nephropathy, *Proc. Soc. Exp. Biol. Med.*, 13(4), A272, 1999.
61. Fanti, P., Sawaya, B.P., Custer, L.J., and Franke, A.A., Serum levels and metabolic clearance of the isoflavones genistein and daidzein in hemodialysis patients, *J. Am. Soc. Nephrol.*, 10, 864-871, 1999.
62. Ceballos-Picot, I., Witko-Sarsat, V., Merad-Boudia, M., Nguyen, A.T., Threvenin, M., Jungers, P., and Descamp-Latscha, B., Glutathione antioxidant system as a marker of oxidative stress in chronic renal failure, *Free Rad. Biol. Med.*, 21, 845-853, 1996.
63. Pereira, B.J.G., Shapiro, L., King, A.J., Fulagas, M.A., Storm, J.A., and Dinerello, C.A., Plasma levels of IL-1-alpha, TNF-alpha and their specific inhibitors in undialysed chronic renal failure, CAPD and hemodialysis patients, *Kidney Intl.*, 45, 890-896, 1994.
64. Ogborn, M.R., Bankovic-Calic, N., Shoesmith, C., Buist, R., and Peeling, J., Soy protein modification of rat polycystic kidney disease, *Am. J. Physiol.*, 274, F541-F549, 1998.
65. Aukema, H.M., Housini, I., and Rawling, J.M., Dietary soy protein effects on inherited polycystic kidney disease are influenced by gender and protein level, *J. Am. Soc. Nephrol.*, 10, 300-308, 1999.
66. Tomobe, K., Philbrick, D.J., Ogborn, M.R., Takahashi, H., and Holub, B.J., Effect of dietary soy protein and genistein on disease progression in mice with polycystic kidney disease, *Am. J. Kidney Dis.*, 31(1), 55-61, 1998.
67. Anderson, J.W., Nutritional management of diabetes mellitus, in Shils, M.E., Olson, J.A., Shike, M., Ross, A.C., and Young, V.A., Eds., *Modern Nutrition in Health and Disease*, Williams & Wilkins, Philadelphia, 1365-1394, 1998.
68. Anderson, J.W., Why do diabetic individuals eat so much protein and fat?, *Med. Exerc. Nutr. Health*, 2, 65-68, 1993.
69. Brezis, M., Silivia, P., and Epstein, F.H., Amino acids induce renal vasodilation in isolated perfused kidney, *Am. J. Physiol.*, 253(F1083), F1090, 1984.
70. Kawata, Y., Mizukami, Y., Fujii, Z., Sakumura, T., Yoshida, K., and Matsuzaki, M., Applied pressure enhances cell proliferation through mitogen-activated protein kinase activation in mesangeal cells, *J. Biol. Chem.*, 273, 16905-16912, 1998.
71. Hirikata, M., Kaname, S., Chung, U.G., Joki, N., Hori, Y., Noda, M., Takuwa, Y., Okazaki, T., Fujita, T., Katoh, T., and Kurokawa, K., Tyrosine kinase dependent expression of TGF-beta by stretch in mesangial cells, *Kidney Int.*, 51, 1028-1036, 1997.
72. Gruden, G., Thomas, S., Burt, D., Lane, S., Chusney, G., Sacks, S., and Viberti, G.C., Mechanical stretch induces vascular permeability factor in human mesangeal cells: mechanism of signal transduction, *Proc. Natl. Acad. Sci.*, 94, 12112-12116, 1997.
73. Huwiler, A., Van Rossum, G., Wartmann, M., and Pfeilschifter, J., Angiotensin II stimulation of stress-activated protein kinases in renal mesangial cells is mediated by the angiotensin AT1 receptor subtype, *Eur. J. Pharmacol.*, 343, 297-302, 1998.
74. Pfeilschifter, J. and Huwiler, A., Nitric oxide stimulates stress-activated protein kinases in glomerular endothelial and mesangial cells, *FEBS Lett.*, 396, 67-70, 1996.

75. Ha, H., Roh, D.D., Kirschenbaum, M.A., and Kamann, V.S., Atherogenic lipoproteins enhance mesangial cell expression of platelet-derived growth factor: role of protein tyrosine kinase and cyclic AMP-dependent protein kinase A, *J. Lab. Clin. Med.*, 131 (456), 465, 1998.
76. Gentile, M.G., Fellin, G., Cofano, F., Fave, A.D., Manna, G., Ciceri, R., Petrini, C., Lavarda, F., Pozzi, F., and D'Amico, G., Treatment of proteinuric patients with a vegetarian soy diet and fish oil, *Clin. Nephrol.*, 40(6), 315-320, 1993.
77. Anthony, M.S., Clarkson, T.B., and Williams, J.K., Effects of soy isoflavones on atherosclerosis: potential mechanisms, *Am. J. Clin. Nutr.*, 68(6 Suppl.), 1390S-1393S, 1998.
78. Kanazawa, T., Osanai, T., Zhang, X.S., Uemura, T., Yin, X.Z., and Onedera, K., Protective effects of soy protein on the peroxidizability of lipoproteins in cerebral vascular diseases, *J. Nutr.*, 125, 639S-646S, 1995.
79. Chen, Z., Zheng, W., Custer, L.J., Dai, Q., Shu, X.O., Jin, F., and Franke, A.A., Usual dietary consumption of soy foods and its correlation with the excretion rate of isoflavonoids in overnight urine samples among Chinese women in Shanghai, *Nutr. Cancer*, 33(1), 82-87, 1999.
80. Albertazzi, P., Pansini, F., Bonaccorsi, G., Zanotti, L., Forini, E., and De Aloysio, D., The effect of dietary soy supplementation on hot flushes, *Obstet. Gynecol.*, 91, 6-11, 1998.
81. McNagny, S.E., Wenger, N.K., and Frank, E., Personal use of postmenopausal hormone replacement therapy by women physicians in the United States, *Ann. Intern. Med.*, 127, 1093-1096, 1997.
82. Washburn, S., Burke, G.L., Morgan, T., and Anthony, M., Effect of soy protein supplementation on serum lipoproteins, blood pressure, and menopausal symptoms in perimenopausal women, *J. Am. Menopause. Soc.*, 6(1), 7-13, 1999.
83. Murkies, A.L., Lombard, C., Strauss, B.J., Wilcox, G., Burger, H.G., and Morton, M.S., Dietary flour supplementation decreases postmenopausal hot flushes: effect of soy and wheat, *Maturitas*, 21, 189-195, 1995.
84. Baird, D.D., Umbach, D.M., Lansdell, L., Hughes, C.L., Setchell, K.D., Weinberg, C.R., Haney, A.F., Wilcox, A.J., and Mclachlan, J.A., Dietary intervention study to assess the estrogenicity of dietary soy among postmenopausal women, *J. Clin. Endocrinol. Metab.*, 80(5), 1685-1690, 1995.
85. National Osteoporosis Foundation. 1996 and 2015 Osteoporosis Prevalence Figures: State by State Report, Washington, D.C., 1997.
86. Nelson, M.E., Fiatarone, M.E., Morganti, C.M., Trice, I., Greenburg, R.A., and Evans, W.J., Effects of high intensity strength training on multiple factors for osteoporotic fractures: a randomized controlled trial, *J. Am. Med. Assoc.*, 272, 1909-1914, 1994.
87. Riggs, B.L., A new option for treating osteoporosis, *N. Engl. J. Med.*, 66, 140-146, 1990.
88. Breslau, N.A., Brinkley, L., Hill, K.D., and Pak, C.Y.C., Relationship of animal protein-rich diet to kidney stone formation and calcium metabolism, *J. Clin. Endocrinol. Metab.*, 66, 140-146, 1988.
89. Scheiber, M.D. and Rebar, R.W., Isoflavones and postmenopausal bone health: a viable alternative to estrogen therapy?, *Menopause*, 6:233-241, 1999.
90. Potter, S., Baum, J.A., Teng, H., Stillman, R.J., and Erdman, J.W., Soy protein and isoflavones: their effects on blood lipids and bone mineral density in postmenopausal women, *Am. J. Clin. Nutr.*, 68, 1375S-1379S, 1998.
91. Ernst, R.L. and Hay, J.W., The U.S. economic and social costs of Alzheimer's revisited, *Am. J. Public Health*, 84, 1261-1264, 1994.

92. Alzheimer's Association. Alzheimer's Disease Statistics Fact Sheet. 1997.
93. Evans, D.A., Estimated prevalence of Alzheimer's disease in the U.S., *Milbank Q.*, (68), 267-289, 1990.
94. American Diabetes Association. Diabetes Facts and Figures. 1999.
95. Shaywitz, S.E., Shaywitz, B.A., Pugh, K.R., Fulbright, R.K., Skudlarski, P., Mencl, W.E., Constable, R.T., Naftolin, F., Palter, S.F., Marchione, K.E., Katz, L., Shankweiler, D.P., Fletcher, J.M., Lacadie, C., Keltz, M., and Gore, J.C., Effect of estrogen on brain activation patterns in postmenopausal women during working memory tasks, *J. Am. Med. Assoc.*, 281, 1197-1202, 1999.
96. Ciocca, D.R. and Vargas Roig, L.M., Estrogen receptors in human nontarget tissues: biological and clinical implications, *Endocrine Rev.*, 16, 35-37, 1995.
97. Sherwin, B.B., Estrogen and cognitive functioning in women, *Proc. Soc. Exp. Biol. Med.*, 217, 17-22, 1998.
98. Yaffe, K., Sawaya, G., Lieberburg, I., and Grady, D., Estrogen therapy in postmenopausal women: effects on cognitive function and dimentia, *J. Am. Med. Assoc.*, 279, 688-695, 1998.
99. Waring, S.C., Rocca, W.A., Peterson, R.C., O'Brien, P.C., Tangalos, E.G., and Kokmen, E., Postmenopausal estrogen replacement therapy and risk of AD, *Neurology*, 52, 965-970, 1999.
100. Kuiper, G.G., Carlsson, B., Grandien, K., Enmark, E., Haggblad, J., Nilsson, S., and Gustafsson, J., Comparison of the ligand binding specificity and transcript tissue distribution of estrogen receptor alpha and beta, *Endocrinology*, 138, 863-870, 1997.
101. Setchell, K.D.R. and Cassidy, A., Dietary isoflavones: biological effects and relevance to human health, *J. Nutr.*, 129, 758S-767S, 1999.
102. White, L., Association of midlife tofu consumption with accelerated brain aging. Third Int. Symp. on the Role of Soy in Preventing and Treating Chronic Disease, 26-27, 1999.
103. Rice, M.M., Graves, A.B., McCurry, S.M., Gibbons, L., Bowen, J., McCormick, W., and Larson, E.B., Tofu consumption and cognition in older Japanese American Men and Women. Third Int. Symp. on the Role of Soy in Preventing and Treating Chronic Disease, 27, 1999.
104. Kim, H., Xia, H., Li, L., and Gewin, J., Modulation of neurodegeneration markers by dietary soy in a primate model of menopause. Third Int. Symp. on the Role of Soy in Preventing and Treating Chronic Disease, 27, 1999.
105. Pan, Y., Anthony, M., and Clarkson, T.B., Effect of estradiol and soy phytoestrogens on choline acetyltransfersase and nerve growth factor mRNA's in the frontal cortex and hippocampus of female rats, *PSEBM*, 221, 118-125, 1999.
106. Weber, K.S., Jacobson, N.A., Setchell, K.D., and Lephart, E.D., Brain aromatase and 5-alpha-reductase, regulatory behaviors and testosterone levels in adult rats on phytoestrogen diets, *Proc. Soc. Exp. Biol. Med.*, 221, 131-135, 1999.

10 Fruits and Vegetables and the Prevention of Oxidative DNA Damage

Kim L. O'Neill, Stephen W. Standage, Bronwyn G. Hughes, and Byron K. Murray

CONTENTS

10.1 INTRODUCTION

Deoxyribonucleic acid (DNA) is found in almost every cell of the human body. This complex molecule governs the development, growth, and activity of every cell therein and is essential to both the life and death of the organism. Changes and mutations to the structure of DNA, introduced by a variety of damages, can disrupt the normal function of the cell and cause many different diseases. Oxidative damage mediated by free radicals is one of the most prevalent insults to DNA integrity and is thought to be a contributing factor in the initiation and progression of a variety of cancers. It has been found that many vegetables and their extracts can play a preventive role in the development of cancer through their antioxidant properties. Popular interest in these developments has led to a massive response by the health-food-supplement industry to provide products touting antioxidant capabilities even though little conclusive evidence has been reached. Because of this, these substances have been the recent subject of intense scientific scrutiny as researchers have attempted to identify the active compounds and elucidate the mechanisms through which they function.

In this chapter, the nature of oxidative DNA damage, the role that vegetables play in disease intervention, and current research topics will be discussed.

0-8493-0038-X/97/$0.00+$.50

10.2 BACKGROUND

DNA is a double-helical molecule made up of two strands that wind around each other in a configuration similar to that of a twisted ladder. The backbone of each strand is made up of five carbon deoxyribose sugars linked together with phosphate groups through phosphodiester bonds. Hydrophobic molecules known as bases are attached to each sugar and directed inward toward the axis of the helix. These bases form hydrogen bonds with the bases on the opposing strand and make up what might be described as the rungs of the ladder. The double helix is held together by these hydrogen bonds and by hydrophobic interactions. In DNA there are four bases: adenine, guanine, cytosine, and thymine, represented, respectively, as A, G, C, and T. In its normal configuration, A binds exclusively to T and G binds exclusively to C. The sequence of these bases on each strand make up what is called the genetic code and it is this code that governs the cellular processes that keep us alive and maintain our health.

Oxidative DNA damage is mediated by substances called free radicals. Free radicals are atoms or molecules that have one or more unpaired electrons in the orbitals of their outer binding shell. These unpaired electrons confer a degree of instability to the radical that is overcome only by filling that orbital with another electron, or by removing the electron that initially inhabited it. Highly electronegative atoms, such as oxygen and nitrogen, cling very tightly to their electrons and are much more likely to acquire electrons than to lose them. The oxygen radicals are commonly known as reactive oxygen species or ROS. Reactive species cause damage to other molecules by stripping them of their electrons in order to fill their own electron orbitals and reach a more stable state. The process of removing an electron from an atom or molecule is called oxidation. The reverse process is called reduction. Those molecules that have their electrons removed by the ROS are thus oxidized and they, as unstable radicals themselves, can strip electrons from yet other molecules. This sets off a chain reaction that can damage lipids, proteins, enzymes, and DNA by changing bond structures, opening rings, removing functional groups, and in the case of DNA, strand breakage. As well, hydrocarbon cross linking in lipid molecules can result in the formation of malondialdehyde, a potent mutagen, which has the ability to translocate to the nucleus and further damage DNA, contributing to cell transformation.

The ROS that induce this oxidative damage come from many endogenous and exogenous sources. Free radicals are produced by the very cellular respiratory mechanisms that create the energy needed for life. In fact, those metabolic pathways that break down the substances taken into the body would not function in the absence of oxygen radicals. For this reason, most life as we know it would cease without the presence of oxygen. As well, specialized cells of the immune system create ROS as part of an "oxidative burst" that they use to destroy invading pathogens. Free radicals can also enter the body from the environment. Cigarette smoke and polluted air have both been shown to carry a great deal of free radicals, as has overcooked meat. Many chemicals and UV light can also generate ROS.

The body has many defense systems to deal with the oxidative stresses that are placed upon it. These include enzymes such as glutathione-*S*-transferase whose function is to catalyze the removal of free radicals from the body, certain proteins called metal chelators that inactivate pro-oxidant metal ions, and various antioxidants absorbed from the diet. Inevitably, some oxidative damage will be created by the free radicals that are not eliminated by these factors. Different excision repair mechanisms correct the damage done to the DNA while other damaged biomolecules are degraded and replaced. None of these mechanisms, however, are one hundred percent foolproof and the damage induced by free radicals can accumulate in the body. This accumulation of oxidative damage is thought to contribute to conditions such as myocardial muscle damage, arteriosclerosis, cancer, cataracts, and even aging.

It has been known for some time that those populations that consume a diet high in fruits and vegetables have better health and suffer far less from cancer and heart disease. Because many vegetable compounds have been shown experimentally to be powerful antioxidants *in vitro*, the scientific community has invested a great deal of time and effort into the research of these substances. In this chapter we will investigate their findings and discuss the applications of the results.

10.3 VITAMINS

Vitamin C (ascorbic acid) and vitamin E (α-tocopherol) both play essential roles in the antioxidant defense of the human body. Vitamin C is a water-soluble component of body fluids while vitamin E is a fat-soluble component of the cellular membrane. Besides its role in the defense against oxidative DNA damage, ascorbic acid plays an essential part in the absorption of iron from the digestive tract by reducing it from ferric iron to ferrous iron. It is also required as a coenzyme for the proper function of several metabolic pathways within the body. The principal function of vitamin E is thought to be antioxidant protection of the cellular membrane, though it may also play a role in membrane stabilization.

Although plants and most animals can synthesize ascorbate from glucose, humans lack the enzyme that completes the terminal step of that pathway, and, for that reason, ascorbate must be obtained from the diet. Vitamin C is provided for in the human diet by a number of fruits and vegetables, with citrus fruits containing the highest concentration of this vitamin. Its importance to the normal function of the body has long been evident from the condition caused by vitamin C deficiency. A disease known as scurvy regularly afflicted armies and navies whose rations were inadequately stocked with the foods that provide the vitamin C they needed. It wasn't until the eighteenth century, when John Lind, a surgeon of the British Royal Navy, added oranges and lemons to the diets of sailors suffering from scurvy, that it was discovered that those fruits would cure and prevent the onset of that sickness.

Ascorbic acid derives its antioxidant functions from its ability to reduce other compounds. Ascorbic acid has two electrons that it donates to radical species, thus stabilizing them and quenching their reactivity. This activity, in itself, prevents oxidative damage, but the process of reducing other compounds oxidizes ascorbic acid to become dehydroascorbate or DHA, which has been shown to arrest the cell cycle at the G2/M DNA damage checkpoint.[1] Recent studies have also shown that vitamin C can upregulate the function of DNA repair enzymes.[2,3] Although the exact mechanisms of these actions are unknown, the effects that they bring about could greatly influence the development of cancer by stopping cellular division long enough for DNA repair enzymes to correct any damage introduced by ROS before the cell continues on to divide.

Because of its water solubility and its ability to enter cells via a Na^{2+}/ascorbic acid cotransporter, vitamin C is ubiquitous in all body fluids. Due to its prevalence in both intra- and extracellular fluids, ascorbic acid can scavenge many kinds of ROS produced from endogenous sources as well as those absorbed from the environment.[4,5] This action confers a great deal of protection against free radical attack on the biomolecules of the body and may be significant for smokers who inhale vast numbers of free radicals in each puff from cigarettes. Although some reports are inconclusive and contradictory,[6,7] it appears that ascorbic acid can be a very effective scavenger of free radicals introduced to the body from cigarette smoke.[8,9]

Another way in which vitamin C is thought to prevent oxidative DNA damage is through its interactions with vitamin E. Vitamin E is a fat-soluble molecule found in many plant oils, with wheat germ oil being the most notable among them. Because of its hydrophobic nature, it forms an important component of the cellular membrane where it protects against lipid peroxidation. ROS introduce damage to the membrane by creating lipid radical chain reactions in the membrane that α-tocopherol quenches. In this process α-tocopherol is oxidized to an inactive state and thus cannot provide further protection against attacks by ROS. Vitamin C recycles vitamin E by reducing it to its active state and in this way reestablishes the antioxidant protection of the cell membrane.[10] Recent studies have shown that dietary vitamin E supplementation can reduce baseline levels of intrinsic DNA damage. As well, it has been shown to be effective against damage done to DNA initiated by both H_2O_2 and ROS created by radiation exposure.[11-13]

Although both vitamin C and vitamin E have been noted for their antioxidant capabilities, it has been known that ascorbate, especially, has the ability to generate free radicals in the presence of metal ions *in vitro*. Indeed, a classic reaction used in the laboratory uses Fe(III), ascorbate, and H_2O_2 to create hydroxyl radicals. Vitamin E can also produce superoxide radicals in the presence of Cu(II) via the reduction of Cu(II) to Cu(I) and the production of H_2O_2 from molecular oxygen.[14] *In vitro* these radicals induce extensive damage to DNA, lipids, and proteins. Because of the pro-oxidant actions of these vitamins, questions have been raised as to whether the nature of vitamin supplementation, as well as vitamin cosupplementation with iron, is truly beneficial.

Much research has been done to discover if those pro-oxidant effects have any relevance physiologically *in vivo*. There is no evidence that excess vitamin supplementation in itself can cause DNA damage. The kidney filters these substances out of the bloodstream and reabsorbs what is needed. The cells that mediate the reabsorption are saturated at a certain concentration and any excess vitamin is simply excreted in the urine. In this manner, the body maintains a constant vitamin level. It is doubtful that any pro-oxidant effects of vitamins would be evident *in vivo,* because the concentration of metal ions in body fluids is tightly regulated. Metal ions are either bound by chelators that inhibit their catalytic action in solution or sequestered by cells and thus not permitted to circulate under normal conditions. Although some studies suggest an initial increase in oxidative DNA damage with initiation of supplementation,[15,16] the great majority show no indication whatsoever that vitamin C or E act as pro-oxidants under physiologic conditions.[17-24] These studies all indicate that vitamins C and E maintain their effectiveness against ROS-induced damage in the presence of metal ions and that any pro-oxidant actions are masked by their antioxidant functions.

10.4 ISOPRENOIDS

Isoprenoids comprise a large family of compounds synthesized from joining multiple numbers of 5-carbon isopentyl building blocks. These compounds include those responsible for fragrances of many plants. For example, myrcene from bay leaves consists of two isoprene units, likewise, limonene from lemon oil. Isoprenoids are also known for their color as well as fragrance. The colors of carrots and tomatoes comes from one group of isoprenoids known as carotenoids. Two carotenoids, lycopene and β-carotene, are responsible for the colors in tomatoes and carrots, respectively. Carotenoids can be found in high quantities in such vegetables as tomatoes, carrots, and spinach as well as in fruits such as peaches and oranges. More than 600 members of the carotenoid family have been identified and several are precursors of vitamin A and retinoic acid. Vitamin A has an essential function as a coenzyme with the protein opsin in the photoreceptor cells of the eye. A deficiency of this factor can cause night blindness, or in more severe, untreated cases, permanent blindness. Vitamin A is also needed for the normal growth of epithelial tissue and bones. Beyond these capacities, isoprenoid molecules have demonstrated antioxidant capabilities *in vitro*, indicating their possible participation in that protective role.

The most distinctive identifier of the carotenoid family is its long chain of 40 carbon atoms, such as in lycopene, linked together by alternating double and single bonds. This chain is often checklisted at one or both ends, as in β-carotene, to form six carbon rings that can be variously substituted. Because of its long hydrophobic chain, members of the carotenoid family are found principally in the cell membrane and bound to hydrophobic amino acid residues of cellular proteins. The hydrophobic nature of carotenoids pose absorption and distribution problems for the human body, whose internal milieu is distinctively aqueous. It is likely for this reason that of the 600 identified members of the carotenoid family, only 34 have been found in human blood.[25]

The proposed antioxidant capacity of these compounds, as well as their ability to induce gap junctions in cells, is thought to play an inhibitory role in cancer. Gap junctions are created by the polymerization of six connexin proteins to form a transmembrane pore between two cells that allows the free interchange of ions and small molecular weight compounds, such as nutrients and important signal molecules. This intercellular signaling has been called gap junction communication and is essential to the normal maintenance of the cell. Tumor-promoting compounds are effective inhibitors of this communication, whereas certain carotenoids can induce the formation of these gap junctions and prevent carcinogenesis in chemically transformed cells.[26] β-carotene demonstrates another very interesting defense against carcinogenesis in its activation of the natural killer (NK) cells of the immune system. These cells perform an essential surveillance function in the body by killing transformed cells. β-carotene supplementation increases the cytotoxicity of NK cells against their cancerous target cells, which can prevent metastasis and tumor formation. This effect is especially marked in elderly men whose NK cell activity has decreased because of age.[27-28] It has also been shown that carotenoid supplementation can enhance DNA repair mechanisms.[29-32] It appears that these functions are independent of any antioxidant actions of the carotenoid molecule.

Increased consumption of fruits and vegetables has been shown to augment the resistance to oxidative damage *in vivo*.[32,33] In addition, *in vitro* carotenoids are effective free-radical scavengers and quench lipid peroxidation reactions efficiently. These properties would indicate their possible use as dietary supplements to prevent oxidative damage, but recent intervention studies presented the scientific community with equivocal, and even contrary, results. The most dramatic example had to do with β-carotene. Several independent studies were undertaken to assess the ability of β-carotene to reduce the occurrence of cancer among smokers and other high-risk populations. These studies found that β-carotene either had no effect on lung cancer or that the incidence of lung cancer in groups taking the supplementation actually increased over those that didn't![34-37] Other studies have also shown that oxidative DNA damage is not significantly affected by supplementation with a single carotenoid above the normal blood serum levels of an individual already consuming a carotenoid-rich diet.[38-40] The greater carotenoid concentration confers no extra protection. Studies, however, that supplement the diet with whole fruits and vegetables or their products, without isolating a single compound, repeatedly demonstrate effective inhibition of oxidative damage.[32,33,41] These results indicate that it is likely that a mixture of various carotenoids and other compounds work synergistically to impart an antioxidant protection to the body. It would greatly profit future researchers to investigate which combinations of molecules confer that protection.

10.5 FLAVONOIDS AND OTHER POLYPHENOLIC COMPOUNDS

Flavonoids are a group of compounds found extensively in the plant kingdom, occurring universally in vascular plants. These compounds can be found in fruits, vegetables, oils, spices, herbs, nuts, seeds, as well as in teas and wines. Literally thousands have been identified and, like the carotenoids, one of their main functions is to provide color to the plant. They are present in the flowers, stems, leaves, and fruits and give them brilliant shades of blue, scarlet, and orange. Unlike the carotenoids, however, flavonoid molecules have a distinctive structure consisting of multiple phenolic rings that are usually substituted by hydroxyl groups. The arrangement of those groups determines in large part the function of the molecule. Because of their ubiquitous nature in the human diet, they have the potential for far greater impact on the oxidative status of an individual than other molecules.

Flavonoids and other polyphenolic compounds can perform very many biological functions. Beyond their antioxidant capacities, they are known to exhibit anti-inflammatory, anti-allergic, antimicrobial, hepatoprotective, and antiviral abilities.

In addition, flavonoid molecules act through a variety of mechanisms to defend the body from ROS-mediated oxidative damage. The first of these is their ability to act as metal cation chelators. When two hydroxyl groups are proximally substituted on the phenol ring, their conformation provides a binding capability that can lock metal ions in an inactive state. This prevents those metal ions from catalyzing the oxidative reactions that damage the cell and its biomolecules. This sort of activity has been observed for years, but recently has been indicated as the main mode of action for quercetin, one of the most prevalent flavonoids in the human diet.[42] Recent studies have elucidated a new nonantioxidant mechanism through which silymarin and other members of the flavonoid family prevent the proliferation of cancer cells.[43,44] Many cancer-inducing factors stimulate tyrosine kinase, an important intracellular signal transduction enzyme, through various growth receptors on the membrane, to initiate changes in the cellular management that can drive a cell to transform. When tyrosine kinase is activated, it initiates a signal cascade terminating in the production of cell growth proteins. Silymarin inhibits tyrosine kinase activity, arrests the cell cycle at the G2/M checkpoint, and stops DNA synthesis and cell growth. These actions provide a potent anticancer weapon that should be explored in further research.

Many flavonoids and polyphenols also have free-radical scavenging capabilities, though their effectiveness varies greatly from one compound to another. Quercetin and various procyanidins derived from grape seed extract have been proven to be powerful scavengers of ROS and inhibitors of carcinogenesis.[45-50] As well, potent polyphenolic compounds have been isolated from olive oil,[51] which likely contribute to the traditionally low levels of prostate and colon cancers in the Mediterranean Basin where olive oil forms a substantial part of the diet. Just as flavonoids and polyphenols resemble vitamin C in their antioxidant properties, they also exhibit pro-oxidant tendencies.[52,53] Those tendencies, however, again seem to be irrelevant under physiologic conditions.[54]

There is a great deal of ongoing investigation in the field of flavonoid and polyphenolic antioxidant research. Researchers are trying to isolate chemicals and components from many different plants to test their effectiveness in reducing oxidative damage. Such things as Brussels sprouts, herbs, green tea, and wine are being studied, though little conclusive evidence as to their ability to prevent oxidative DNA damage has been reached. Compounds need to be identified, and their actions understood, before any claims that they improve health or prevent disease can be made.

10.6 ORGANOSULFUR COMPOUNDS

Another group of plant compounds that are pharmacologically active is the organosulfur group that naturally occur in *Allium* species, including garlic, onions, leeks, and shallots.[55,56] Garlic has a long history of containing medicinally active ingredients such as the organosulfur compounds that have been reported to have numerous beneficial health effects including protection from oxidative damage.[57-59]

10.7 RESEARCH CHALLENGES

Research in all areas of antioxidant defense has increased exponentially in recent years. Despite all the work, there currently exist several challenges to the studies performed in this field. These difficulties exist not only in the compounds and reactions being examined, which in themselves are highly complex, but in the very tests and procedures used to study them. One of the greatest difficulties in conducting this kind of research is that there is no way to directly measure the amount of DNA damage done to the body as a whole by free radicals. Nor are there ways to directly measure the amount of protection afforded by a specific supplement. Researchers must use indicators, called biomarkers, that merely help them infer what is going on within the body. Oxidized bases such as 8OHdG (8-hydroxydeoxyguanosine), the oxidized product of guanine, is an example of a biomarker. When the DNA is damaged by free radicals, these compounds are cut out of the DNA by various excision repair mechanisms and can be measured in either the blood or the urine. These are not direct measures, though, of DNA damage because they represent only a balance between the rate at which those bases are being oxidized and the rate at which they are being repaired. For example, if an oxidative stress were placed on a cell, ROS damage would accumulate in the DNA, but if DNA repair mechanisms were not functioning, no oxidized bases would be detected as biomarkers. In addition, if DNA repair mechanisms were upregulated in other cells, oxidized bases would be detected from the repair of previously damaged DNA even though those cells were not under current oxidative stress. Both of these scenarios can lead to faulty conclusions by the researcher.

The tests themselves are prone to error. HPLC (High Performance Liquid Chromatography) and GC/MS (Gas Chromatography/Mass Spectroscopy), the two tests that measure these products, though exquisitely sensitive, are prone to variation themselves. Small procedural discrepancies between one lab and another will frequently result in differences in the data. A slightly more effective way of measuring oxidative damage is to draw lymphocytes from the blood and run a single-cell gel electrophoresis or comet assay. This technique allows the researcher to literally visualize the damage done to the DNA of each lymphocyte.[60] However, because each lab uses different equipment and because the criteria used to score the damage done to the cell are not conserved between research groups, many discrepancies arise here as well. The scientific community has not established a way to rate the damage equally and this creates, at times, a problem of arbitrary units. Thus, results can be compared and trends seen within a study, but comparisons between studies are hindered. The very act of running any of these tests can introduce artifactual damage into the DNA that can skew the data and lead to false conclusions.

Finally, in intervention studies that use whole vegetables or vegetable products without isolating a specific substance, it is difficult for the researcher to ascertain if the observed results were caused by a single compound or many working synergistically. These are a few of the current obstacles that hinder the progress of our understanding of oxidative DNA damage. Future research whose focus is to develop a more direct measure of oxidative damage would profit this field of study. Despite these hurdles, modern science is quickly gaining insight and understanding of the sources of oxidative DNA damage and its prevention.

10.8 CONCLUSION

Vegetables and fruits provide a wealth of protective substances that defend against the oxidative species that attack our DNA from both within and without. Though we do not yet understand all of the mechanisms by which the DNA damage or defense is mediated, much has been discovered. Many substances found in fruits and vegetables play a protective role against free-radical oxidation and the development of cancer that can ensue because of it. For that reason, it is important to incorporate generous portions of fruits and vegetables in our diet.

REFERENCES

1. Bijur, G.N., Briggs, B., Hitchcock, C.L., and Williams, M.V., Ascorbic acid-dehydroascorbate induces cell cycle arrest at G2/M DNA damage checkpoint during oxidative stress, *Environ. Mol. Mutagen.*, 1999; 33(2): 144-52.
2. Cooke, M.S., Evans, M.D., Podmore, I.D., Herbert, K.E., Mistry, N., Mistry, P., Hickenbotham, P.T., Hussieni, A., Griffiths, H.R., and Lunec, J., Novel repair action of vitamin C upon *in vivo* oxidative DNA damage, *FEBS Lett.*, 1998; 439(3): 363-7.
3. Konopacka, M., Widel, M., and Rzeszowska-Wolny, J., Modifying effect of vitamins C, E and beta-carotene against gamma-ray-induced DNA damage in mouse cells, *Mutat. Res.*, 1998; 417(2-3): 85-94.
4. Panayiotidis, M. and Collins, A.R., Ex vivo assessment of lymphocyte antioxidant status using the comet assay, *Free Rad. Res.*, 1997; 27(5): 533-7.
5. Sweetman, S.F., Strain, J.J., and McKelvey-Martin V.J., Effect of antioxidant vitamin supplementation on DNA damage and repair in human lymphoblastoid cells, *Nutr. Cancer*, 1997; 27(2): 122-30.
6. Prieme, H., Loft, S., Nyyssonen, K., Salonen, J.T., and Poulsen, H.E., No effect of supplementation with vitamin E, ascorbic acid, or coenzyme Q10 on oxidative DNA damage estimated by 8-oxo-7,8-dihydro-2'-deoxyguanosine excretion in smokers, *Am. J. Clin. Nutr.*, 1997; 65(2): 503-7.
7. Lee, B.M., Lee, S.K., and Kim, H.S., Inhibition of oxidative DNA damage, 8-OhdG, and carbonyl contents in smokers treated with antioxidants (vitamin E, vitamin C, beta-carotene and red ginseng), *Cancer Lett.*, 1998; 132(1-2): 219-27.
8. Howard, D.J., Ota, R.B., Briggs, L.A., Hampton, M., and Pritsos, C.A., Oxidative stress induced by environmental tobacco smoke in the workplace is mitigated by antioxidant supplementation, *Cancer Epidemiol. Biomarkers. Prev.*, 1998; 7(11): 981-8.
9. Duthie, S.J., Ma, A., Ross, M.A., and Collins, A.R., Antioxidant supplementation decreases oxidative DNA damage in human lymphocytes, *Cancer Res.*, 1996; 56(6): 1291-5.
10. May, J.M., Is ascorbic acid an antioxidant for the plasma membrane?, *FASEB J.*, 1999; 13(9): 995-1006.

11. Slamenova, D., Horvathova, E., Kosikova, B., Ruzekova, L., and Labaj, J., Detection of lignin biopolymer- and vitamin E-stimulated reduction of DNA strand breaks in H2O2- and MNNG-treated mammalian cells by the comet assay, *Nutr. Cancer*, 1999; 33(1): 88-94.
12. Hughes, C.M., Lewis, S.E., McKelvey-Martin, V.J., and Thompson, W., The effects of antioxidant supplementation during Percoll preparation on human sperm DNA integrity, *Hum. Reprod.*, 1998; 13(5): 1240-7.
13. Lunec, J., Podmore, I.D., Griffiths, H.R., Herbert, K.E., Mistry, N., and Mistry, P., Effects of vitamin E supplementation on *in vivo* oxidative DNA damage, Dizdaroglu, M., Karakaya, A.E., Eds., *Advances in DNA Damage and Repair: Oxygen Radical Effects, Cellular Protection, and Biological Consequences*, New York, Kluwer Academic/Plenum Press, 283-294, 1999.
14. Yamashita, N., Murata, M., Inoue, S., Burkitt, M.J., Milne, L., and Kawanishi, S., α-Tocopherol induces oxidative damage to DNA in the presence of copper(II) ions, *Chem. Res. Toxicol.*, 1998; 11(8): 855-62.
15. Paolini, M., Pozzetti, L., Pedulli, G.F., Marchesi, E., and Cantelli-Forti, G., The nature of prooxidant activity of vitamin C, *Life Sci.*, 1999; 64(23): PL 273-8.
16. Rehman, A., Collis, C.S., Yang, M., Kelly, M., Diplock, A.T., Halliwell, B., and Rice-Evans, C. The effects of iron and vitamin C co-supplementation on oxidative damage to DNA in healthy volunteers, *C*, 1998; 246(1): 293-8.
17. Gerster, H., High-dose vitamin C: a risk for persons with high iron stores?, *Int. J. Vitam. Nutr. Res.*, 1999; 69(2): 67-82.
18. Yang, M., Collis, C.S., Kelly, M., Diplock, A.T., and Rice-Evans, C., Do iron and vitamin C co-supplementation influence platelet function or LDL oxidizability in healthy volunteers?, *Eur. J. Clin. Nutr.*, 1999; 53(5): 367-74.
19. Crott, J.W. and Fenech, M., Effect of vitamin C supplementation on chromosome damage, apoptosis and necrosis ex vivo, *Carcinogenesis*, 1999; 20(6): 1035-41.
20. Collis, C.S., Yang, M., Diplock, A.T., Hallinan, T., and Rice-Evans, C.A., Effects of co-supplementation of iron with ascorbic acid on antioxidant--pro-oxidant balance in the guinea pig, *Free Rad. Res.*, 1997; 27(1): 113-21.
21. Berger, T.M., Polidori, M.C., Dabbagh, A., Evans, P.J., Halliwell, B., Morrow, J.D., Roberts, L.J., II, and Frei, B., Antioxidant activity of vitamin C in iron-overloaded human plasma, *J. Biol. Chem.*, 1997; 272(25): 15656-60.
22. Lucesoli, F. and Fraga, C.G., Oxidative stress in testes of rats subjected to chronic iron intoxication and alpha-tocopherol supplementation, *Toxicology,* 1999; 132(2-3): 179-86.
23. Bartfay, W.J., Hou, D., Brittenham, G.M., Bartfay, E., Sole, M.J., Lehotay, D., and Liu, P.P., The synergistic effects of vitamin E and selenium in iron-overloaded mouse hearts, *Can. J. Cardiol.*, 1998; 14(7): 937-41.
24. Carr, A. and Frei, B., Does vitamin C act as a pro-oxidant under physiological conditions?, *FASEB J.,* 1999; 13(9): 1007-24.
25. Khachik, F., Spangler, C., Smith, J.C., Jr., Identification, quantification and relative concentrations of carotenoids and their metabolites in human milk and serum, *Anal. Chem.*, 1997; 69(10): 1873-81.
26. Stahl, W., Nicolai, S., Briviba, K., Hanusch, M., Broszeit, D., Peters, M., Martin, H.D., and Sies, H., Biological activities of natural and synthetic carotenoids: Induction of gap junctional communication and singlet oxygen quenching, *Carcinogenesis*, 1997; 18(1): 89-92.

27. Carlos, T.F., Riondel, J., Mathieu, J., Guiraud, P., Mestries, J.C., and Favier, A., β-Carotene enhances natural killer cell activity in athymic mice, *In Vivo*, 1997; 11: 87-91.
28. Santos, M., Meydani, S.N., Leka, L., Wu, D., Fotouhi, N., Meydani, M., Hennekens, C.H., Gaziano, J.M., Natural killer cell activity in elderly men is enhanced by β-carotene supplementation, *Am. J. Clin. Nutr.*, 1996; 63:772-7.
29. Sheng, Y., Pero, R.W., Olson, A.R., Bryngellsson, C., and Hua, J., DNA repair enhancement by a combined supplement of carotenoids, nicotinamide and zinc, *Cancer Detect. Prev.*, 1998; 22(4): 284-92.
30. De Flora, S., Bagnasco, M., and Vainio, H., Modulation of genotoxic and related effects by carotenoids and vitamin A in experimental models: mechanical issues, *Mutagenesis*, 1999; 14(2): 153-72.
31. Pool-Zobel, B.L., Bub, A., Muller, H., Wollowski, I., and Rechkemmer, G., Consumption of vegetables reduces genetic damage in humans: first results of a human intervention trial with carotenoid-rich foods, *Carcinogenesis*, 1997; 18(9): 1847-1850.
32. Pool-Zobel, B.L., Bub, A., Leigibel, U.M., Treptow-van Lishaut, S., and Rechkemmer, G., Mechanisms by which vegetable consumption reduces genetic damage in humans, *Cancer Epidemiol. Biomarkers Prev.*, 1998; 7(10): 891-899.
33. Cao, G., Booth, S.L., Sadaeski, J.A., and Prior, R.L., Increases in human plasma antioxidant capacity after consumption of controlled diets high in fruit and vegetables, *Am. J. Clin. Nutr.,* 1998; 68: 1081-7.
34. Rowe, P.M., Beta-carotene takes a collective beating, *Lancet*, 1996; 347: 249.
35. Omen, S.G., et.al., Effects of a combination of beta carotene and vitamin A on lung cancer and cardiovascular disease, *N. Engl. J. Med.*, 1996; 234(18): 1150-5.
36. Von Poppel, G., Poulsen, H., Loft, S., and Verhagen, H., No influence of beta carotene on oxidative DNA damage in male smokers, *J. Nat. Cancer Inst.*, 1995; 87(4): 310-1.
37. α-Tocopherol, β-Carotene Prevention Study Group. The effect of vitamin E and beta carotene on the incidence of lung cancer and other cancers in male smokers, *N. Engl. J. Med.*, 1994; 330(15): 1029-35.
38. Collins, A.R., Gedik, C.M., Olmedilla, B., Southon, S., and Bellizzi, M., Oxidative DNA damage measured in human lymphocytes: large differences between sexes and between countries, and correlations with heart disease mortality rates, *FASEB J.*, 1998; 12(13): 1397-400.
39. Lowe, G.M., Booth, L.A., Young, A.J., and Bilton, R.F., Lycopene and beta-carotene protect against oxidative damage in HT29 cells at low concentrations but rapidly lose this capacity at higher doses, *Free Rad. Res.*, 1999; 30(2): 141-51.
40. Collins, A.R., Olmedilla, B., Southon, S., Granado, F., and Duthie, S.J., Serum carotenoids and oxidative DNA damage in human lymphocytes, *Carcinogenesis*, 1998; 19(12): 2159-62.
41. Riso, P., Pinder, A., Santangelo, A., and Porrini, M., Does tomato consumption effectively increase the resistance of lymphocyte DNA oxidative damage?, *Am. J. Clin. Nutr.*, 1999; 69(4): 712-8.
42. Sestili, P., Guidarelli, A., Dacha, M., and Cantoni, O., Quercetin prevents DNA single strand breakage and cytotoxicity caused by tert-butylhydroperoxide: free radical scavenging versus iron chelating mechanism, *Free Rad. Biol. Med.*, 1998; 25(2): 196-200.

43. Ahmad, N., Gali, H., Javed, S., and Agarwal, R., Skin cancer chemopreventive effects of a flavonoid antioxidant silymarin are mediated via impairment of receptor tyrosine kinase signaling and perturbation in the cell cycle progression, *Biochem. Biophys. Res. Commun.*, 1998; 247(2): 294-301.
44. Liang, Y., Huang, Y., Tsai, S., Lin-Shiau, S., Chen, C., and Lin, J., Suppression of inducible cyclooxygenase and inducible nitric oxide synthase by apigenin and related flavonoids in mouse macrophages, *Carcinogenesis*, 1999; 20(10): 1945-1952.
45. Noroozi, M., Angerson, W.J., and Lean M.E., Effects of flavonoids and vitamin C on oxidative DNA damage to human lymphocytes, *Am. J. Clin. Nutr.*, 1998; 67: 1210-8.
46. Duthie, S.J. and Dobson, V.L., Dietary flavonoids protect human colonocyte DNA from oxidative attack in vitro, *Z. Ernahrungswiss*, 1999; 38(1): 28-34.
47. Zhao, J., Wang, J., Chen, Y., and Agarwal, R., Anti-tumor-promoting activity of a polyphenolic fraction isolated from grape seeds in the mouse skin two-stage intitiation–promotion protocol and identification of procyanidin b5-3'-gallate as the most effective antioxidant constituent, *Carcinogenesis*, 1999; 20(9): 1737-1745.
48. Lean, M.E., Norooz, M., Kelly, I., Burns, J., Talwar, D., Sattar, N., and Crozier, A., Dietary flavonols protect diabetic human lymphocytes against oxidative damage to DNA, *Diabetes*, 1999; 48(1): 176-81.
49. Duthie, S.J., Collins, A.R., Duthie, G.G., and Dobson, V.L., Quercetin and myricetin protect against hydrogen peroxide-induced DNA damage (strand breaks and oxidised pyrimidines) in human lymphocytes, *Mutat. Res.*, 1997; 393(3): 223-31.
50. Musonda, C.A. and Chipman, J.K., Quercetin inhibits hydrogen peroxide (H_2O_2)-induced NF-kappaB DNA binding activity and DNA damage in HepG2 cells, *Carcinogenesis*, 1998; 19(9): 1583-9.
51. Visioli, F., Bellomo, G., and Galli, C., Free radical scavenging properties of olive oil polyphenols, *Biochem. Biophys. Res. Commun.*, 1998; 247(1): 60-64.
52. Yamashita, N., Tanemura, H., and Kawanishi, S., Mechanism of oxidative DNA damage induced by quercetin in the presence of Cu(II), *Mutat. Res.*, 1999; 425(1): 107-15.
53. Moran, J.F., Klucas, R.V., Grayer, R.J., Abian, J., and Becana, M., Complexes of iron with phenolic compounds from soybean nodules and other legume tissues: prooxidant and antioxidant properties, *Free Rad. Biol. Med.*, 1997; 22(5): 861-70.
54. Ohshima, H., Yoshie, Y., Auriol, S., and Gilibert, I., Antioxidant and pro-oxidant actions of flavonoids: effects on DNA damage induced by nitric oxide, peroxynitrite and nitroxyl anion, *Free Rad. Biol. Med.*, 1998; 25(9): 1057-65.
55. Fenwick, G.R. and Hanley, A.B., The genus *Allium*, *CRC Crit., Rev. Food Sci. Nutr.*, 1985; 22: 199.
56. Fenwick, G.R. and Hanley, A.B., The genus *Allium*, Part 2, *CRC Crit., Rev. Food Sci. Nutr.*, 1985; 22: 273.
57. Siegers, C.P., Robke, A., and Pentz, R., Effects of garlic preparations on superoxide production by phorbol ester activated granulocytes, *Phytomedicine*, 1999; 6: 13-26.
58. Munday, J.S., James, K.A., Fray, L.M., Kirkwood, S.W., and Thompson, K.G., Daily supplementation with aged garlic extract, but not raw garlic, protects low density lipoprotein against in vitro oxidation, *Atherosclerosis*, 1999; 143: 399-404.
59. Dwivedi, C., John, L.M., Schmidt, D.S., and Engineer, F.N., Effects of oil-soluble organosulfur compounds from garlic on doxorubicin-induced lipid peroxidation, *Anticancer Drugs*, 1998; 9: 291-4.
60. Fairbairn, D.W., Olive, P.L., and O'Neill, K.L., The comet assay: a comprehensive review, *Mutat. Res.*, 1995; 339: 37-59.

11 Health Benefits of Fruits and Vegetables: The Protective Role of Phytonutrients

John A. Wise

CONTENTS

11.1 INTRODUCTION

For the past two decades there has been increasing recognition of the health benefits of consuming diets rich in fruits and vegetables. Early studies by Wattenberg[1] focused awareness on the potential role of dietary constituents in prevention of cancer. In animal studies, he investigated the inhibition of several chemically induced cancers by a wide range of natural compounds in human food.[2] In 1982, the Food and Nutrition Board of the National Academy of Sciences examined the role of diet and cancer, concluding that important phytonutrients present in foods may decrease the risk of cancer.[3] Subsequently, numerous research studies of different types have demonstrated a strong association between phytonutrients from fruits and vegetables

0-8493-0038-X/97/$0.00+$.50

TABLE 11.1
Reduction of Chronic Disease Risk Associated with Consumption of Fruit and Vegetables

Disease	Ref.
Cancer	10–12
Cardiovascular Disease	13–21
Stroke	20–22
Osteoporosis	23–25
Macular Degeneration	26–29
Cataracts	30–31
Neurodegeneration	32–38
Alzheimer's Disease	
Parkinson's Disease	
Amyotrophic Lateral Sclerosis	
Diabetes	39–43

and the reduction in the risk of not only cancer, but of several chronic diseases.[4-7] These include coronary heart disease, stroke, vascular pathologies, neurodegenerative diseases, diabetes, hypertension, cataracts, macular degeneration, and osteoporosis (Table 11.1).

The majority of studies associating degenerative health conditions to low consumption of fruits and vegetables are found in the epidemiological literature. However, a more limited number of experimental dietary studies in humans rely on intermediate end points related to disease risk by using biological markers.[8,9] These biomarkers also serve as important corollaries between studies in animal models and cell cultures, and nutritional epidemiological studies. The ability of phytonutrients from fruits and vegetables to provide protective effects are related to modulation of biomarkers, which reflect mechanisms of action and will be considered later.

11.2 HEALTH BENEFITS OF FRUITS AND VEGETABLES: EPIDEMIOLOGICAL EVIDENCE

The correlative evidence for the protective effect of fruits and vegetables comes from case-control and cohort studies. In a recent review of epidemiological studies it was concluded that consumption of greater quantities of fruits and vegetables is associated consistently with reduced risk of cancer. Block et al. reviewed over 200 studies investigating the relationship between fruit and vegetable intake and various cancers.[10] It was reported that statistically significant protective effects of fruit and vegetable consumption were found in 128 of the 156 dietary studies reporting relative risk. For most cancer sites, individuals consuming low amounts of fruit and vegetables had about twice the risk of cancer compared to those with a higher intake. More recently, studies examining individual vegetable consumption reported decreases in cancer risk. Giovannucci and Clinton reported that consumption of tomatoes reduced prostate cancer in men, primarily attributable to the active constituent, lycopene,[11] and broccoli sprouts have been shown to possess inhibitors against chemical carcinogens.[12]

The benefit of fruits and vegetables for stroke and cardiovascular prevention has been identified with dietary fiber for over three decades. These studies demonstrated that dietary fiber in fruits and vegetables lowered total cholesterol and LDL, thereby reducing coronary heart disease (CHD) risk.[13-16] Recently, there have been new studies showing the benefit of nonfiber components for lowering cardiovascular and stroke risk. Hertog and colleagues have presented a series of papers from their epidemiological studies in The Netherlands. These studies, which span over 25 years, demonstrate a clear relationship between flavonoid intake and CHD and stroke prevention.[17-20] In their seven-country study, the average intake of antioxidant flavonoids was inversely related to mortality from CHD in the 16 cohorts.[19] It was reported that 25% of the variance in CHD rates was attributable to flavonoid intake. In a previous study, dietary flavonoid intake was assessed in 805 elderly men, ages 65 to 84, over 5 years. Flavonoid intake was significantly inversely associated with mortality from CHD and modestly associated with myocardial infarction.[17] The consumption of apples, tea, and onions was found to be associated with lower CHD risk in this elderly population. In a prospective study of over 34,000 postmenopausal women in a mid-western U.S. state, total flavonoid intake was associated with decreased deaths from CHD.[21]

Hertog and colleagues also investigated the impact of flavonoid intake on the risk of stroke. Dietary flavonoid consumption among individuals was ranked by quartiles with the higher the quartile of flavonoid intake reflecting the lower the risk of stroke.[20] More recently, questionnaire survey data from the Nurses' Health Study (NHS) and the Health Professional's Follow-up Study (HPFS) were analyzed to determine the incidence of ischemic stroke in relation to fruit and vegetable intake.[22] This data set consisted of over 170,000 male and female health professionals with an age range of 35 to 75 years. Citrus fruits and fruit juices as well as cruciferous and green leafy vegetables were inversely associated with ischemic stroke in both cohorts. The authors concluded that no single constituent within a fruit and vegetable diet could be linked to their findings. They suggest that it is more realistic to expect that synergistic effects related to dietary fiber, flavonoids, potassium, folate, and lifestyle contributed to the observed risk reduction.

Several papers now report that higher fruit and vegetable consumption is associated with reduced osteoporosis and better bone health. In 1999, Tucker et al. reviewed data from the original cohort from the Framingham Heart Study.[23] This information was collected over a four-year period and showed that both potassium and magnesium intake from fruits and vegetables were highly correlated to bone mineral density (BMD). In fact, fruit and vegetable intake was associated with greater BMD at three sites for men and two sites for women. New and colleagues in the U.K. corroborated these findings.[24] A total of 65 women were screened for menses cycle, endocrine and hormonal status, and lifestyle. After successful enrollment in the study, the women underwent measures of bone mass, bone marker metabolism (e.g., serum pyridinoline, deoxypyridinoline, osteocalcin), and dietary intake by a food-frequency questionnaire. Low intakes of beta-carotene, potassium, magnesium, and vitamin C from dietary sources were associated with increased bone resorption and poorer bone health. The authors indicated that the negative relationship found between vitamin C intake and bone resorption was important due to ascorbic acid's role in the hydroxylation of proline and lysine residues. Hydroxylysine is involved in normal cross-linking in collagen fiber formation. This may explain earlier data indicating that women aged 55 to 64 who used vitamin C supplements for greater than 10 years had higher bone mineral density than nonusers.[25]

The use of generalized cohort surveys provides information pertaining to long-term diet and lifestyle trends and the impact on health. In particular, the first National Health and Nutrition Examination Survey (NHANES) in 1971 and 1972 was instrumental in identifying factors pertaining to age-related macular degeneration. It was this study that reported the benefit of eating foods rich in vitamin A.[26] A multicenter study using five ophthalmology centers in the U.S. reported that those in the top quintile of carotenoid intake had a 43% lower risk for age-related macular degeneration.[27] It was the specific carotenoids (e.g., lutein and zeaxanthin) found in green leafy vegetables that provided the strongest association with this risk reduction. It has been recently reported that fruits and vegetables of various colors and varieties contain appreciable amounts of lutein and zeaxanthin, which are thought to help combat the onset of age-related macular degeneration.[28]

Besides macular degeneration, cataract formation is another common malady associated with aging. Anderson et al.[29] postulated that many ocular diseases are related to free-radical-induced lipid peroxidation. These authors suggested that individuals limit the amount of direct sunlight exposure to the eyes and encourage increased consumption of fruits and vegetables.

One epidemiological study examined the relationship between antioxidant nutrient status and risk for senile cataracts. Those in the upper percentiles of vitamin C, vitamin E, and carotenoid consumption exhibited lower risk of cataracts, both cortical and subcapsular.[30] It was observed that people consuming fewer than 3.5 servings of fruits and vegetables per day had an increased risk for both types of cataracts. The benefit of consuming dietary lutein and zeaxanthin was reported in a recent study from 36,644 U.S. health professionals.[31] Individuals in the highest quintile of lutein and zeaxanthin intake had a 19% lower risk for cataracts. Specifically, broccoli and spinach were most consistently associated with a lower risk.

While not definitive, there is increasing evidence that reactive oxygen species (ROS) are important in neurodegenerative diseases. There is some basic evidence that free-radical damage is responsible for this degeneration but newer evidence suggests that mediators associated with pro-inflammatory genes may be even more influential.[32] In particular, Alzheimer's Disease is thought to result from inflammatory mechanisms within the microglial cells.[33] Suggestive evidence has been derived from AD patients using anti-inflammatory drugs, which are reported to slow the progression of AD.[34] Neuroprotection is thought to occur from free-radical scavenging such as is associated with vitamin E and other antioxidants.[35] Moreover, oxidative damage is linked to the pathogenesis of neuronal degeneration in amyotrophic lateral sclerosis[36] and Parkinson's disease.[37] In fact, postmortem evidence from Parkinson's patients supports the involvement of oxidative stress. Impaired mitochondrial function, alterations in superoxide dismutase and reduced glutathione, and damage to lipids, proteins, and DNA were reported.[37] While fruit and vegetable consumption has not been shown to correlate positively with mental function, one study showed that low blood levels of riboflavin and folic acid correlated with lower scores on the Halstead-Reitan Categories Test.[38] This nonverbal test is a measure of abstract thinking ability.

Likewise, there have been recent developments in the use of antioxidants for diabetes. It is well documented that diabetics are exposed to a high level of oxidative stress, which leads to organ dysfunction and pathology. One purported mechanism is the role that reactive oxygen species (ROS) play in pancreatic beta-cell death. Ho and Bray[39] reported that pancreatic-specific ROS production plays a critical role by activating the transcription factor, NFKappaB. The ability of antioxidants to inhibit NFKappaB activation is paramount for the prevention of beta-cell death. In mice, it was found that supplementation with vitamins C and E preserved *in vivo* pancreatic beta-cell function.[40] In a diabetic rat model, lipophilic scavengers such as vitamin E, alpha-lipoic acid, and n-acetyl-cysteine were found to reduce or prevent nerve conduction deficit.[41] These findings in regards to preservation of pancreas function are supported by epidemiological studies in humans. A group of 1122 subjects underwent an oral glucose tolerance test, and their food consumption was assessed using a food-frequency questionnaire.[42] Fruit consumption did not provide benefit, but vegetable consumption elicited an inverse relationship with the risk of nondiagnosed noninsulin-dependent diabetes (NIDDM). Moreover, this association was maintained even after adjustment for age, gender, and family history.

A recent study investigated diet patterns between Hispanic Americans consuming a plant-based diet vs. those consuming a meat-based diet in the hopes of identifying patterns of diabetic onset.[43] As would be expected, those individuals consuming a plant-based diet exhibited more favorable blood lipid profiles and lower blood pressures. In addition, these individuals had lower fasting insulin and glucose levels, suggesting lower risk for Type 2 diabetes.

11.3 PHYTONUTRIENTS ASSOCIATED WITH HEALTH PROMOTION

The association of fruit and vegetable consumption and the delay or prevention of chronic disease appears to be attributable to the biological activity of constituent nutrients. Fruits and vegetables are a rich source of vitamins, trace minerals, and dietary fiber as well as a wide variety of biologically active compounds. Due to the botanically diverse families found in dietary fruits and vegetables, over 10,000 bioactive phytonutrients have been identified and are an integral part of the human diet.[44-46] Major classes of phytonutrients include carotenoids, polyphenols, anthocyanins, flavonoids, isothiocyanates, sulfides, and phytosterols[44-46] (Table 11.2). This broad range of natural compounds appears to have dozens of biological functions, which may be overlapping and complementary. Interest in phytonutrients has resulted in identifying mechanisms of action at the cellular or molecular level for many of these compounds (Table 11.3).

TABLE 11.2
Major Phytonutrient Classes from Fruits and Vegetables Associated with Health Promotion

- Carotenoids
- Glucosinolates/Isothiocyanates
- Polyphenols
  - Flavonoids
    - Anthocyanins
    - Bioflavonoids
    - Proanthocyanidins
  - Non-Flavonoids
- Phytoestrogens
- Phenolics/Cyclic Compounds
- Saponins
- Phytosterols
- Sulfide and Thiols

TABLE 11.3
Mechanisms of Action of Phytonutrients Which May Confer Disease Prevention Effects

- Generalized Protective Mechanisms
  - Antioxidative protection
  - Reduction in DNA Damage
  - Improved Immune Function
  - Modulation of Hormones
- Condition-Specific Protection
  - Cancer
    - Modulation of Detoxification Enzymes
    - Inhibition of tumor promotion
    - Blocking angiogenesis
    - P53 Gene Activation
  - Cardiovascular Disease and Stroke
    - Protection of LDL Cholesterol
    - Superoxide Quenchers
    - Nitric Oxide Synthetase Inducers
    - Alteration of Cholesterol Metabolism
    - Homocysteine Control
    - Decreased Platelet Aggregation
    - Control of Blood Pressure
  - Osteoporosis
  - Macular Degeneration and Cataracts

11.4 GENERALIZED PROTECTIVE MECHANISMS

11.4.1 ANTIOXIDATIVE PROTECTION

The antioxidant defense system is essential for protection of cell structures and macromolecules from damage by free radicals, which largely result from normal metabolic processes. This defense system generally declines with age and can be compromised by various forms of oxidative stress resulting from exposure to smoke, drugs, environmental pollutants, radiation, and physical exercise. Current understanding of the antioxidant defense system reveals a highly complex, interactive, multifactorial network which includes vitamins C and E; β-carotene and other carotenoids; enzyme antioxidants dependent on zinc, copper, selenium, or manganese such as superoxide dismutase, glutathione peroxidases; the tripeptide glutathione, alpha lipoic acid; and very likely, numerous phytonutrients. Complex recycling and regeneration reactions must occur to optimize protection from free radicals. Moreover, deficiencies or imbalances may compromise these interactions as well.

Fruits and vegetables are very good sources for nearly all these important antioxidants, and in addition contain thousands of phytonutrients (see Table 11.2). The most widely studied nutrients found in fruits and vegetables are β-carotene, vitamin C, and vitamin E. Their role as antioxidants for exerting a protective effect *in vivo* as well as a preventative role in CVD and cancer has been well established. When disease outcomes of five large studies were correlated with plasma levels of these nutrients, the quintiles with the highest level of β-carotene (>0.22 μg/ml), α-tocopherol (>12.9 μg/ml), and vitamin C (>8.8 μg.ml) showed the lowest risk for both cancer and CVD.[47,48] It is significant that plasma levels conferring the lowest risk compared favorably with various biomarkers representing intermediate end points for risk assessment. The ability of smooth muscle cells to modify LDL cholesterol *ex vivo* was completely inhibited when LDL was derived from plasma with >9.5 ug/ml of vitamin C or vitamin E levels greater than 12.9 μg/ml. And the acute rise in plasma and LDL reactive oxygen species (TBARS) due to smoking 6 cigarettes in 90 min could be eliminated by vitamin C levels of 9.5 μg/ml or 15.1 μg/ml of vitamin E.[47]

Many of these compounds are known to be good antioxidants *in vitro* and are thought to be protective *in vivo* against oxidative damage to cellular components.[49-51] Flavonoids and other phenolic compounds appear to be antioxidants that contribute to the high antioxidant capacity observed in certain fruits and vegetables.[52] Furthermore, some flavonoids have been shown to have many times greater antioxidant capacity than vitamins C or E.[53a] The effects of feeding elderly women strawberries, spinach, red wine, or vitamin C was determined by three methods which measure the antioxidant capacity of serum.[51] A single meal including strawberries, spinach, or red wine increased serum antioxidant capacity to an extent equivalent or greater than a large dose of vitamin C (1250 mg). These increases were attributed to the antioxidant properties of flavonoids and polyphenols, which were effectively absorbed from the single serving.

Similar results were found in a recent study[53b] which showed the total antioxidant activity of a medium-sized apple (150 g) to be equivalent to 2250 mg of vitamin C while the actual vitamin C content of the apple was less than 10 mg. This activity was obtained from whole apple extracts, which demonstrated strong inhibition of human tumor cell proliferation *in vitro*, and was attributed to the phenolic acids and flavonoids present.

Another study examined the effects of supplementing fruit and vegetable extracts over a four-week period. The capsule supplement contained dried fruit juice extracts from oranges, apples, pineapples, papayas, cranberries, and peaches while the vegetable juice extract was from carrots, parsely, beets, broccoli, kale, cabbage, spinach, and tomatoes. Serum lipid peroxide levels decreased from 16.85 to 3.13 μmol/l in the first week and remained unchanged through week 4. Measurement of carotenoids and alpha-tocopherol showed significant increases in plasma levels in the first week, demonstrating the effective uptake of important phytonutrients using this delivery form.[54]

11.4.2 Reduction of DNA Damage

Damage to DNA occurs mainly through free-radical attacks on DNA bases, resulting in base alteration and strand breaks, and possible mutations. Antioxidants have been shown to provide protection against damage in a variety of human studies. In a double blind, placebo-controlled trial in smokers and nonsmokers, a significant decrease in cellular base damage in lymphocyte DNA was demonstrated using a daily supplement of β-carotene (25 mg), vitamin C (100 mg), and α-tocopherol (280 mg).[55] In another study, 23 healthy men consumed a low carotenoid diet for two weeks while supplementing with carrot and tomato juices (33 ml/d) and spinach powder (10 g/d). All subjects demonstrated decreased lymphocyte DNA strand breaks.[56] In the carrot juice intervention, DNA base oxidation was also reversed. In a study using a cross-over design, 10 women (two groups of five) consumed either a tomato-free diet or a diet containing tomato puree standardized to 16.5 mg of lycopene per day for 21 days each.[57] DNA damage in lymphocytes was measured at 0, 21, and 42 days. All subjects demonstrated significant reductions in DNA damage after 21 days of tomato consumption and this protection was correlated with plasma lycopene levels.

A recent study employed supplementation with mixed fruit and vegetable juice extracts in a group of 20 elderly volunteers (mean age = 68). Supplements were taken twice daily for 80 days and resulted in approximately an average four-fold decrease in damage to peripheral lymphocyte DNA. All subjects showed protective effects of supplementation, with similar reduction in DNA damage in both smokers and nonsmokers.[58]

11.4.3 Improved Immune Function

The human immune system plays an indispensable role in protecting against various disease-causing agents as well as mutant or malignant cells. It functions through a complex system of highly interactive cells and bioactive compounds produced by these cells. Many factors can adversely affect immune functions including stress, environmental exposures, aging, and nutritional deficiencies. In fact, essential nutrients and an array of phytonutrients found in fruits and vegetable have been shown to affect almost every aspect of the immune system.[59] Two studies examined the effect of a multivitamin and mineral supplement on immune functions in healthy elderly individuals. Both studies were double blind and placebo controlled, with a duration of 12 months. Chandra[60] demonstrated that the supplement group (n = 48) had increased levels of certain T-cell subsets and natural killer cells, enhanced B-cell activity, increased interleukin-2 production, and higher antibody response and natural killer cell activity. These subjects also had significantly less illness due to infections during the year than the placebo group (n = 48).

In the second study, delayed-hypersensitivity skin test (DHST) responses were measured to a panel of seven recall antigens.[61] The DHST responses were significantly improved in the supplement group (n = 29) but not the placebo group (n = 27), and serum status of multiple nutrients increased in the supplement group but not the placebo group. Using vitamin E supplementation alone for 235 days, DHST response was also improved in healthy elderly individuals compared to the placebo group.[62]

Several studies have demonstrated that supplementation with beta-carotene produced major changes in immune cell numbers or activity levels, at least in elderly subjects. Watson et al.[63] reported that T-helper cells, natural killer cells (NK), and cells with interleukin-2 (IL-2) and transferrin receptors were all substantially increased with two months of β-carotene supplementation and that this response was dose dependent (30 mg or greater per day). In a study in elderly men (aged 65 to 85) over 10–12 years, 50 mg of β-carotene on alternate days resulted in 1.6-fold greater NK cell activity relative to a placebo group.[64] There was no increase in NK cells, IL-2 receptors, or IL-2 production in a group of middle-aged men (51 to 64). The influence of β-carotene on patients with oral leukoplakia was examined after supplementing 30 mg/day.[65] Observed responses included alterations of abnormal epithelial cells and increased plasma levels of tumor necrosis factor-alpha. Selenium, an essential trace mineral, was supplemented to selenium-replete humans with 200 μg/d of sodium selenite for 8 weeks.[66] Increases in IL-2 receptors, cloned expansion, and activity of T-lymphocyte cells were correlated with selenium supplementation in the absence of a selenium-deficient status.

Flavonoids that have demonstrated activity in the human body are particularly abundant in fruits and vegetables. Although information is limited on the absorption, distribution, metabolism, and excretion of these compounds in humans, measurable plasma concentrations are achieved from dietary sources and appear to have meaningful biological activities. A variety of experiments with selected flavonoids have shown anti-allergenic, anti-inflammatory, antiviral, and antioxidant activities, as reviewed by Middleton.[67] As an example, apigenin and related flavonoids were shown to inhibit the activities of inducible cyclooxygenase and inducible nitric oxide synthetase, both involved in antigen-stimulated inflammatory responses. Inhibition occurred by suppression of messenger RNA and protein synthesis; the same mechanism was observed for apigenin inhibition of nuclear factor-kB.

Plant sterols and sterolins are found in fruits and vegetables, and have been shown to have immunomodulatory properties.[68] The phytosterol mixture of beta-sitosterol (BSS) and its glycoside (BSSG) was studied in animals and human clinical trials, and appears to target T-helper lymphocytes, the Th1 and Th2 cells, helping to normalize their functioning, and resulting in improved T-lymphocyte and NK cell activity. Overactive antibody responses, such as those found in autoimmune diseases and allergies, have been reduced by BSS/BSSG administration.

Inserra et al. examined the effects of supplementation with fruit and vegetable extracts on immune functions in elderly (n = 53; ages 60–86; mean = 68 years) subjects.[69] Supplements consisted of two capsules containing mixed fruit extracts from apples, oranges, pineapples, papaya, cranberries, and peaches; and two mixed vegetable extract capsules from carrots, parsley, beets, broccoli, kale, cabbage, spinach, and tomatoes. Subjects consumed a total of four capsules per day for 80 days. The study group had 13 smokers and more than one-half the subjects (n = 30) were taking a multivitamin/mineral supplement, which they continued during the study. Supplements significantly increased serum levels of lutein/zeaxanthin, lycopene, α-carotene, β-carotene, and α-tocopherol. In addition, significant increases in the spontaneous proliferation of peripheral blood monocytes (PBM) and natural killer (NK) cell cytotoxicity at three effector:target ratios were observed for nonsmokers, but not for smokers. IL-2 production from stimulated PBM cells was significantly increased in both smokers and nonsmokers.

A number of phytochemicals possess estrogenic activity in sufficient concentrations, and hence are known as phytoestrogens; these include certain isoflavones (e.g., genistein, daidzein, biochanin A), lignans (precursors to equol), and coumestans.[70,71] The richest natural dietary sources of the estrogenic isoflavones are soy products, while flax products are exceptionally rich in estrogenic lignans. Since soy-based diets can impede cancer induction and growth in rodents, and human populations which traditionally eat soy-rich diets are characterized by greatly decreased risk for many "Western" cancers, considerable attention has focused on the possibility that the estrogenic isoflavones may be responsible for much of this protection.[72-74] Flax-based diets also show cancer-retardant activity in rodents.[75,76] Other rodent studies show that phytoestrogen-rich soy diets can have a favorable impact on bone density, and soy supplements are thus being examined as possible aids to bone health.[77,78] A further application for dietary phytoestrogens currently under investigation is the use of these compounds in the management of menopausal symptoms as an alternative to hormone replacement therapies.[79-81]

Finally, since estrogenic activity appears to reduce risk for cardiovascular disease, in part by improving serum lipid profiles, and soy-based diets are known to lower elevated serum cholesterol in humans, the utility of phytoestrogens for vascular protection is being explored.[80,82-84]

11.4.4 Modulation of Hormones

Whether ordinary dietary intakes of phytoestrogen-rich foods can significantly modulate human estrogen activity *in vivo* — either by a direct agonist effect or by a partial agonist effect that might reduce net estrogenic activity under some circumstances — is a matter of considerable controversy. With respect to the estrogenic isoflavones, they occur in foods primarily in conjugated forms that are not efficiently absorbed. Moreover, first-pass hepatic metabolism results in rapid conjugation of most of the free isoflavones that are absorbed, such that serum-free isoflavone concentrations in people eating soy-rich diets are in the low nanomolar range.[85,86] Since the estrogenic potency of isoflavones is several orders of magnitude lower than that of estradiol, it is questionable whether the ingestion of isoflavones from natural foods could result in significant estrogenic activity. In fact, when estrogenic effects on reproductive physiology are monitored, soy-based supplements usually have been found to lack estrogenic activity.[87,88] Moreover, it should be noted that the many studies showing that isoflavones can retard cell growth *in vitro* — at least in part by inhibiting tyrosine kinase activity — utilized micromolar concentrations of these compounds, and thus have no evident nutritional relevance.

Nonetheless, some rodent studies indicate that phytoestrogen-rich soy protein concentrates have greater cancer retardant activity than phytoestrogen-poor concentrates. More recently, a handful of reports indicate that nutritionally relevant doses of soy phytoestrogens, administered with or without soy protein, can retard cancer spread in rodents, in part owing to the inhibition of angiogenesis.[89,90] One of the most intriguing of these studies noted that plasma IGF-I levels — which can modulate both cancer development and angiogenesis — were notably reduced in rats consuming isoflavone-enriched soy protein.[91] Since orally administered estrogens likewise can decrease IGF-I levels, the possibility arises that dietary phytoestrogens could exert protective estrogenic effects on the liver — prior to their conjugation — despite an absence of significant systemic estrogenic activity. It is of course also conceivable that phytoestrogens are achieving protective effects by mechanisms unrelated to estrogen receptors; for example, isoflavones have direct antioxidant activity, and, like other polyphenols, may have gene inductive effects via antioxidant response elements.[92,93] Beneficial effects of phytoestrogen-rich soy concentrates on vascular reactivity in monkeys have also been reported recently.[82-84] Presumably, future clinical and animal studies with phytoestrogen concentrates will enable us to reach a judicious understanding of the true potential of dietary phytoestrogens for health protection.

11.5 CONDITION-SPECIFIC MECHANISMS OF ACTION

11.5.1 CANCER

Phase II enzymes — A number of classes of phytochemicals — including the isothiocyanates, indoles, and dithiolthiones derived from the breakdown of glucosinolates (found in cruciferous vegetables), various phenolic compounds, and coumarins — act to enhance tissue levels of so-called phase II detoxifying enzymes.[94-97] The primary function of this category of enzymes is to conjugate a variety of xenobiotic compounds with glutathione, enabling their efficient urinary excretion. Among the compounds detoxified by these enzymes are many electrophilic compounds — activated mutagens — that can interact with DNA to form covalent adducts which can give rise to heritable mutations. Thus, phytochemicals which are efficient phase II inducers have antimutagenic activity, and can block the initiation stage of carcinogenesis. Phase II inducers appear to work by activating still poorly characterized transcription factors that bind to specific response elements — known as "electrophile response elements" or "antioxidant response elements" — in the promoter regions of the genes for phase II enzymes, stimulating the transcription of these genes.[94] How phytochemicals achieve this activation is still obscure. However, information pertaining to phase I suppressors is clearer. These so-called phase I detoxifying enzymes — also known as mixed-function oxidase or cytochrome P-450 enzymes — expedite the excretion of hydrophobic xenobiotic compounds by adding hydroxyl or epoxide groups that render them more water soluble and often prepare them for conjugation by phase II enzymes. Unfortunately, phase I metabolism converts certain compounds to reactive electrophiles that have mutagenic activity. Curiously, many of the glucosinolate derivatives which induce phase II enzymes, also have the ability to suppress the activity of certain phase I enzymes.[96,98-101] This decreased activity results primarily from decreased enzyme expression — in part attributable to reduced enzyme half-life rather than allosteric inhibition.

Direct carcinogen inactivation — Certain phytochemicals can bind covalently to activated mutagens, rendering them innocuous. This mechanism has been demonstrated in *in vitro* systems — whether it is of significant importance *in vivo* is open to question. In one well-known instance of this effect, vitamin C in the gastric juice can interact with dietary nitrite in a way that prevents the spontaneous formation of nitrosamines.[102,103] This mechanism is believed to underlie the protective impact of vitamin C-rich foods on gastric cancer risk.

AP-1 antagonists — Certain phytochemicals, most notably polyphenols such as those found in green tea, impact cancer induction in the promotional stage, after initiating mutations have already occurred. Initiated preneoplastic cells are highly prone to apoptotic or programmed cell death; promoting agents act in various ways to block apoptosis in these cells, increasing the chance that they will eventually give rise to a malignant tumor.[104-107] Conversely, antipromotional agents such as polyphenols tend to encourage the apoptotic process.[108-112] One of the characteristic effects of promoting agents is to activate the AP-1 transcription factors that play a central role in promoting cell growth and blocking apoptosis. Recent studies show that green tea polyphenols (e.g., epigallocatchin gallate) act to inhibit the activation of AP-1; the mechanism of this effect is still controversial.[113-115] Since AP-1 also plays important roles in inducing the proteolytic activities required for cell migration, metastasis, and angiogenesis, inhibitors of AP-1 activation have the additional potential to slow the spread of preexisting cancers. Indeed, in animal studies green tea polyphenols have recently shown growth retardant, antimetastatic and anti-angiogenic activities.[116-119]

Inhibitors of isoprene metabolism — Natural isoprenoid compounds, derived from a metabolic pathway in which the enzyme HMG-CoA reductase is rate limiting, play a key role in supporting cell proliferation and preventing apoptosis.[120,121] In particular, synthesis of the isoprenoid dolichyl phosphate is required to enable transfer of IGF-I receptors to the cell surface, where they can mediate IGF-I activity.[122,123] In most cell lines and many cancers, IGF-I activity is crucial for cell cycle progression and prevention of apoptosis.[124-126] Thus, inhibition of dolichyl phosphate synthesis can slow cell multiplication and encourage apoptosis in many preneoplastic and neoplastic cell lines.[120] A number of phytochemical isoprenoids — including tocotrienols and lycopene — have the ability to suppress expression of HMG-CoA reductase by posttranscriptional mechanisms;[127-129] this in turn decreases dolichyl phosphate production, reduces the cell surface expression of IGF-I receptors, and thus decreases IGF-I activity. In animal models, phytochemical isoprenoids have been shown to exert antipromotional activity, as well as to slow the growth of preexisting tumors.[127,128] Conceivably, the substantial cancer protection associated with tomato consumption as shown in epidemiological studies reflects the ability of lycopene to interfere with endogenous synthesis of isoprenoids.[130]

Angiogenesis inhibitors — Agents that inhibit angiogenesis have antipromotional activity and can slow the growth of existing cancers. The recently demonstrated ability of green tea polyphenols to inhibit angiogenesis in rabbit corneas may reflect its activity as an AP-1 antagonist,[119] as discussed above. Since IGF-I activity is required for effective angiogenesis,[131] one might expect inhibitors of isoprene metabolism such as lycopene or tocotrienols to be anti-angiogenic; however, the impact of these agents on angiogenesis has not yet been studied.

Flavonoids can suppress cancer growth or induction by impeding cell cycle progression and promoting apoptosis — Flavonoids and other phytochemicals derived from fruits, vegetables, and herbs have the potential to inhibit cancer induction and growth by interfering with signaling pathways required for cell cycle progression and suppression of apoptosis. Thus, cell culture studies indicate that various flavonoids can inhibit induction of ornithine decarboxylase,[132,133] and are directly inhibitory to tyrosine kinases,[134,135] protein kinase C,[136,137] and phosphatidylinositol-3-kinase.[138,139] Flavonoids can also interfere with arachidonate metabolism; certain lipoxygenase products act as growth factors or promote metastatic behavior in some cancers, while cyclooxygenase products are believed to contribute to the induction of colon and breast cancers. *In vitro*, certain flavonoids have been shown to inhibit lipoxygenases,[140,141] whereas others can inhibit one or both types of cyclooxygenases.[142,143] Flavonoids have also been shown to upregulate apoptosis in cancer cell lines.[144,145] In some instances, this effect is associated with increased activation of p53 or its downstream mediator p21/WAF.[145,146] Inhibition of the mitogenic signaling enzymes, cited in the preceding paragraph, could be expected not only to retard cell cycle progression, but would also be likely to promote apoptosis.

11.5.2 Vascular Health

Antioxidants and LDL metabolism — Many phytochemicals — most notably polyphenols and flavonoids, as well as ascorbic acid — have potent antioxidant activity owing to the presence of hydroxyl groups that can readily donate one electron. These antioxidants have the potential to protect LDL particles from oxidation, and thus lessen their atherogenicity. Indeed, several clinical studies demonstrate that phytochemical-rich diets can protect LDL.[147-153] Although vitamin C is not as effective as vitamin E in blocking LDL oxidation, it is able to recycle oxidized vitamin E to its reduced antioxidant form, thus potentiating the protection afforded by vitamin E.[154-157]

Superoxide quenchers — Superoxide produced by the endothelium, vascular smooth muscle, or intimal macrophages can destroy the protective nitric oxide generated by the vascular endothelium, converting it to the highly toxic peroxynitrite radical in the process. Vitamin C, as well as certain polyphenols, can quench superoxide by electron donation, thus sparing nitric oxide.[158,159] Since vascular nitric oxide has anti-atherosclerotic, vasodilatory, antithrombotic, and anti-inflammatory effects,[160] agents which protect it from superoxide can have a broad favorable impact on vascular health.

Nitric oxide synthase inducers — Phytochemicals also can promote effective nitric oxide activity by inducing the endothelial enzyme which generates it. This may be achieved through inhibition of isoprene metabolism;[161,162] thus, isoprenoid compounds such as tocotrienols and lycopene which downregulate HMG-CoA reductase have the potential to induce endothelial nitric oxide synthase. Conceivably, the reported ability of tocotrienols to promote regression of carotid atheroma is mediated by this mechanism.[163] There is also recent evidence that certain polyphenols can increase the expression of nitric oxide synthase in endothelial cells;[164] this suggests that dietary polyphenols may provide this benefit. For example, this might rationalize the protective impact of heavy green tea ingestion on stroke risk in Japan.[165]

Potassium — Although all natural foods contain potassium, fruits and vegetables are the richest dietary sources — on a per calorie basis — of this underappreciated electrolyte. The demonstrated ability of potassium-rich diets to lower elevated blood pressure stems, at least in part, from potassium's natriuretic activity — that is, it promotes renal excretion of sodium, decreasing the adverse impact of salted diets on blood pressure regulation.[166,167] In addition, the modest increase in serum potassium achievable with high-potassium diets has a hyperpolarizing effect on vascular endothelium, the net effect of which is to boost endothelial nitric oxide generation while suppressing production of superoxide.[168-171] This latter activity implies that potassium can be viewed as an important antioxidant nutrient. Epidemiological studies reveal that increased potassium intakes can reduce risk for heart attack and especially stroke, even when they do not influence blood pressure.

Inhibitors of cholesterol synthesis — The phytochemical isoprenoids which down-regulate HMG-CoA reductase have the evident ability to suppress cholesterol synthesis and thus lower serum cholesterol. This is a well-known property of tocotrienols,[172,173] and has recently been demonstrated with high intakes of lycopene as well.[129] Certain flavonoids such as hesperidin (from citrus fruits) likewise can inhibit HMG-CoA reductase, though the mechanism of this is not clear.[174,175]

Bile acid binders — Fruits and vegetables are often rich sources of soluble fiber. Many soluble fibers can prevent the efficient absorption of lipid micelles in the digestive tract, thus expediting the fecal loss of bile acids. The resulting deficiency of bile acids triggers hepatic induction of 7-alpha-hydroxylase, the rate-limiting enzyme for the conversion of cholesterol to bile acids. This in turn drains the hepatic cholesterol pool and induces increased expression of hepatic LDL receptors, resulting in a lowering of serum LDL cholesterol.[176-178] The cholesterol-lowering activity of adequate dietary intakes of soluble fibers has been demonstrated repeatedly in clinical trials.[179-182] Potentially, soluble fiber can also lower cholesterol by giving rise to propionic acid in the colon; this compound is absorbed, and can somehow decrease hepatic HMG-CoA reductase activity.[183] However, since the net effect of soluble fiber is to increase this activity, it is unlikely that propionic acid is the chief mediator of the cholesterol-lowering action of soluble fiber.

Homocysteine control — Fruits and vegetables are major dietary sources of the vitamins folate and pyridoxine, which play central roles in homocysteine metabolism.[184-188] Deficiencies of these vitamins lead to elevations of homocysteine, which is toxic to vascular endothelium.[189-191] Elevated homocysteine is linked to increased risk for heart attack, stroke, peripheral atherosclerosis, and venous thromboembolism,[184] whereas increased serum levels of folate and pyridoxine tend to correlate with lower homocysteine levels and decreased vascular risk.[192-194] Fruit and vegetable intake has been correlated inversely with serum homocysteine in several studies.[196-198]

Control of blood pressure — Hypertension is a risk factor for cardiovascular disease and stroke and is one of the most prevalent chronic conditions in the U.S., affecting 24% of the adult population and 32% of African Americans.[199] Dietary recommendations have long been used for blood pressure control — namely, weight loss or maintenance and sodium restriction; and more recently increasing dietary intake of potassium, calcium, and magnesium.

The Dietary Approaches to Stop Hypertension (DASH) trial, conducted at four medical centers, compared the affects of three dietary patterns on blood pressure.[200] For a period of 8 weeks participants ate either a fruits and vegetables diet (8 to 10 servings per day), a combination diet consisting of fruits and vegetables plus low-fat dietary products, or a control diet similar to the typical American food intake. Both the fruits and vegetables diets and the combination diet significantly lowered blood pressure compared to the control diet. Further analysis of a subgroup in the study indicated that health-related quality of life improved in the treatment groups but not the control group.[201] In another substudy in African Americans, blood pressure was significantly lowered by the combination diet and to a lesser extent by the fruit and vegetable diet.[202] When nutritional factors were examined in relation to hypertension among 41,541 U.S. female nurses, a diet rich in fruits and vegetables was associated with reduced blood pressure. Dietary fiber and magnesium, but not calcium and potassium, were inversely associated with systolic and diastolic blood pressure.[203] Garlic consumption has also been correlated with reduction in blood pressure, possibly by a direct relaxant effect on smooth muscle.[204] Hypertensive patients who had guava added to their diets (500 to 1000 g/d for 4 weeks), showed significant decreases in mean systolic and diastolic pressures.[205]

11.5.3 Osteoporosis

Alkaline buffering — Diets rich in sulfydryl amino acids — such as those high in animal proteins — are metabolized to yield sulfuric acid; this strong acid is buffered by dissolution of bone matrix, which releases phosphates. If the diet can provide this buffering activity, bone can be spared.[206-208] The chief sources of buffering activity in foods are salts of potassium, magnesium, and calcium; as fruits and vegetables tend to be rich in potassium and magnesium, especially on a per-calorie basis, they can be expected to provide excellent buffering activity for bone protection.

Indeed, recent epidemiology has correlated increased intakes of potassium, magnesium — and fruits and vegetables — with greater bone density.[23,24]

Potassium natriuresis — Dietary salt, for reasons that remain unclear, decreases the renal retention of calcium, leading to increased urinary calcium loss. Thus, heavily salted diets are associated with lesser bone density and increased fracture risk.[209-213] As noted above, dietary potassium promotes renal sodium excretion, and this counteracts the impact of salted diets on calcium retention.[214,215] Diets rich in fruits and vegetables — and thus in potassium salts — therefore provide specific protection from the adverse impacts of both animal protein and salt on bone density.

Vitamin K — This vitamin, most richly supplied by dark green leafy vegetables, is needed for the proper posttranslational modification (glutamate carboxylation) of certain proteins, such as osteocalcin, that play a role in the bone mineralization process.[216,217] In epidemiological studies, dietary vitamin K intakes as well as serum markers of vitamin K status correlate with greater bone density and/or reduced fracture risk,[218-221] whereas some studies find that long-term use of the anticoagulant warfarin, which antagonizes the biochemical activity of vitamin K, is associated with increased fracture risk.[222] Several studies in humans or animals demonstrate a favorable effect of supplemental vitamin K on markers of bone formation and/or resorption.[223-226]

Vitamin C — The role of vitamin C in bone mineralization involves hydroxylation reactions required for cross-linking in the bone matrix and amidation of calcitonin, a thyroid peptide hormone necessary for bone calcium deposition. In one study, serum ascorbic acid levels in 20 hip fracture patients were found to be nearly one half the serum levels present in 20 matched pair controls.[227] Another study, which measured bone mineral density (spine and hip) in 775 postmenopausal women, showed a positive association with vitamin C intake and bone mineral density in individuals who also had dietary calcium intakes of 500 mg daily.[228] In postmenopausal women who had not used estrogen replacement therapy, long-term intake of approximately 400 mg of vitamin C daily was associated with increased bone mineral density.[25] Smoking is also a known risk factor for hip fracture, and in a large prospective study of 66,651 women, smokers were stratified into two categories (high/low) for intake of vitamin C and vitamin E.[229] After adjustments for major osteoporosis risk factors, low intake of vitamin C increased hip fracture risk 2.1-fold, low intake of vitamin E increased risk 2.7-fold and low intake of vitamins C and E increased risk fourfold. The vitamin E effect is not clear but could be attributed to a generalized antioxidant sparing of vitamin C.

11.5.4 Macular Degeneration and Cataracts

Macular pigment — In plant chloroplasts, the carotenoids lutein and zeaxanthin, which are quenchers of singlet oxygen, function to protect membranes from photooxidative damage. Mammals have copied this strategy, accumulating these carotenoids in the macula as protective antioxidants.[230–233] Epidemiology indicates that risk for age-related macular degeneration is substantially lower in individuals who regularly consume foods rich in lutein/zeaxanthin — most notably spinach.[27]

Increased serum levels of these carotenoids are also correlated with lesser risk for macular degeneration.[232]

11.6 OVERVIEW

There is clearly a large and growing volume of epidemiological evidence pointing to diets rich in fruits and vegetable as notably protective with respect to vascular health, stroke, bone density, and risks for diabetes, macular degeneration, and many types of cancer. Furthermore, the likelihood that these epidemiological associations reflect causative relationships is heightened by recent research defining plausible cellular mechanisms whereby the nutrients and phytochemicals in fruits and vegetables may exert their protective effects. Thus, the growing consensus that increased intakes of fruits and vegetables are highly desirable is completely concordant with the findings of recent biomedical research.

REFERENCES

1. Wattenberg, L.W., Chemoprevention of cancer, *Cancer Res.*, 45: 1-6, 1985.
2. Wattenberg, L.W., Inhibition of carcinogenesis by minor nutrient constituents of the diet, *Proc. Nutr. Soc.*, 49: 173-183, 1990.
3. Committee on Diet, Nutrition and Cancer, Inhibitors of carcinogenesis in *Diet, Nutrition and Cancer*, Washington, D.C., National Academy Press; pp.358-370, 1982.
4. Middleton, E., Jr. and Kandaswami, C., The impact of plant flavonoids on mammalian biology: implications for immunity, inflammation and cancer, in *The Flavonoids: Advances in Research Since 1986*, Harborne, J.B., Ed., New York, Chapman and Hall, pp.620-652, 1994.
5. Howard, B.V. and Kritchevsky, D., Phytochemicals and cardiovascular disease, *Circulation*, 95: 2591-2593, 1997.
6. Tribble, D.L., Antioxidant consumption and risk of coronary heart disease: emphasis on vitamin C, vitamin E and beta-carotene, *Circulation*, 99: 591-595, 1999.
7. Anderson, J.J.B. and Garner, S.C., The effects of phytoestrogens on bone, *Nutr. Res.*, 17: 1617-1632, 1997.
8. Fahey, J.W, Clevidence, B.A., and Russel, R.M., Methods for assessing the biological effects of specific plant components, *Nutr. Rev.*, 57(9): S34-S40,1999.
9. Lampe, J.W., Health effects of vegetables and fruit: assessing mechanism of actions in human experimental studies, *Am. J. Clin. Nutr.*, 70(3S): 475S-490S, 1999.
10. Block, G., Patterson, B., and Subar, A., Fruit, vegetables, and cancer prevention: a review of the epidemiological evidence, *Nutr. Cancer*, 18(1): 1-29, 1992.
11. Giovannucci, E. and Clinton, S.K., Tomatoes, lycopene, and prostrate cancer, *Proc. Soc. Exp. Biol. Med.*, 218(2): 129-139, 1998.
12. Fahey, JW, Zhang, Y., and Talalay, P., Broccoli sprouts: an exceptionally rich source of inducers of enzymes that protect against chemical carcinogens, *Proc. Natl. Acad. Sci. USA*, 94(19): 10367-10372, 1997.
13. Trowell, H., Ischemic heart disease and dietary fiber, *Am. J. Clin. Nutr.*, 25(9):926-932, 1972.
14. Kritchevsky, D. and Story, J.A., Fiber, hypercholesteremia and atherosclerosis, *Lipids*, 13(5): 366-369, 1978.
15. Jenkins, D.J., Dietary fibre, diabetes, and hyperlipidemia, Progress and prospects, *Lancet*, 2(8155): 1287-1290, 1979.

16. Menotti, A., Diet, cholesterol and coronary heart disease, A perspective. *Acta Cardiol.*, 54(3): 169-172, 1999.
17. Hertog, M.G., Feskens, E.J., Hollmand, P.C., Katan, M.B., and Kromhout, D., Dietary antioxidant flavonoids and risk of coronary heart disease: the Zutphen Elderly Study, *Lancet*, 342(8878):1007-1011, 1993.
18. Hertog, M.G., Hollman, P.C., Katan, M.B., and Kromhout, D., Intake of potentially anticarcinogenic flavonoids and their determinations in adults in the Netherlands, *Nutr. Cancer*, 20(1): 21-29, 1993.
19. Hertog, M.G., Kromhout, D., Aravnis, C., Blackburn, H., Buzina, R., et al., Flavonoid intake and long-term risk of coronary heart disease and cancer in the seven-country study, *Arch. Intern. Med.*, 155(5): 381-386, 1995.
20. Keli, S.O., Hertog, M.G., Feskens, E.J., and Kromhout, D., Dietary flavonoids, antioxidant vitamins and incidence of stroke: the Zutphen study, *Arch. Intern. Med.*, 156(6):637-642, 1996.
21. Yochum, L., Kusky, L.H., Meyer, K., and Folsom, A.R., Dietary flavonoid intake and risk of cardiovascular disease in postmenopausal women, *Am. J. Epidemiol.*, 149(10): 943-949, 1999.
22. Joshipra, K.J., Ascherio, A., Manson, J.E., Stampfer, M.J., Rimm, E.G., Speizer, F.E., Hennekens, C.H., Spiegelman, D., and Willett, W.C., Fruit and vegetable intake in relation to risk of ischemic stroke, *J. Am. Med. Assoc.*, 282(13): 1233-1239, 1999.
23. Tucker, K.L., Hannan, M.T., Chen, H., Cupples, L.A., Wilson, P.W., and Kiel, D.P., Potassium, magnesium and fruit and vegetable intake are associated with greater bone mineral density in elderly men and women, *Am. J. Clin. Nutr.*, 69(4): 727-736, 1999.
24. New, S.A., Robins, S.P., Campbell, M.K., Martin, J.C., Garton, J.C., Garton, M.J., Bolton-Smith, C., et al., Dietary influences of bone mass and bone metabolism: further evidence of a positive link between fruit and vegetable consumption and bone health, *Am. J. Clin. Nutr.*, 71:142-151, 2000.
25. Leveille, S.G., LaCroix, A.Z., Koepsell, T.D., Beresford, S.A., Van Belle, G., and Buchner, D.M., Dietary vitamin C and bone mineral density in postmenopausal women in Washington state, USA, *J. Epidemiol. Commun. Health*, 51(5): 479-485, 1997.
26. Goldberg, J., Flowerdew, G., Smith, E., Brody, J.A., and Tso, M.O., Factors associated with age-related macular degeneration. An analysis of data from the first National Health and Nutrition Examination Survey, *Am. J. Epidemiol.*, 128(4): 700-710, 1988.
27. Seddon, J.M., Ajani, U.A., Sperduto, R.D., et al., Dietary carotenoids, vitamin A, C and E and advanced age-related macular degeneration, *J. Am. Med. Assoc.*, 272: 1413-1420, 1994.
28. Sommerburg, O., Keunen, J.E., Bird, A.C., and van Juijk, F.J., Fruits and vegetables that are sources for lutein and zeaxanthin: the macular pigment in human eyes, *Br. J. Ophthalmol.*, 82(8): 907-910, 1998.
29. Anderson, R.E., Kretzer, F.L., and Rapp, L.M., Free radicals and ocular disease, *Adv. Exp. Med. Biol.*, 366:73-86, 1994.
30. Jacques, P.F. and Chylack, L.T., Jr., Epidemiological evidence of a role for the antioxdant vitamins and carotenoids in cataract prevention, *Am. J. Clin. Nutr.*, 53(1S): 352S-355S, 1991.
31. Brown, L., Rimm, E.B., Seddon, J.M., Giovannucci, E.L., et al., A prospective study of carotenoid intake and risk of cataract extraction in U.S. men, *Am. J. Clin. Nutr.*, 70(4): 517-524, 1999.
32. Floyd, R.A., Antioxidants, oxidative stress and degenerative neurological disorders, *Proc. Soc. Exp. Biol. Med.*, 222(3): 236-245, 1999.

33. Aisen, P.S., Inflammation and Alzheimer's disesae: mechanism and therapeutic strategies, *Gerontology*, 43(1-2): 143-149, 1997.
34. Aisen, P.S., Inflammation and Alzheimer disease, *Mol. Chem. Neuropathol.*, 28(1-3): 83-88, 1996.
35. Behl, C., Vitamin E and other antioxidants in neuroprotection, *Int. J. Vitam. Nutr. Res.*, 69(3): 213-219, 1999.
36. Ferrante, R.J., Browne, S.E., Shinobu, L.A., Bowling, A.C., Baik, M.J., MacGarvey, U., et al., Evidence of increased oxidative damage in both sporadic and familial amyotrophic lateral sclerosis, *J. Neurochem.*, 69(5): 2064-2074, 1997.
37. Jenner, P. and Olanow, C.W., Oxidative stress and the pathogenesis of Parkinson's disease, *Neurology*, 47(6S): S161-S170, 1996.
38. Goodwin, J.S., Goodwin, J.M., and Garry, P.J., Association between nutritional status and cognitive functioning in a healthy elderly population, *J. Am. Med. Assoc.*, 249(21): 2917-2921, 1983.
39. Ho, E. and Bray, T.M., Antioxidants, NFKappaB activation, and diabetogenesis, *Proc. Soc. Exp. Biol. Med.*, 222(3): 205-213, 1999.
40. Kento, H., Kajimoto, Y., Miyagawa, J., Matsuoka, T., Fujitani, Y., et al., Beneficial effects of antioxidants in diabetes: possible protection of pancreatic beta-cells against glucose toxicity, *Diabetes*, 48(12): 2398-2406, 1999.
41. Cameron, N.E. and Cotter, M.A., Effects of antioxidants on nerve and vascular dysfunction in experimental diabetes, *Diabetes Res. Clin. Pract.*, 45(2-3): 137-146, 1999.
42. Williams, D.E., Wareham, N.J., Cox, B.D., Byrne, C.D., Hales, C.N., and Day, N.E., Frequent salad vegetable consumption is associated with a reduction in the risk of diabetes mellitus, *J. Clin. Epidemiol.* 52(4): 329-335, 1999.
43. Alexander, H., Lockwood, L.P., Harris, M.A., and Melby, C.L., Risk factors for cardiovascular disease and diabetes in two groups of Hispanic Americans with differing dietary habits, *J. Am. Coll. Nutr.*, 18(2): 127-136, 1999.
44. Harborne, J.B., *The Flavonoids: Advances in Research Since 1986*, London: Chapman and Hall, 1993.
45. Harborne, J.B., *Methods in Plant Biochemistry. I. Plant Phenolics*, London: Academic Press, 1989.
46. Bravo, L., Polyphenols: Chemistry, dietary sources, metabolism and nutritional significance, *Nutr. Rev.*, 56(11): 317-333, 198.
47. Stahelin, H.B., Gey, K.F., Eicholzer, M., et al., Plasma antioxidant vitamins and subsequent cancer mortality in the 12-year follow-up of the prospective Basel Study, *Am. J. Epidemiol.*, 133: 766-775, 1991.
48. Gey, K.F., Ten-year retrospective on the antioxidant hypothesis of arteriosclerosis: Threshold plasma levels of antioxidant micronutrients related to minimum cardiovascular risk, *Nutr. Biochem.*, 6:206-236, 1995.
49. Wang, H., Cao, G., and Prior, R.L., Total antioxidant capacity of fruits, *J. Agric. Food Chem.*, 44:701-705, 1996.
50. Cao, G., Sofic E., and Prior, R.L., Antioxidant capacity of tea and common vegetables, *J. Agric. Food Chem.*, 44:3426-3431, 1996.
51. Cao, G., Russell, R.M., Lischner, N., and Prior, R.L., Serium antioxidant capacity is increased by consumption of strawberries, red wine or vitamin C in elderly women, *J. Nutr.*, 128: 2383-2390, 1998.

52. Guo, C., Cao, G., Sofic, E., and Prior, R.L., High performance liquid chromatography coupled with coulometric array detection of electroactive components in fruits and vegetables: Relationship to oxygen radical absorbance capacity, *J. Agric. Food Chem.*, 45: 1787-1796, 1997.
53a. Cao, G., Sofic, E., and Prior, R.L., Antioxidant and prooxidant behavior of flavonoids: Structure-activity relationships, *Free Rad. Biol. Med.*, 22:749-760, 1997.
53b. Eberhardt, M.V., Lee, C.Y., and Liu, R.H. Nutrition: antioxidant activity of fresh apples, *Nature*, 405: 903-904, 2000.
54. Wise, J.W., Morin, R.J., Sanderson, R., and Blum, K., Changes in plasma carotenoid, alpha-tocopherol, and lipid peroxide levels in response to supplementation with concentrated fruit and vegetable extracts: a pilot study, *Curr. Ther. Res.*, 57: 445-461, 1996.
55. Duthie, S.J., Ma, A., Ross, M.A., and Collins, A.R., Antioxidant supplementation decreases oxidative DNA damage in human lymphocytes, *Cancer Res.*, 56:1291-1295, 1996.
56. Pool-Zobel, B.L., Bub, A., Muller, H., Wollowski, I., and Rechkemmer, G., Consumption of vegetables reduces genetic damage in humans: first results of a human intervention trial with carotenoid-rich foods, *Carcinogenesis*, 18:1847-1850, 1997.
57. Riso, P., Pinder, A., Santangelo, A., and Porrini, M., Does tomato consumption effectively increase the resistance of lymphocyte DNA to oxidative damage, *Am. J. Clin. Nutr.,* 69:712-718, 1999.
58. Smith, M.J., Inserra, P.F., Watson, R.R., Wise, J.A., and O'Neill K.L., Supplementation with fruit and vegetable extracts may decrease DNA damage in the peripheral lymphocytes of an elderly population, *Nutr. Res.*, 19(10): 1507-1518, 1999
59. Kubena, K.S. and McMurray, D.N., Nutrition and the immune system: a review of the nutrient-nutrient interactions, *J. Am. Diet. Assoc.*, 96:1156-1164, 1996.
60. Chandra, R.K., Effect of vitamin and trace-element supplementation on immune responses and infection in elderly subjects, *Lancet*, 340(8828):1124-1127, 1992.
61. Bogden, J.D., Bendich, A., Kemp, F.W., et al., Daily micronutrient supplements enhance delayed-hypersensitivity skin test responses in older people, *Am. J. Clin. Nutr.* 60: 437-447, 1994.
62. Meydani, S.N., Meydani, M., Blumberg, J.B., et al., Vitamin E supplementation and in vivo immune response in healthy subjects, *J. Am. Med. Assoc.*, 277: 1380-1386, 1997.
63. Watson, R.R., Prabhala, R.H., Plezia, P.M., and Alberts, D.S., Effect of beta-carotene on lymphocytes subpopulations in elderly humans: evidence for a dose-response relationship, *Am. J. Clin. Nutr.*, 53: 90-94, 1991.
64. Santos, M.S., Meydani, S.N., Leka, L., et al., Natural killer cell activity in elderly men is enhanced by β-carotene supplementation, *Am. J. Clin. Nutr.*, 64:772-777, 1996.
65. Prabhala, R.H., Braune, L.M., Garewal, H.S., and Watson, R.R., Influence of beta-carotene on immune functions, *Ann. NY Acad. Sci.*, 691:262-263, 1993.
66. Roy, M., Kiremidjian-Schumacher, L., Wishe, H.I., Cohen, M.W., and Stotzky, G., Supplementation with selenium and human immune cell functions. I. Effect on lymphocyte proliferation and interleukin 2 receptor expression, *Biol. Trace Elem. Res.*, 41(1-2): 103-114, 1994.
67. Middleton, E.J., Effect of plant flavonoids on immune and inflammatory cell function, *Adv. Exp. Med. Biol.*, 439:175-182, 1998.
68. Bouic, P.J. and Lamprecht, J.H., Plant sterols and sterolins: a review of their immune-modulating properties, *Altern. Med. Rev.*, 4(3): 170-177, 1999.

69. Inserra, P.L., Shuguan, J., Solkoff, D., Lee, J., Zhang, Z., Xu, M., Hesslink, R., Jr., Wise, J., and Watson, R.R., Immune function in elderly smokers and nonsmokers improves during supplementation with fruit and vegetable extracts, *Intern. Med.*, 2(1): 3-10, 1999.
70. Kurzer, M.S. and Xu, X., Dietary phytoestrogens, *Annu. Rev. Nutr.*, 17:353-381, 1997.
71. Mazur, W., Phytoestrogen content in foods, *Baillieres Clin. Endocrinol. Metab.*, 12(4):729-742, 1998.
72. Messina, M.J., Persky, V., Setchell, K.D., and Barnes, S., Soy intake and cancer risk: a review of the *in vitro* and *in vivo* data, *Nutr. Cancer,* 21:113-131, 1994.
73. Messina, M. and Barnes, S., The role of soy products in reducing risk of cancer, *J. Natl. Cancer Inst.*, 83:541-546, 1991.
74. Barnes, S., Effect of genistein on in vitro and in vivo models of cancer, *J. Nutr.,* 125:777S-783S, 1995.
75. Thompson, L.U., Experimental studies on lignans and cancer, *Baillieres Clin. Endocrinol. Metab.,* 12:691-705, 1998.
76. Serraino, M. and Thompson, L.U., The effect of flaxseed supplementation on the initiation and promotional stages of mammary tumorigenesis, *Nutr. Cancer,* 17:153-159, 1992.
77. Scheiber, M.D. and Rebar, R.W., Isoflavones and postmenopausal bone health: a viable alternative to estrogen therapy?, *Menopause,* 6:233-241, 1999.
78. Anderson, J.J. and Garner, S.C., Phytoestrogens and bone, *Baillieres Clin. Endocrinol. Metab.,* 12:543-557, 1998.
79. Ramsey, L.A., Ross, B.S., and Fischer, R.G., Phytoestrogens and the management of menopause [In Process Citation], *Adv. Nurse Pract.,* 7:26-30, 1999.
80. Washburn, S., Burke, G.L., Morgan, T., and Anthony, M., Effect of soy protein supplementation on serum lipoproteins, blood pressure, and menopausal symptoms in perimenopausal women [see comments], *Menopause,* 6:7-13, 1999.
81. Clarkson, T.B., Anthony, M.S., Williams, J.K., Honore, E.K., and Cline, J.M., The potential of soybean phytoestrogens for postmenopausal hormone replacement therapy, *Proc. Soc. Exp. Biol. Med.,* 217:365-368, 1998.
82. Clarkson, T.B. and Anthony, M.S., Phytoestrogens and coronary heart disease, *Baillieres Clin. Endocrinol. Metab.,* 12:589-604, 1998.
83. Wagner, J.D., Cefalu, W.T., Anthony, M.S., Litwak, K.N., Zhang, L., and Clarkson, T.B., Dietary soy protein and estrogen replacement therapy improve cardiovascular risk factors and decrease aortic cholesteryl ester content in ovariectomized cynomolgus monkeys, *Metabolism,* 46:698-705, 1997.
84. Honore, E.K., Williams, J.K., Anthony, M.S., and Clarkson, T.B., Soy isoflavones enhance coronary vascular reactivity in atherosclerotic female macaques, *Fertil. Steril.,* 67:148-154, 1997.
85. Barnes, S., Evolution of the health benefits of soy isoflavones, *Proc. Soc. Exp. Biol. Med.,* 217:386-392, 1998.
86. Adlercreutz, H., Markkanen, H., and Watanabe, S., Plasma concentrations of phytooestrogens in Japanese men, *Lancet,* 342:1209-1210, 1993.
87. Cline, J.M., Paschold, J.C., Anthony, M.S., Obasanjo, I.O., and Adams, M.R., Effects of hormonal therapies and dietary soy phytoestrogens on vaginal cytology in surgically postmenopausal macaques, *Fertil. Steril.,* 65:1031-1035, 1996.
88. Anthony, M.S., Clarkson, T.B., Hughes, C.L.J., Morgan, T.M., and Burke, G.L., Soybean isoflavones improve cardiovascular risk factors without affecting the reproductive system of peripubertal rhesus monkeys, *J. Nutr.,* 126:43-50, 1996.

89. van A., I., Feskens, E.J., Bowles, C.H., and Kromhout, D., Body iron stores and mortality due to cancer and ischaemic heart disease: a 17-year follow-up study of elderly men and women, *Int. J. Epidemiol.,* 24:665-670, 1995.
90. Zhou, J.R., Mukherjee, P., Gugger, E.T., Tanaka, T., Blackburn, G.L., and Clinton, S.K., Inhibition of murine bladder tumorigenesis by soy isoflavones via alterations in the cell cycle, apoptosis, and angiogenesis, *Cancer Res.* 58:5231-5238, 1998.
91. Zhou, J.R., Gugger, E.T., Tanaka, T., Guo, Y., Blackburn, G.L., and Clinton, S.K., Soybean phytochemicals inhibit the growth of transplantable human prostate carcinoma and tumor angiogenesis in mice, *J. Nutr.,* 129:1628-1635, 1999.
92. Lee, S.K., Song, L., Mata-Greenwood, E., Kelloff, G.J., Steele, V.E., and Pezzuto, J.M., Modulation of in vitro biomarkers of the carcinogenic process by chemopreventive agents, *Anticancer Res.,* 19:35-44, 1999.
93. Fei, P., Matwyshyn, G.A., Rushmore, T.H., and Kong, A.N., Transcription regulation of rat glutathione S-transferase Ya subunit gene expression by chemopreventive agents, *Pharm. Res.,* 13:1043-1048, 1996.
94. Prestera, T. and Talalay, P., Electrophile and antioxidant regulation of enzymes that detoxify carcinogens, *Proc. Natl. Acad. Sci. USA,* 92:8965-8969, 1995.
95. Talalay, P., Fahey, J.W., Holtzclaw, W.D., Prestera, T., and Zhang, Y., Chemoprotection against cancer by phase 2 enzyme induction, *Toxicol. Lett.*, 82-83:173-179, 1995.
96. Zhang, Y. and Talalay, P., Anticarcinogenic activities of organic isothiocyanates: chemistry and mechanisms, *Cancer Res.*, 54:1976s-1981s, 1994.
97. Fahey, J.W., Zhang, Y. and Talalay, P., Broccoli sprouts: an exceptionally rich source of inducers of enzymes that protect against chemical carcinogens, *Proc. Natl. Acad. Sci. USA,* 94:10367-10372, 1997.
98. Stresser, D.M., Bjeldanes, L.F., Bailey, G.S., and Williams, D.E., The anticarcinogen 3,3'-diindolylmethane is an inhibitor of cytochrome P-450, *J. Biochem. Toxicol.*, 10:191-201, 1995.
99. Barcelo, S., Gardiner, J.M., Gescher, A., and Chipman, J.K., CYP2E1-mediated mechanism of anti-genotoxicity of the broccoli constituent sulforaphane [see comments], *Carcinogenesis*, 17:277-282, 1996.
100. Schmiedlin-Ren, P., Edwards, D.J., Fitzsimmons, M.E., He, K., Lown, K.S., Woster, P.M., et al., Mechanisms of enhanced oral availability of CYP3A4 substrates by grapefruit constituents. Decreased enterocyte CYP3A4 concentration and mechanism-based inactivation by furanocoumarins, *Drug Metab. Dispos.,* 25:1228-1233, 1997.
101. Brady, J.F., Li, D.C., Ishizaki, H., and Yang, C.S., Effect of diallyl sulfide on rat liver microsomal nitrosamine metabolism and other monooxygenase activities, *Cancer Res.,* 48:5937-5940, 1988.
102. Mirvish, S.S., Grandjean, A.C., Reimers, K.J., Connelly, B.J., Chen, S.C., Morris, C.R., et al., Effect of ascorbic acid dose taken with a meal on nitrosoproline excretion in subjects ingesting nitrate and proline, *Nutr. Cancer*, 31:106-110, 1998.
103. Vermeer, I.T., Moonen, E.J., Dallinga, J.W., Kleinjans, J.C., and van Maanen, J.M., Effect of ascorbic acid and green tea on endogenous formation of N-nitrosodimethylamine and N-nitrosopiperidine in humans, *Mutat. Res.*, 428:353-361, 1999.
104. Wright, S.C., Zhong, J., and Larrick, J.W., Inhibition of apoptosis as a mechanism of tumor promotion, *FASEB J.*, 8:654-660, 1994.
105. Schulte-Hermann, R., Grasl-Kraupp, B., and Bursch, W., Tumor development and apoptosis, *Int. Arch. Allergy Immunol.*, 105:363-367, 1994.

106. Stincombe, S., Buchmann, A., Bock, K.W., and Schwarz, M., Inhibition of apoptosis during 2,3,7,8-tetrachlorodibenzo-p-dioxin-mediated tumour promotion in rat liver, *Carcinogenesis*, 16:1271-1275, 1995.
107. Schulte-Hermann, R., Bursch, W., Grasl-Kraupp, B., Mullauer, L., and Ruttkay-Nedecky, B., Apoptosis and multistage carcinogenesis in rat liver, *Mutat. Res.*, 333:81-87, 1995.
108. McCarty, M.F., Selenium, calcium channel blockers, and cancer risk--the Yin and Yang of apoptosis?, *Med. Hypotheses*, 50:423-433, 1998.
109. Ahmad, N., Feyes, D.K., Nieminen, A.L., Agarwal, R., and Mukhtar, H., Green tea constituent epigallocatechin-3-gallate and induction of apoptosis and cell cycle arrest in human carcinoma cells, *J. Natl. Cancer Inst.*, 89:1881-1886, 1997.
110. Hibasami, H., Komiya, T., Achiwa, Y., Ohnishi, K., Kojima, T., Nakanishi, K., et al., Induction of apoptosis in human stomach cancer cells by green tea catechins, *Oncol. Rep.*, 5:527-529, 1998.
111. Yang, G.Y., Liao, J., Kim, K., Yurkow, E.J., and Yang, C.S., Inhibition of growth and induction of apoptosis in human cancer cell lines by tea polyphenols, *Carcinogenesis*, 19:611-616, 1998.
112. Paschka, A.G., Butler, R., and Young, C.Y., Induction of apoptosis in prostate cancer cell lines by the green tea component, (-)-epigallocatechin-3-gallate, *Cancer Lett.*, 130:1-7, 1998.
113. Dong, Z., Ma, W., Huang, C., and Yang, C.S., Inhibition of tumor promoter-induced activator protein 1 activation and cell transformation by tea polyphenols, (-)-epigallocatechin gallate, and theaflavins, *Cancer Res.*, 57:4414-4419, 1997.
114. Chung, J.Y., Huang, C., Meng, X., Dong, Z., and Yang, C.S., Inhibition of activator protein 1 activity and cell growth by purified green tea and black tea polyphenols in H-ras-transformed cells: structure-activity relationship and mechanisms involved [In Process Citation], *Cancer Res.*, 59:4610-4617, 1999.
115. Barthelman, M., Bair, W.B., Stickland, K.K., Chen, W., Timmermann, B.N., and Valcic, S., et al., (-)-Epigallocatechin-3-gallate inhibition of ultraviolet B-induced AP-1 activity, *Carcinogenesis*, 19:2201-2204, 1998.
116. Wang, Z.Y., Huang, M.T., Ho, C.T., Chang, R., Ma, W., Ferraro, T., et al., Inhibitory effect of green tea on the growth of established skin papillomas in mice, *Cancer Res.*, 52:6657-6665, 1992.
117. Liao, S., Umekita, Y., Guo, J., Kokontis, J.M., and Hiipakka, R.A., Growth inhibition and regression of human prostate and breast tumors in athymic mice by tea epigallocatechin gallate, *Cancer Lett.*, 96:239-243, 1995.
118. Conney, A.H., Lu, Y., Lou, Y., Xie, J., and Huang, M., Inhibitory effect of green and black tea on tumor growth, *Proc. Soc. Exp. Biol. Med.*, 220:229-233, 1999.
119. Cao, Y. and Cao, R., Angiogenesis inhibited by drinking tea [letter], *Nature*, 398:381, 1999.
120. Doyle, J.W. and Kandutsch, A.A., Requirement for mevalonate in cycling cells: quantitative and temporal aspects, *J. Cell Physiol.*, 137:133-140, 1988.
121. Keyomarsi, K., Sandoval, L., Band, V., and Pardee, A.B., Synchronization of tumor and normal cells from G1 to multiple cell cycles by lovastatin, *Cancer Res.*, 51:3602-3609, 1991.

122. Carlberg, M., Dricu, A., Blegen, H., Wang, M., Hjertman, M., Zickert, P., et al., Mevalonic acid is limiting for N-linked glycosylation and translocation of the insulin-like growth factor-1 receptor to the cell surface. Evidence for a new link between 3-hydroxy-3-methylglutaryl-coenzyme a reductase and cell growth, *J. Biol. Chem.*, 271:17453-17462, 1996.
123. Dricu, A., Wang, M., Hjertman, M., Malec, M., Blegen, H., Wejde, J., et al., Mevalonate-regulated mechanisms in cell growth control: role of dolichyl phosphate in expression of the insulin-like growth factor-1 receptor (IGF-1R) in comparison to Ras prenylation and expression of c-myc, *Glycobiology*, 7:625-633, 1997.
124. Baserga, R., Porcu, P., Rubini, M., and Sell, C., Cell cycle control by the IGF-1 receptor and its ligands, *Adv. Exp. Med. Biol.*, 343:105-112, 1993.
125. Baserga, R., Resnicoff, M., and Dews, M., The IGF-I receptor and cancer, *Endocrine*, 7:99-102, 1997.
126. Parrizas, M., Saltiel, A.R., and LeRoith, D., Insulin-like growth factor 1 inhibits poptosis using the phosphatidylinositol 3'-kinase and mitogen-activated protein kinase pathways, *J. Biol. Chem.*, 272:154-161, 1997.
127. Elson, C.E. and Yu, S.G., The chemoprevention of cancer by mevalonate-derived constituents of fruits and vegetables, *J. Nutr.*, 124:607-614, 1994.
128. Elson, C.E., Peffley, D.M., Hentosh, P., and Mo, H., Isoprenoid-mediated inhibition of mevalonate synthesis: potential application to cancer, *Proc. Soc. Exp. Biol. Med.*, 221:294-311, 1999.
129. Parker, R.A., Pearce, B.C., Clark, R.W., Gordon, D.A., and Wright, J.J., Tocotrienols regulate cholesterol production in mammalian cells by post-transcriptional suppression of 3-hydroxy-3-methylglutaryl-coenzyme A reductase, *J. Biol. Chem.*, 268:11230-11238, 1993.
130. Fuhrman, B., Elis, A., and Aviram, M., Hypocholesterolemic effect of lycopene and beta-carotene is related to suppression of cholesterol synthesis and augmentation of LDL receptor activity in macrophages, *Biochem. Biophys. Res. Commun.*, 233:658-662, 1997.
131. Smith, L.E., Kopchick, J.J., Chen, W., Knapp, J., Kinose, F., Daley, D., et al., Essential role of growth hormone in ischemia-induced retinal neovascularization, *Science*, 276:1706-1709, 1997.
132. Bomser, J.A., Singletary, K.W., Wallig, M.A., and Smith, M.A., Inhibition of TPA-induced tumor promotion in CD-1 mouse epidermis by a polyphenolic fraction from grape seeds, *Cancer Lett.*, 135(2): 151-157, 1999.
133. Dragsted, L.O., Strube, M., and Larsen, J.C., Cancer-protective factors in fruits and vegetables: biochemical and biological background, *Pharmacol. Toxicol.*, 72(1S): 116-135, 1993.
134. Richter, M., Ebermann, R., and Marian, B., Quercetin-induced apoptosis in colorectal tumor cells: possible role of EGF receptor signaling, *Nutr. Cancer*, 34:88-99, 1999.
135. Ramdas, L. and Budde, R.J., The instability of polyhydroxylated aromatic protein tyrosine kinase inhibitors in the presence of manganese, *Cancer Biochem. Biophys.* 16:375-385, 1998.
136. Lin, J.K., Chen, Y.C., Huang, Y.T., and Lin-Shiau, S.Y., Suppression of protein kinase C and nuclear oncogene expression as possible molecular mechanisms of cancer chemoprevention by apigenin and curcumin, *J. Cell Biochem.*, (Suppl. 28-29):39-48, 1997.
137. Ferriola, P.C., Cody, V., and Middleton, E.J., Protein kinase C inhibition by plant flavonoids. Kinetic mechanisms and structure-activity relationships, *Biochem. Pharmacol.*, 38:1617-1624, 1989.

138. Gamet-Payrastre, L., Manenti, S., Gratacap, M.P., Tulliez, J., Chap, H., and Payrastre, B., Flavonoids and the inhibition of PKC and pI 3-kinase, *Gen. Pharmacol.*, 32:279-286, 1999.
139. Agullo, G., Gamet-Payrastre, L., Manenti, S., et al., Relationship between flavonoid structure and inhibition of phosphatidylinositol 3-kinase: a comparison with tyrosine kinase and protein kinase C inhibition, *Biochem. Pharmacol.,* 53:1649-1657, 1997.
140. You, K.M., Jong, H.G., and Kim, H.P., Inhibition of cyclooxygenase/lipoxygenase from human platelets by polyhydroxylated/methoxylated flavonoids isolated from medicinal plants, *Arch. Pharm. Res.,* 22:18-24, 1999.
141. De Groot, H. and Rauen, U., Tissue injury by reactive oxygen species and the protective effects of flavonoids, *Fundam. Clin. Pharmacol.*, 12:249-255, 1998.
142. Liang, Y.C., Huang, Y.T., Tasi, S.H., Lin-Shiau, S.Y., Chen, C.F., and Lin J.K., Suppression of inducible cyclooxygenase and inducible nitric oxide synthase by apigenin and related flavonoids in mouse macrophages, *Carcinogenesis*, 20:1945-1952, 1999.
143. Kim, H.P., Mani, I., Iversen, L., and Ziboh, V.A., Effects of naturally-occurring flavonoids and biflavonoids on epidermal cyclooxygenase and lipoxygenase from guinea-pigs, *Prostaglandins Leukot. Essential Fatty Acids*, 58:17-24, 1998.
144. Kuntz, S., Wenzel, U., and Daniel, H., Comparative analysis of the effects of flavonoids on proliferation, cytotoxicity and apoptosis in human colon cell lines, *Eur. J. Nutr.,* 38:133-142, 1999.
145. Bai, F., Matsui, T., Ohtani-Fujita, N., Matsukawa, Y., Ding, Y., and Sakai, T., Promoter activation and following induction of the p21/WAF1 gene by flavone is involved in G1 phase arrest in A549 lung adenocarcinoma cells, *FEBS Lett.*, 437: 61-64, 1998.
146. Plaumann, B., Fritsche, M., Rimpler, H., Brander, G., and Hess, R.D., Flavonoids activate wild-type p53, *Oncogene*, 13:1605-1614, 1996.
147. Abbey, M., Noakes, M., and Nestel, P.J., Dietary supplementation with orange and carrot juice in cigarette smokers lowers oxidation products in copper-oxidized low-density lipoproteins, *J. Am. Diet. Assoc.*, 95:671-675, 1995.
148. Abu-Amsha, R., Croft, K.D., Puddey, I.B., Proudfoot, J.M., and Beilin, L.J., Phenolic content of various beverages determines the extent of inhibition of human serum and low-density lipoprotein oxidation *in vitro*: identification and mechanism of action of some cinnamic acid derivatives from red wine, *Clin. Sci. (Colch.),* 91:449-458, 1996.
149. Hininger, I., Chopra, M., Thurnham, D.I., Laporte, F., Richard, M.J., Favier, A., et al., Effect of increased fruit and vegetable intake on the susceptibility of lipoprotein to oxidation in smokers, *Eur. J. Clin. Nutr.,* 51:601-606, 1997.
150. Pearson, D.A., Tan, C.H., German, J.B., Davis, P.A., and Gershwin, M.E., Apple juice inhibits human low density lipoprotein oxidation, *Life Sci.*, 64:1913-1920, 1999.
151. Aviram, M. and Fuhrman, B., Polyphenolic flavonoids inhibit macrophage-mediated oxidation of LDL and attenuate atherogenesis, *Atherosclerosis*, 137 (Suppl.):S45-S50, 1998.
152. Nigdikar, S.V., Williams, N.R., Griffin, B.A., Howard, A.N., Consumption of red wine polyphenols reduces the susceptibility of low-density lipoproteins to oxidation in vivo [see comments], *Am. J. Clin. Nutr.,* 68:258-265, 1998.
153. Stein, J.H., Keevil, J.G., Wiebe, D.A., Aeschlimann, S., and Folts, J.D., Purple grape juice improves endothelial function and reduces the susceptibility of LDL cholesterol to oxidation in patients with coronary artery disease, *Circulation*, 100:1050-1055, 1999.
154. Kagan, V.E., Serbinova, E.A., Forte, T., Scita, G., and Packer, L., Recycling of vitamin E in human low density lipoproteins, *J. Lipid. Res.,* 33:385-397, 1992.

155. Tribble, D.L., Thiel, P.M., van den Berg, J.J., and Krauss R.M., Differing alpha-tocopherol oxidative lability and ascorbic acid sparing effects in buoyant and dense LDL, *Arterioscler. Thromb. Vasc. Biol.*, 15:2025-2031, 1995.
156. Thomas, S.R., Neuzil, J., Mohr, D., and Stocker, R., Coantioxidants make alpha-tocopherol an efficient antioxidant for low-density lipoprotein, *Am. J. Clin. Nutr.*, 62:1357S-1364S, 1995.
157. Frei, B., Keaney, J.F.J., Retsky, K.L., and Chen, K., Vitamins C and E and LDL oxidation, *Vitam. Horm.*, 52:1-34, 1996.
158. Taddei, S., Virdis, A., Ghiadoni, L., Magagna, A., and Salvetti, A., Vitamin C improves endothelium-dependent vasodilation by restoring nitric oxide activity in essential hypertension, *Circulation*, 97:2222-2229, 1998.
159. Dudgeon, S., Benson, D.P., MacKenzie, A., Paisley-Zyszkiewicz, K., and Martin. W., Recovery by ascorbate of impaired nitric oxide-dependent relaxation resulting from oxidant stress in rat aorta, *Br. J. Pharmacol.*, 125:782-786, 1998.
160. Cannon, R.O., Role of nitric oxide in cardiovascular disease: focus on the endothelium [published erratum appears in *Clin. Chem.*, 1998 Sep;44(9):2070], *Clin. Chem.*, 44:1809-1819, 1998.
161. Endres, M., Laufs, U., Huang, Z., Nakamura, T., Huang, P., Moskowitz, M.A., et al., Stroke protection by 3-hydroxy-3-methylglutaryl (HMG)-CoA reductase inhibitors mediated by endothelial nitric oxide synthase, *Proc. Natl. Acad. Sci.* USA, 95:8880-8885, 1998.
162. Laufs, U. and Liao, J.K., Post-transcriptional regulation of endothelial nitric oxide synthase mRNA stability by Rho GTPase, *J. Biol. Chem.*, 273:24266-24271, 1998.
163. Tomeo, A.C., Geller, M., Watkins, T.R., Gapor, A., and Bierenbaum, M.L., Antioxidant effects of tocotrienols in patients with hyperlipidemia and carotid stenosis, *Lipids*, 30:1179-1183, 1995.
164. Ramasamy, S., Drummond, G.R., Ahn, J., Storek, M., Pohl, J., and Parthasarathy, S., et al., Modulation of expression of endothelial nitric oxide synthase by nordihydroguaiaretic acid, a phenolic antioxidant in cultured endothelial cells, *Mol. Pharmacol.*, 56:116-123, 1999.
165. Sato, Y., Nakatsuka, H., Watanabe, T., Hisamichi, S., Shimizu, H., and Fujisaku, S., et al., Possible contribution of green tea drinking habits to the prevention of stroke, *Tohoku J. Exp. Med.*, 157:337-343, 1989.
166. Smith, S.R., Klotman, P.E., and Svetkey, L.P., Potassium chloride lowers blood pressure and causes natriuresis in older patients with hypertension, *J. Am. Soc. Nephrol.*, 2:1302-1309, 1992.
167. Mano, M., Sugawara, A., Nara, Y., Nakao, K., Horie, R., Endo, J., et al., Potassium accelerates urinary sodium excretion during salt loading without stimulating atrial natriuretic polypeptide secretion, *Clin. Exp. Pharmacol. Physiol.*, 19:795-801, 1992.
168. McCabe, R.D., Bakarich, M.A., Srivastava, K., and Young, D.B., Potassium inhibits free radical formation, *Hypertension*, 24:77-82, 1994.
169. Young, D.B., Lin, H., and McCabe, R.D., Potassium's cardiovascular protective mechanisms, *Am. J. Physiol.*, 268:R825-R837, 1995.
170. Yang, B.C., Li, D.Y., Weng, Y.F., Lynch, J., Wingo, C.S., and Mehta, J.L., Increased superoxide anion generation and altered vasoreactivity in rabbits on low-potassium diet, *Am. J. Physiol.*, 274:H1955-H1961, 1998.
171. Raij, L., Luscher, T.F., and Vanhoutte, P.M., High potassium diet augments endothelium-dependent relaxations in the Dahl rat, *Hypertension*, 12:562-567, 1988.

172. Qureshi, A.A., Qureshi, N., Wright, J.J., Shen, Z., Kramer, G., Gapor, A., et al., Lowering of serum cholesterol in hypercholesterolemic humans by tocotrienols (palmvitee), *Am. J. Clin. Nutr.*, 53:1021S-1026S, 1991.
173. Qureshi, A.A., Bradlow, B.A., Brace, L., Manganello, J., Peterson, D.M., and Pearce, B.C., et al., Response of hypercholesterolemic subjects to administration of tocotrienols, *Lipids*, 30:1171-1177, 1995.
174. Monforte, M.T., Trovato, A., Kirjavainen, S., Forestieri, A.M., Galati, E.M., and Lo, C.R., Biological effects of hesperidin, a citrus flavonoid (Note II): hypolipidemic activity on experimental hypercholesterolemia in rat, *Farmaco*, 50:595-599, 1995.
175. Bok, S.H., Lee, S.H., Park, Y.B., Bae, K.H., Son, K.H., Jeong, T.S., et al., Plasma and hepatic cholesterol and hepatic activities of 3-hydroxy-3-methyl-glutaryl-CoA reductase and acyl CoA: cholesterol transferase are lower in rats fed citrus peel extract or a mixture of citrus bioflavonoids, *J. Nutr.*, 129:1182-1185, 1999.
176. Kritchevsky, D., Dietary fibre and lipid metabolism, *Int. J. Obesity*, 11(Suppl. 1) 33-43, 1987.
177. Kishimoto, Y., Wakabayashi, S., and Takeda, H., Hypocholesterolemic effect of dietary fiber: relation to intestinal fermentation and bile acid excretion, *J. Nutr. Sci. Vitaminol.* (Tokyo), 41:151-161, 1995.
178. Matheson, H.B., Colon, I.S., and Story, J.A., Cholesterol 7 alpha-hydroxylase activity is increased by dietary modification with psyllium hydrocolloid, pectin, cholesterol and cholestyramine in rats, *J. Nutr.*, 125:454-458, 1995.
179. Broekmans, W.M.R., Klopping-Ketelaars, I.A.A., Schuurman, R.W.C. et al., Fruits and vegetables increase plasma carotenoids and vitamins and decrease homocysteine in humans, *J. Nutr.*, 130:1578-1583, 2000.
180. Truswell, A.S., Dietary fibre and blood lipids, *Curr. Opin. Lipidol.*, 6:14-19, 1995.
181. Anderson, J.W., Dietary fibre, complex carbohydrate and coronary artery disease, *Can. J. Cardiol.*, 11(Suppl. G) 55G-62G, 1995.
182. Coats, A.J., The potential role of soluble fibre in the treatment of hypercholesterolaemia, *Postgrad. Med. J.*, 74:391-394, 1998.
183. Levrat, M.A., Favier, M.L., Moundras, C., Remesy, C., Demigne, C., and Morand, C., Role of dietary propionic acid and bile acid excretion in the hypocholesterolemic effects of oligosaccharides in rats, *J. Nutr.*, 124:531-538, 1994.
184. Prasad, K., Homocysteine, a risk factor for cardiovascular disease, *Int. J. Angiol.*, 8:76-86, 1999.
185. Naurath, H.J., Joosten, E., Riezler, R., Stabler, S.P., Allen, R.H., and Lindenbaum, J., Effects of vitamin B12, folate, and vitamin B6 supplements in elderly people with normal serum vitamin concentrations, *Lancet*, 346:85-89, 1995.
186. Selhub, J., Jacques, P.F., Wilson, P.W., Rush, D., and Rosenberg, I.H., Vitamin status and intake as primary determinants of homocysteinemia in an elderly population, *J. Am. Med. Assoc.*, 270:2693-2698, 1993.
187. Ubbink, J.B., The role of vitamins in the pathogenesis and treatment of hyperhomocyst(e)inaemia, *J. Inherit. Metab. Dis.*, 20:316-325, 1997.
188. van den Berg, M., Franken, D.G., Boers, G.H., Blom, H.J., Jakobs, C., Stehouwer, C.D., et al., Combined vitamin B6 plus folic acid therapy in young patients with arteriosclerosis and hyperhomocysteinemia, *J. Vasc. Surg.*, 20:933-940, 1994.
189. Tawakol, A., Omland, T., Gerhard, M., Wu, J.T., and Creager, M.A., Hyperhomocyst(e)inemia is associated with impaired endothelium-dependent vasodilation in humans, *Circulation*, 95:1119-1121, 1997.
190. Bellamy, M.F., McDowell, I.F., Ramsey, M.W., Brownlee, M., Bones, C., Newcombe, R.G., et al., Hyperhomocysteinemia after an oral methionine load acutely impairs endothelial function in healthy adults, *Circulation*, 98:1848-1852, 1998.

191. Upchurch, G.R.J., Welch, G.N., Fabian, A.J., Freedman, J.E., Johnson, J.L., Keaney, J.F.J., et al., Homocyst(e)ine decreases bioavailable nitric oxide by a mechanism involving glutathione peroxidase, *J. Biol. Chem.,* 272:17012-17017, 1997.
192. Robinson, K., Mayer, E.L., Miller, D.P., Green, R., van Lente, F., Gupta, A., et al., Hyperhomocysteinemia and low pyridoxal phosphate. Common and independent reversible risk factors for coronary artery disease, *Circulation*, 92:2825-2830, 1995.
193. Folsom, A.R., Nieto, F.J., McGovern, P.G., Tsai, M.Y., Malinow, M.R., Eckfeldt, J.H., et al., Prospective study of coronary heart disease incidence in relation to fasting total homocysteine, related genetic polymorphisms, and B vitamins: the Atherosclerosis Risk in Communities (ARIC) study [see comments], *Circulation*, 98:204-210, 1998.
194. Chasan-Taber, L., Selhub, J., Rosenberg, I.H., Malinow, M.R., Terry, P., Tishler, P.V., et al., A prospective study of folate and vitamin B6 and risk of myocardial infarction in US physicians, *J. Am. Coll. Nutr.,* 15:136-143, 1996.
195. Tucker, K.L., Selhub, J., Wilson, P.W., and Rosenberg, I.H., Dietary intake pattern relates to plasma folate and homocysteine concentrations in the Framingham Heart Study, *J. Nutr.,* 126:3025-3031, 1996.
196. Oshaug, A., Bugge, K.H., and Refsum, H., Diet, an independent determinant for plasma total homocysteine. A cross sectional study of Norwegian workers on platforms in the North Sea, *Eur. J. Clin. Nutr.,* 52:7-11, 1998.
197. Kato, I., Dnistrian, A.M., Schwartz, M., Toniolo, P., Koenig, K., Shore, R.E., et al., Epidemiologic correlates of serum folate and homocysteine levels among users and non-users of vitamin supplement, *Int. J. Vitam. Nutr. Res.,* 69:322-329, 1999.
198. Brouwer, I.A., van Dusseldorp, M., West, C.E., Meyboom, S., Thomas, C.M., Duran, M., et al., Dietary folate from vegetables and citrus fruit decreases plasma homocysteine concentrations in humans in a dietary controlled trial, *J. Nutr.,* 129:1135-1139, 1999.
199. Burt, V.L., Whelton, P., Roccella, E.J., et al., Prevalence of hypertension in the US adult population: results from the Third National Health and Nutrition Examination Survey, 1988-1991, *Hypertension*, 25:305-313, 1995.
200. Appel, L.J., Moore, T.J., Obarzanek, E., et al., A clinical trial of the effects of dietary patterns of blood pressure, *N. Engl. J. Med.,* 336: 1117-1124, 1997.
201. Plaisted, C.S., Lin, P.H., Ard, J.D., McClure, M.L., and Svetkey, L.P., The effects of dietary patterns on quality of life: a substudy of the dietary approaches to stop hypertension (DASH) randomized clinical trial, *J. Am. Diet. Assoc.*, 99: S84-89, 1999.
202. Svetkey, L.P., Simons-Morton, D., Vollmer, W.M., Appel, L.J., Conlin, P.R., Ryan, D.H., Ard, J., and Kennedy, B.M., Effects of dietary patterns on blood pressure: subgroup analysis of the Dietary Approaches to Stop Hypertension (DASH) randomized clinical trial, *Arch. Intern. Med.,* 159(3): 285-293, 1999.
203. Ascherio, A., Hennekens, C., Willett, W.C., Sacks, F., Rosner, B., Manson, J., Witteman, J., and Stampfer, M.J., Prospective study of nutritional factors, blood pressure and hypertension among US women, *Hypertension*, 27(5): 1065-1072, 1996.
204. Reuter, H.D., Koch, H.P., and Lawson, L.D., Therapeutic effects and applications of garlic and its preparations. In Koch H.P. and Lawson L.D., Eds., *Garlic: The Science and Therapeutic Applications of* Allium Sativum L. *and Related Species*, Baltimore: Williams & Wilkins, 1996:135-212.
205. Singh, R.B., Rastogi, S.S., Singh, N.K., Ghosh, G., Gupta, S., and Niaz, M.A., Can guava fruit intake decrease blood pressure and blood lipids?, *J. Hum. Hypertens.,* 7(1):33-38, 1993.
206. Wachman, A. and Bernstein, D.S., Diet and osteoporosis, *Lancet*, 1:958-959, 1968.

207. Breslau, N.A., Brinkley, L., Hill, K.D., and Pak, C.Y., Relationship of animal protein-rich diet to kidney stone formation and calcium metabolism, *J. Clin. Endocrinol. Metab.,* 66:140-146, 1988.
208. Marsh, A.G., Sanchez, T.V., Michelsen, O., Chaffee, F.L., and Fagal, S.M., Vegetarian lifestyle and bone mineral density, *Am. J. Clin. Nutr.,* 48:837-841, 1988.
209. Goulding, A., Fasting urinary sodium/creatinine in relation to calcium/creatinine and hydroxyproline/creatinine in a general population of women, *N Z Med. J.,* 93:294-297, 1981.
210. Goulding, A. and Campbell, D., Dietary NaCl loads promote calciuria and bone loss in adult oophorectomized rats consuming a low calcium diet, *J. Nutr.,* 113:1409-1414, 1983.
211. Goulding, A. and Campbell, D.R., Effects of oral loads of sodium chloride on bone composition in growing rats consuming ample dietary calcium, *Miner. Electrolyte Metab.,* 10:58-62, 1984.
212. McParland, B.E., Goulding, A., and Campbell, A.J., Dietary salt affects biochemical markers of resorption and formation of bone in elderly women, *Br. Med. J.,* 299:834-835, 1989.
213. Mizushima, S., Tsuchida, K., and Yamori, Y., Preventive nutritional factors in epidemiology: interaction between sodium and calcium, *Clin. Exp. Pharmacol. Physiol.,* 26:573-575, 1999.
214. Lemann, J.J., Gray, R.W., and Pleuss, J.A., Potassium bicarbonate, but not sodium bicarbonate, reduces urinary calcium excretion and improves calcium balance in healthy men, *Kidney Int.,* 35:688-695, 1989.
215. Lemann, J.J., Pleuss, J.A., Gray, R.W., and Hoffmann, R.G., Potassium administration reduces and potassium deprivation increases urinary calcium excretion in healthy adults [corrected] [published erratum appears in *Kidney Int.,* 1991 Aug;40(2):388], *Kidney Int.,* 39:973-983, 1991.
216. Booth, S.L., Skeletal functions of vitamin K-dependent proteins: not just for clotting anymore, *Nutr. Rev.,* 55:282-284, 1997.
217. Ferland, G., The vitamin K-dependent proteins: an update, *Nutr. Rev.,* 56:223-230, 1998.
218. Binkley, N.C. and Suttie, J.W., Vitamin K nutrition and osteoporosis, *J. Nutr.,* 125:1812-1821, 1995.
219. Jie, K.G., Bots, M.L., Vermeer, C., Witteman, J.C., and Grobbee, D.E., Vitamin K status and bone mass in women with and without aortic atherosclerosis: a population-based study, *Calcif. Tissue Int.,* 59:352-356, 1996.
220. Kanai, T., Takagi, T., Masuhiro, K., Nakamura, M., Iwata, M., and Saji, F., Serum vitamin K level and bone mineral density in post-menopausal women, *Int. J. Gynaecol. Obstet.,* 56:25-30, 1997.
221. Feskanich, D., Weber, P., Willett, W.C., Rockett, H., Booth, S.L., and Colditz, G.A., Vitamin K intake and hip fractures in women: a prospective study, *Am. J. Clin. Nutr.,* 69:74-79, 1999.
222. Philip, W.J., Martin, J.C., Richardson J.M., Reid D.M., Webster J., Douglas A.S., Decreased axial and peripheral bone density in patients taking long-term warfarin, *Q. J. Med.,* 88:635-640, 1995.
223. Knapen, M.H., Hamulyak, K., and Vermeer, C., The effect of vitamin K supplementation on circulating osteocalcin (bone Gla protein) and urinary calcium excretion, *Ann. Intern. Med.,* 111:1001-1005, 1989.

224. Vermeer, C., Gijsbers, B.L., Craciun, A.M., Groenen-van Dooren, M.M., and Knapen, M.H., Effects of vitamin K on bone mass and bone metabolism, *J. Nutr.,* 126:1187S-1191S, 1996.
225. Craciun, A.M., Wolf, J., Knapen, M.H., Brouns, F., and Vermeer, C., Improved bone metabolism in female elite athletes after vitamin K supplementation, *Int. J. Sports. Med.,* 19:479-484, 1998.
226. Matsunaga, S., Ito, H., and Sakou, T., The effect of vitamin K and D supplementation on ovariectomy-induced bone loss [In Process Citation], *Calcif. Tissue Int.,* 65:285-289, 1999.
227. Falch, J.A., Mowe, M., and Bohmer, T., Low levels of serum ascorbic acid in elderly patients with hip fractures, *Scand. J. Clin. Lab. Invest.*, 58(3), 225-228, 1998.
228. Hall, S.L. and Greendale, G.A., The relation of dietary vitamin C intake to bone mineral density: results from the PEPI study, *Calcif. Tiss. Int.*, 63(3), 183-189, 1998.
229. Melhus, H., Michaelsson, K., Holmberg, L., Wolk, A., and Ljunghall, S., Smoking, antioxidant vitamins, and the risk of hip fracture, *J. Bone Min. Res.*, 14(1), 129-135, 1999.
230. Handelman, G.J., Dratz, E.A., Reay, C.C., and van Kuijk, J.G., Carotenoids in the human macula and whole retina, *Invest. Ophthalmol. Vis. Sci.,* 29:850-855, 1988.
231. Schalch, W., Carotenoids in the retina — a review of their possible role in preventing or limiting damage caused by light and oxygen, *EXS*, 62:280-298, 1992.
232. Snodderly, D.M., Evidence for protection against age-related macular degeneration by carotenoids and antioxidant vitamins, *Am. J. Clin. Nutr.*, 62:1448S-1461S, 1995.
233. Sujak, A., Gabrielska, J., Grudziski, W., Borc, R., Mazurek, P., et al., Lutein and zeaxanthin as protectors of lipid membranes against oxidative damage: the structural aspects, *Arch. Biochem. Biophys*. 371:301-307, 1999.

Section III

Herbs and Health

12 Herbal Remedies that Promote Health and Prevent Disease

Winston J. Craig

CONTENTS

12.1 INTRODUCTON

The annual sale of botanical products has grown to be a multimillion dollar business. Today we are witnessing a great deal of interest in the use of herbal remedies. Some consumers have become dissatisfied with conventional medicine. They perceive it

0-8493-0038-X/97/$0.00+$.50

as impersonal and expensive, and conventional drug therapy often has undesirable side effects. For many Americans, the medicinal use of plant extracts seems to be a more natural, less expensive way, and involving therapies that are more gentle and largely without side effects.

Plants have always played a significant role in maintaining the health and improving the quality of human life. Many Western drugs owe their origin to plant extracts. For example, reserpine, which is widely used for the treatment of high blood pressure, was originally extracted from the plant *Rauwolfia serpentina* while digitalis, used as a heart stimulant, was derived from the foxglove plant (*Digitalis purpurea*). The American Indians also utilized a number of native herbs for medicinal purposes. Self-prescribed herbal preparations are commonly consumed today for a whole host of common ailments or conditions, such as anxiety, arthritis, colds, coughs, constipation, declining mental acuity, depression, fever, headaches, infections, insomnia, intestinal disorders, premenstrual syndrome, stress, ulcers, and weakness.

Culinary herbs to flavor foods have also been grown and used since antiquity. For most of these herbs, the flavor is provided by the aromatic ingredients in their essential oils and oleoresins. Many of these compounds are terpenoids and they have an important physiological activity that protects the consumer against disease. While these herbs are generally consumed in small amounts, it is interesting to note that they contain similar health-promoting phytochemicals as do fruits and vegetables (see Table 12.1). Flavoring soups, stews, entrees, and other dishes with herbs such as basil, caraway, cilantro, coriander, cumin, dill, oregano, rosemary, sage, thyme, and other herbal seasonings provides a wide variety of important phytochemicals and permits us to reduce our salt intake. There is clearly a botanical and chemical similarity between many of the herbal seasonings and conventional vegetables in the human dietary.

12.2 HERBAL RELIEF FOR THE GASTROINTESTINAL SYSTEM

12.2.1 Help for Problems of the Digestive System

The dried rhizome of ginger (*Zingiber officianale*) has a long history of use as a flavoring agent. More recently, it has aroused interest because of its effectiveness for indigestion, loss of appetite, the treatment of nausea, and preventing the symptoms of motion sickness. Ginger promotes the secretion of saliva and gastric juices as well as bile.[2] It also increases peristalsis and the tone of the intestinal tract. The activity of ginger is due to its volatile oil, which contains the sesquiterpenes zingiberene and bisabolene and the pungent gingerols. New research showed that about six compounds appear to be important (especially [10]-shogaol) to provide the antiemetic activity of ginger.[3] In the same study, eugenol and methyl eugenol in cloves were also found to be very effective as anti-emetics. Modest amounts of ginger appear to be safe since no toxic or unpleasant side effects have been reported.[4]

TABLE 12.1
Phytochemicals Found in Herbs

Phytochemical	Herbal Source of Phytochemical[1]
Carotenoids	Green leafy herbs, paprika, rose hips
Coumarins	Alfalfa, aniseed, chamomile, fenugreek, parsley, red clover
Curcuminoids	Ginger, turmeric
Flavonoids	Chamomile, ginkgo, hawthorn, licorice root, milk thistle, nettles, passionflower, rosemary, thyme
Lignans	Flaxseed, milk thistle, schizandra
Phthalides	Anise, caraway, cilantro, cumin, dill, fennel, parsley
Phytosterols	Nettles, pumpkin seeds, saw palmetto
Phenolic acids	Echinacea, rosemary, sage, St. John's wort, thyme
Polyacetylenes	Anise, caraway, cilantro, cumin, dill, fennel, parsley
Saponins	Alfalfa, black cohosh, ginseng, horse-chestnut, licorice root, snakeroot
Sulfides	Chives, garlic, leeks, onions
Terpenes	Basil, buchu, ginkgo, juniper, lemon grass, oregano, peppermint, rosemary, sage, thyme

The dried inner bark of slippery elm (*Ulmus fulva*) has a high content of mucilages. The soothing properties of these mucilages make it useful for treating inflammation or ulceration of the stomach or intestinal tract, colitis, and irritated mucous membranes.[2] The leaves and flowering tops of peppermint (*Mentha piperita*) provide a volatile oil rich in menthol. This oil promotes gastric secretions and has a spasmolytic effect on the smooth muscle of the digestive system. This latter activity explains its use as an effective treatment for irritable bowel syndrome.[5] Excessive use of the oil, however, can produce toxic effects.

German chamomile (*Matricaria recutita L.*) is marketed in Europe for a wide variety of ailments. It is used effectively both internally and externally for its anti-inflammatory, antispasmodic, and antibacterial properties.[4] Chamomile tea is used to relieve gastrointestinal spasms, indigestion, peptic ulcers, and menstrual cramps. To be effective, chamomile tea must be made from the fresh herb. Compresses, rinses, or gargles are used to treat hemorrhoids, inflammations, and irritations of the skin, mouth, gums, and throat. The blue-colored oil obtained from chamomile contains many terpenoids and flavonoids which provide the anti-inflammatory and antispasmodic effects. The major activity of chamomile is believed to be provided by alpha-bisabolol, which comprises about 13% of the essential oil.[6] People allergic to flowers in the daisy family may suffer allergic reactions with chamomile.

Licorice (*Glycyrrhiza glabra*) is useful for the treatment of peptic and duodenal ulcers. The flavonoids in licorice root (liquiritin, isoliquiritin, liquiritigenin, isoliquiritigenin) are thought to be responsible for its anti-ulcer activity.[7] The active and major constituent of the rhizomes and roots is glycyrrhizin, a triterpenoid glycoside which possesses anti-inflammatory and anti-allergic properties, due to its ability to block prostaglandin metabolism.[4] Licorice also has pronounced expectorant and effective cough suppressant properties. In large doses, licorice can produce serious side effects including edema, high blood pressure, excessive potassium excretion, and heart failure. Hence, the elderly and those suffering cardiovascular disease or kidney problems should exercise caution when using licorice. Furthermore, what appears to be licorice may in fact contain no licorice at all, since its flavor can be mimicked by anise.

Turmeric (*Curcuma domestica*), the yellow food coloring used in curry and other foods, is useful for stimulating bile production, for liver and gallbladder complaints, and a loss of appetite.[2] The essential oil of turmeric contains a mixture of tumerones and atlantones and zingiberene. The yellow curcuminoids in turmeric are known to possess appreciable anti-inflammatory, antimicrobial, and antitumor properties.[8] Teas made from the dried leaves of blackberry (*Rubus fruticosus*), blueberry (*Vaccinium corymbosum*), and raspberry (*Rubus idaeus*) are useful for the treatment of diarrhea.[4] The leaves are very rich in tannins which provide astringency and the antidiarrheal effect. The dried blueberry fruits have also been used for simple diarrhea. On the other hand, fresh blueberries can exert a laxative effect. The teas made from the leaves of these berries are also effectively used as a mouthwash for treating sore mouth and an inflamed throat.

Fennel seeds (*Foeniculum vulgare*) are known to stimulate gastrointestinal motility and are useful for treating digestive disorders such as mild, spastic disorders of the upper gastrointestinal tract and flatulence. Fennel (with its anise-like flavor) possesses anti-inflammatory, antispasmodic, and expectorant properties. The essential oil of fennel is rich in *trans*-anethole, fenchone, and estragole, terpenoids which possess a secrolytic action on the respiratory tract.[2]

12.2.2 Laxatives

In today's society many people do not drink sufficient water, do not exercise regularly, and consume diets with insufficient fiber. The result is often constipation and irregularity. Millions of dollars are spent on various laxatives, especially by the elderly, to provide relief from constipation. There are a number of plant-based laxatives available to the consumer. The bulk-producing herbs act in much the same way as a high-fiber diet. Another group of herbs that contain anthraquinones stimulate intestinal motility and promote water and electrolyte accumulation in the colon. This latter group of laxatives can reduce the natural bowel function and lead to reliance upon laxatives.[4] Psyllium, cascara sagrada, or senna are all commonly utilized in many over-the-counter laxative preparations.

The most popular of the bulk-forming laxatives is *Plantago psyllium*. The seeds and husks of psyllium, being high in mucilage, swell to many times their original volume when contact is made with water. The use of psyllium will therefore increase the volume of the intestinal contents and facilitate evacuation of the bowels. Although psyllium is a safe and effective laxative, a small percentage of people experience allergic reactions.[4] Since psyllium can expand its volume to many times its original size, care must be taken not to overdose. Intestinal obstructions may occur in cases of improper use. The use of *Plantago* seeds has also been suggested as a useful method to achieve weight loss. Recently, it was shown that 20 g of psyllium consumed with 200 ml of water 3 hours before a meal, and then again immediately before the meal, can produce a significant increase in the feeling of satisfaction and fullness.[9] In addition, there was a significant reduction in calorie and fat consumption (up to 15 g less fat consumed per day).

Another common laxative is cascara sagrada, the dried, aged bark of *Rhamnus purshiana*, a small tree of the Pacific Northwest belonging to the Buckthorn family. Cascara is fairly mild-acting, producing only minor effects on the small intestine and therefore has a low risk of dependence. The active constituents in cascara are a mixture of four cascarosides as well as minor amounts of other anthraquinone glycosides. Large doses or long-term use of cascara may cause chronic diarrhea and inflammation of the colon. Nursing mothers should avoid using cascara since the anthraquinones in cascara are expressed in the mother's milk and these will adversely affect the infant.[4,10]

Another widely used stimulant laxative that contains anthraquinones is senna. Senna consists of the dried leaflets of either *Cassia acutifolia* Delile (Alexandria senna) or *Cassia angustifolia* Vahl (Tinnevelley senna), small shrubs of the pea family. The leaves and pods of senna contain a family of anthraquinones called sennosides which stimulate the colon and provide the desired laxative action. The leaves are safer to use than the pods since the pods contain about twice the level of active compounds. Senna acts much like cascara. However, senna induces more intestinal muscle contractions and may cause nausea, cramping, and dehydration. Being a potent purgative, senna should be used carefully.[10,11] Nevertheless, senna is more commonly used than cascara since it is less expensive. Senna should not be used for more than a week at a time, since dependency will result and the bowels will become very sluggish with extensive use of the herb. Chronic use of senna can also lead to fluid and electrolyte imbalance.[4,10]

12.2.3 Liver Protecton from Milk Thistle

Milk thistle (*Silybum marianum*), a native of the Mediterranean region, is cultivated for its culinary, medicinal, and ornamental purposes. The young, tender leaves, rich in flavonoids, are used in salads while the ripe black seeds are roasted and used as a coffee substitute. A complex mixture of flavonolignans, called silymarin (4 to 6% of the ripe seeds), have been isolated from the seeds of milk thistle. Silymarin includes silybin, isosilybin, dehydrosilybin, silydianin, silychristin, and other flavonolignans. Silymarin is known to protect against liver damage caused by the deadly *Amanita phalloides* (death cap) mushroom.[12] Numerous studies have demonstrated the efficacy and safety of silymarin for treatment of liver disease such as alcohol-induced cirrhosis. Silymarin appears to help stabilize liver cell membranes to prevent entry of toxic substances, and also stimulates the regenerative ability of the liver and the formation of new hepatocytes by promoting protein synthesis.[2] Preparations of silymarin are also used for treatment of chronic hepatitis as well as protection of the liver against environmental toxins. Milk thistle teas are ineffective since silymarin is very poorly soluble in water. Furthermore, oral use requires a concentrated product since silymarin is poorly absorbed from the gastrointestinal tract.

12.3 HERBS FOR THE UROGENITAL SYSTEM

12.3.1 Assistance for the Kidneys

Herbal diuretics function by promoting blood flow in the kidneys and hence increase the volume of urine produced. These herbs may also be useful for the treatment of kidney infections and inflammation of the urinary tract, or for the prevention of kidney stones.[4] A number of herbal preparations have also been widely used as diuretics to treat premenstrual syndrome and other conditions. Extracts of goldenrod, buchu, juniper, parsley, bearberry, and stinging nettle appear to be modestly effective diuretics that may be used safely in moderation.[11]

The most effective herbal product that safely acts as a diuretic is goldenrod (*Solidago* sp.). It is widely used in Europe to treat inflammations of the urinary tract. In addition, goldenrod also has anti-inflammatory and antibacterial activity. While there are over 130 species of goldenrod, most of them have similar diuretic activities. The active constituents of goldenrod include flavonoids, tannins, and saponins.[4] Buchu (*Barosma betulina*), a small shrub indigenous to South Africa, is useful for its diuretic properties. Its leaves, which have a peppermint odor, are rich in flavonoids and contain an aromatic oil rich in terpenoids such as diosphenol, limonene, and menthone. Buchu leaf is used to treat inflammations and infections of the kidney, bladder, and urinary tract.[2]

The dried ripe berries of the juniper tree (*Juniperus communis*) have a useful diuretic function. Juniper is also useful for urinary tract infections and inflammations, kidney and bladder stones, and digestive disorders such as heartburn and bloating.[2] The diuretic effect of juniper results from its content of terpinen-4-ol and other monoterpenes in the essential oil of the berries. These compounds seem to increase the glomerular filtration rate in the kidney. Juniper berries are potentially the most toxic of the diuretic herbs. Long-term use or an overdosage may cause kidney damage characterized by albuminuria or renal hematuria.[4] Parsley (*Petroselinum crispum*) is widely used as a garnish. The leaves and roots of parsley are useful for the treatment of infections of the urinary tract, and for kidney and bladder stones. Parsley contains substantial levels of a variety of phytochemicals — furocoumarins, terpenoids, flavonoids, and phthalides. The active constituents in the essential oil of parsley seeds include apiol and myristicin.[4]

A tea made from the dried leaves of bearberry or uva ursi (*Arctostaphylos uva-ursi*) has diuretic and strong astringent qualities. Bearberry is also very effective against urinary tract infections. Antibacterial action results from the presence of two phenolic glycosides, hydroquinone glucuronides and hydroquinone sulfate esters, formed in the body from arbutin, a natural constituent of bearberry. One drawback of uva ursi is that it is effective only if the urine is alkaline.[4] Prolonged use of uva ursi is not recommended since large and frequent doses can cause vomiting, convulsions, and other side effects.[4,7]

The ovate leaves and fibrous stems of stinging nettle (*Urtica dioica*) are covered with tiny, hollow, silica-tipped hairs which release the irritant formic acid and histamine when touched. However, the stinging irritant can be tamed by cooking or drying. Nettle juice or the dried leaves of *U. dioica* possess diuretic activity, possibly due to their high flavonoid content.[2] Nettles find use in the treatment of urinary tract infections and kidney stones. An extract of the root of stinging nettles has proven useful for increasing the volume of urine and maximum urinary flow, while decreasing residual urine, especially in men with a mildly enlarged prostate.[2]

Additional herbs that possess some degree of diuretic activity include the dandelion (*Taraxacum officinale*), hibiscus (*Hibiscus sabdariffa* L.), horsetail (*Equisetum arvense* L.), and rose hips (*Rosa canina*). Horsetail, a silica-rich, hollow-stemmed perennial, exerts a weak diuretic activity due to the presence of several flavonoid glycosides and a saponin. The dried leaves and root of the dandelion that are harvested before the flowering season can stimulate bile flow and diuresis. The activity of the leaves results from the presence of a number of sesquiterpene lactones and flavonoids.[2]

12.3.2 Cranberry Cure

Cranberry juice is useful for reducing bacterial infections of the bladder. The antibacterial effect of cranberries was thought to result from the acidity of the urine produced when cranberries or cranberry beverage was consumed. Recently, cranberry juice was shown to inhibit by about 80% the adherence of *E. coli* bacteria to the mucosal surface of the urinary tract.[4] Both cranberry and blueberry juices actually contain the inhibitory substance. Bacteriuria, which is common in elderly women, usually occurs without any symptoms. When elderly women were given either 300 ml of cranberry juice or a placebo every day for 6 months it was found that the women taking the cranberry were only one-half as likely to develop bacteriuria with pyuria compared with those not using the cranberry juice. During the study, the women consuming the cranberry juice were twice as likely to make the transition from being infected to being noninfected on successive months.[13] These effects were unrelated to the acidity of the women's urine.

12.3.3 Relief for the Prostate

Extracts of the fruit of saw palmetto have been used for the treatment of benign hypertrophy (enlargement) of the prostate (BHP). The active substances in saw palmetto provide such beneficial effects as increased urinary flow, increased ease in commencing urination, reduced residual urine, and decreased frequency of urination.[4] Within three months, 90% of BHP patients who used saw palmetto considered the herbal therapy successful.[14]

The root of stinging nettle (*Urtica dioica*) has been shown to provide symptomatic relief of urinary difficulties in men with benign enlargement of the prostate.[15] A dose of 4 to 6 g per day of *U. dioica* is used to increase the volume of urine produced and diminish the urge to void during the night. French researchers observed that men with prostate enlargement who daily consumed stinging nettle root extract greatly reduced the frequency of nocturia, especially in patients with less severe conditions. The steroids stigmast-4-en-3-one, stigmasterol, and campesterol in stinging nettle root were observed to strongly inhibit the Na^+,K^+-ATPase activity of the prostate which may subsequently suppress prostate cell metabolism and growth.[16]

The enzyme aromatase mediates the conversion of androgens to estrogens, which has been implicated in promoting prostate growth. The potential inhibition of aromatase by stinging nettle components is currently being studied.[17]

Pumpkin seeds (*Cucurbita pepo*), which are very rich in a variety of phytosterols, has shown promise for treating BHP. Regular use of ground seeds relieves the difficulties associated with an enlarged prostate, without reducing the enlargement.[2] A number of European studies have reported the efficacy of the bark from the African prune tree (*Pygeum africanum*) for treatment of BHP. After 1 to 2 months of daily treatment with *P. africanum* extract, men over 50 years of age with enlarged prostates experienced less need for nighttime urination, an improved urinary flow and volume, and a reduced postvoiding residual volume. Clinical benefits were even maintained for one month after treatment.[18]

12.4 HERBAL HELP FOR DIABETICS

Diabetes is a disease characterized by inappropriate hyperglycemia. The unregulated blood sugar can result from either a deficiency of insulin or a reduction in its effectiveness. Noninsulin-dependent diabetics may use oral hypoglycemic agents to stimulate the pancreas to produce more insulin. Careful dietary habits and exercise are essential components in the management of diabetes. Nevertheless, a few herbs have shown promise for assisting in the management of diabetes.

Bitter melon (*Momordica charantia*) is a green, cucumber-shaped tropical fruit with gourd-like bumps, that is eaten unripe like a vegetable. Clinical trials with type II diabetics has established that use of the bitter melon extract can effectively lower blood sugar levels and improve glucose tolerance in diabetics.[19,20] Bitter melon contains a mixture of steroids which have a potent hypoglycemic effect. Recent experiments found that polypeptide-p isolated from the fruit could mimic insulin activity.[21]

Animal and human studies have shown that consumption of fenugreek seeds (*Trigonella foenum graecum*) can lower blood sugar levels in diabetics.[22,23] Research in India found that glucose tolerance improved, urinary glucose excretion decreased 70%, and insulin responses were reduced in diabetics after defatted fenugreek was used for 10 days.[22] Total serum cholesterol, LDL cholesterol, and triglyceride levels, but not HDL cholesterol, all significantly decreased about 20% when fenugreek was added to the diet. These changes in blood lipids are important factors for a diabetic who usually has elevated blood lipids. A daily use of 25–100 mg of fenugreek seeds could serve as an effective supportive therapy in the management of diabetes. New research has found that the soluble dietary fiber is partly responsible for the blood sugar-lowering effect of fenugreek.[24]

Recent studies have shown that gurmar (*Gymnema sylvestre*), a native plant of the forests of India, can effectively be used in the management of type I and II diabetes mellitus. Gymnema contains certain components that block the sensation of sweetness when applied to the tongue, but it does not block absorption of sugar. An extract of the leaves of *G. sylvestre* reduces insulin requirements or oral hypoglycemic drug dosage, improves fasting blood glucose levels, and improves blood glucose control by enhancing the action of insulin and possibly by regenerating the beta cells of the pancreas.[25,26] These effects are observed in diabetics only, but not in healthy volunteers.

A number of other herbs show potential for the management of hyperglycemia. Subjects who consumed bread containing 25% flaxseed meal (*Linum usitatissimum*) showed almost 30% improvement in a glucose tolerance test compared with those who ate plain bread.[27] Flax seed is known to be very rich in soluble fiber. An extract from cinnamon (*Cinnamomum zeylanicum*) has been found to potentiate insulin activity.[28] For centuries, ginseng (*Panax ginseng*) has been used to treat diabetes by practitioners of traditional Chinese medicine. In a double-blind, placebo-controlled study, patients with type II diabetes who took 200 mg of ginseng for 8 weeks experienced improved fasting blood glucose levels and improved glycated hemoglobin levels.[29] Preliminary studies have reported antihyperglycemic activity or improved glucose tolerance from a number of other herbs including garlic, onions, bay leaves, cloves, coriander, cumin, cloves, juniper berries, prickly pear cactus, turmeric, and ivy gourd leaves.[30-33] Further research is warranted to validate these findings and discover if there is any clinical significance to the hypoglycemic effects of these herbs.

12.5 HERBS FOR CARDIOVASCULAR PROBLEMS

A plant-based diet rich in fruits, vegetables, whole grains, and legumes and low in saturated fat along with regular aerobic exercise is a regime recommended for anyone with an elevated risk of cardiovascular disease. In addition, there are a few herbs available that provide some help for persons with hyperlipidemia, an abnormal tendency to form blood clots, an impaired blood flow, hypertension, or other cardiovascular problems.

12.5.1 HYPOLIPIDEMIC AND ANTI-CLOTTING AGENTS

Garlic (*Allium sativum* L.), with its rich content of sulfur compounds, has been shown effective for a variety of cardiovascular problems. The major sulfur compound in garlic is allicin, which is released when intact cells of a clove are cut or crushed. Regular use of garlic can be useful in lowering the risk of heart attacks and strokes since it lowers both total and LDL cholesterol levels and triglyceride levels, without affecting HDL cholesterol levels.[34,35] On average, one-half to one clove of garlic per day reduces hypercholesterolemia by about 10% of the initial value.[34] Garlic also increases fibrinolytic activity and inhibits platelet aggregation due in part to the presence of ajoenes, allyl methyl trisulfide, vinyldithiins, and other sulfur compounds produced from the breakdown of allicin.[35-37] Bordia and co-workers have identified two components of garlic oil, diallyl trisulfide and to a lesser degree diallyl disulfide, which inhibit both platelet aggregation and platelet thromboxane formation.[38] Ali and Thomson found that the daily ingestion of 3 g of garlic for 6 months resulted in an 80% decrease in serum thromboxane B_2 as well as a 20% decrease in coronary heart disease in middle-aged men.[39] A number of studies have shown that garlic also lowers either systolic or diastolic blood pressure and protects the elastic properties of the aorta.[35] A meta-analysis of eight clinical trials suggested that patients with mild hypertension may benefit from a regular use of garlic.[40]

The odor-modified garlic extract (*Kyolic*) has been found to be just as effective as fresh garlic for lowering blood cholesterol levels.[41] On the other hand, the dried garlic is less effective than fresh garlic or not active at all. A clinical trial also found a steam-distilled garlic oil preparation was ineffective in treating patients with moderate hypercholesterolemia.[42] The beneficial properties of garlic are typically seen when substantial amounts are used over a period of time. Onions (*Allium cepa* L.) may also be considered to be natural anticlotting agents since they possess sulfur compounds, such as α-sulfinyl disulfides, with fibrinolytic activity and can strongly inhibit the arachidonic acid cascade in platelets and suppress platelet aggregation.[35,36,43]

Some hypercholesterolemic patients have received benefit from the use of psyllium (*Plantago psyllium*), a rich source of soluble fiber. A daily intake of 10 g of psyllium for 4 months produced a mean decrease in blood cholesterol levels of 10 to 15 mg/dl and LDL cholesterol levels of 13 mg/dl, respectively.[44]

The use of flaxseed flour (*Linum usitatissimum*) may also lower both blood cholesterol and LDL cholesterol levels due to its very low saturated fat content, high content of polyunsaturated fat and phytosterols, and mucilage content.[27] Fifteen patients with elevated blood cholesterol levels who regularly consumed ground flaxseed experienced about a 10% decrease in total cholesterol and LDL cholesterol levels as well as a substantial decrease in platelet aggregation, while their HDL cholesterol and triglyceride levels did not significantly change.[45]

The sweet-smelling resin (guggulu) of *Commiphora mukul*, a small, thorny myrrh tree native to India has been used to treat lipid disorders. Gugulipid, the lipid soluble extract of guggulu, has both hypolipidemic and anti-inflammatory properties and contains a mixture of diterpenes, sterols, and phenolic acids. The guggulsterones in gugulipid are regarded as the major cholesterol-lowering compounds, since they stimulate the metabolism of LDL cholesterol by the liver.[39] In a double-blind crossover study using gugulipid, cholesterol and triglyceride levels dropped 11 and 17%, respectively, compared with decreases of 10 and 22% achieved with the drug clofibrate.[46] Gugulipid tolerance was very high and adverse effects were minimal. However, persons should not take gugulipid at the same time as conventional drugs since gugulipid does decrease the bioavailability of diltiazem and propranolol, two conventional cardiovascular drugs.[47]

Terpenoids found in common herbs are reported to have cholesterol-suppressive effects.[48,49] Hypercholesterolemic subjects consuming lemon grass oil (*Cymbopogon citratus*), rich in geraniol and citral, experienced a drop in their cholesterol levels over a 3-month period.[50] Studies using powdered fenugreek seeds (*Trigonella foenum graecum*) showed that hypercholesterolemic subjects experienced a significant reduction of LDL cholesterol and triglyceride levels without any change in HDL levels.[51,52] A nonsaponin fraction has been discovered in the root of Asian ginseng (*Panax ginseng*) that inhibits platelet aggregation by potently inhibiting thromboxane A_2 production.[53] Some research groups have shown that the seed oil of evening primrose (*Oenothera biennis*) may favorably alter blood lipid levels, decrease platelet adhesiveness, and increase blood clotting time.[54, 55] Evening primrose oil contains substantial amounts (7 to 10%) of gamma-linolenic acid, a precursor of important prostaglandins. Ginger extracts are known to exhibit a strong inhibitory effect on thromboxane synthesis and platelet aggregation while having no effect on blood lipid levels. The inhibitory effect is largely due to the presence in the ginger extract of two labdane diterpene dialdehydes.[56]

12.5.2 Improved Blood Flow

Anthocyanins, the water-soluble pigments responsible for the red, mauve, purple, or blue color of most flowers and fruits, find use for the treatment of vascular disorders and capillary fragility.[1] Extracts of grape seed (*Vitis vinifera* L.) and also pycnogenol, an extract from the bark of coastal French pine trees, are rich in anthocyanidins. These polyphenolic compounds provide protection against LDL oxidation and show promise for the treatment of vascular disorders.[4,57] An extract of the seeds of horse-chestnut (*Aesculus hippocastanum*) increases venous flow and venous tone and is used for the symptomatic relief of chronic venous insufficiency. The extract improves a number of symptoms including a decrease in pain and tiredness, and lower leg edema.[58] The active compound in horse-chestnut is escin, a triterpene glycoside with antioxidant properties that inhibits the activity of lysosomal enzymes thought to increase the permeability of blood vessel walls.[4] An extract of the rhizomes of butcher's broom (*Ruscus aculeatus*), a short evergreen shrub from the Mediterranean region, is also helpful for treating venous insufficiency. The active components of butcher's broom are believed to be two steroidal saponins, ruscogenin and neurogenin.[11]

A concentrated extract of the leaves of the Ginkgo tree has become very popular for improving cerebral blood flow. *Ginkgo biloba* extract, due to its vasodilating effect and enhancement of blood flow, appears to be helpful in elderly patients with conditions such as memory loss, dizziness, depression, confusion, and other ailments resulting from cerebral insufficiency.[4,59-61] The active constituents in Gingko, which are thought to be flavone glycosides and diterpenoids (gingkolides), inhibit the activity of the platelet activating factor.

The flavonoid-rich herb hawthorn can also improve blood flow. The leaves, fruits, and flowers of hawthorn (*Crataegus* spp.) are widely used in Europe for improving the pumping capacity of the heart and for the treatment of angina. Hawthorn causes dilation of the smooth muscles of the coronary vessels, increases blood flow, and reduces the tendency for angina.[4] The proanthocyanidins which inhibit the biosynthesis of thromboxane A_2 are considered the active principles in the flower heads of hawthorn (*Crataegus oxyacantha*).[62] Patients with chronic heart disease that were given 600 mg/d of a hawthorn extract had lower blood pressure and heart rate, and less shortness of breath when exercising, compared with those not receiving the hawthorn.[63]

12.5.3 Protecton Against LDL Oxidation

Flavonoids are very effective antioxidants and they protect LDL cholesterol from oxidation as well as inhibiting platelet aggregation.[64-66] A Dutch study found that the flavonoid intake from fruit, vegetables, and tea was inversely associated with heart disease mortality, and incidence of heart attack and stroke over a five-year period. Those who had the highest consumption of flavonoids had 60% less mortality from heart disease and 70% lower risk of stroke than the low-flavonoid consumers.[67,68] Data from the Seven Countries Study revealed an inverse relationship between the average flavonoid intake and age-adjusted mortality from heart disease after 25 years of follow-up.[69] Some of the commonly used herbs that are rich in flavonoids include chamomile, dandelion, ginkgo, green tea, hawthorn, licorice, passionflower, milk thistle, onions, rosemary, sage, and thyme. In addition to flavonoids, these herbs also contain a variety of phenolic compounds, such as caffeic, chlorogenic, and ferulic acids, which can inhibit atherosclerosis.[70]

Either licorice extract (free of glycyrrhizinic acid) or the isoflavan glabridin in licorice root, have been shown to significantly inhibit the oxidation of LDL and the extent of atherosclerotic lesions.[71] During the study, the total and LDL cholesterol levels and blood coagulation remain unchanged. Since glabridin was less active than the whole licorice extract it would appear that licorice contains a number of other phenolic antioxidants such as licochalcones. Several epidemiological studies have suggested that drinking either green or black tea may lower blood cholesterol and blood pressure levels and provide a degree of protection against cardiovascular disease.[72] Some of these changes may be due to the capacity of green tea catechins and gallate esters to reduce intestinal cholesterol absorption as well as lowering the blood's coagulative ability. Tea flavonoids, the catechins in green tea leaves, or the theaflavins (catechin dimers) in black tea leaves, also inhibit LDL oxidation.[73] Of the catechins, epigallocatechin gallate provided the most protection and was more protective than vitamin E, while the theaflavins exerted even stronger inhibitory effects than catechins.

12.6 HERBAL HELP FOR THE IMMUNE SYSTEM

A number of herbal products are known to facilitate enhancement of the immune system. These include *Echinacea*, garlic, cat's claw, astragalus, licorice, and other herbs. Flavonoid-rich and carotenoid-rich herbs may be expected to enhance the immune system.[4] Before the introduction of sulfa drugs, *Echinacea* (purple coneflower) was commonly used to treat infections due to its anti-inflammatory and immunostimulatory activity. *Echinacea* can promote the activity of lymphocytes, increase phagocytosis, and induce interferon production.[4] *Echinacea* preparations can help prevent colds as well as reduce the severity and duration of flu symptoms.[74] Taking *Echinacea* when symptoms first appear may shorten the duration of a common cold by as much as one-third, from 10 days to 7 days.[75] In another study, students who took *Echinacea* had 15% fewer colds and 27% fewer recurrent infections, compared with placebo.[75] *Echinacea* typically loses its effectiveness if taken daily on a continuous basis. It is best taken at the onset of cold or flu symptoms and continued for about two weeks. The activity of *Echinacea* is believed to be provided by certain polysaccharides and isobutylamides.[1]

When HIV-positive patients were daily given 200 mg or more of glycyrrhizin, the triterpenoid saponin in licorice root (*Glycyrrhiza glabra* L.), their helper T-cell counts increased, helper-to-suppressor T-cell ratios improved, and liver function improved within 2 months.[76] Glycyrrhizin and its aglycone, glycyrrhetinic acid, have been reported to induce interferon activity and augment natural killer cell activity.[77] There are also reports that the chalcones in licorice possess antiviral activity against the human immunodeficiency virus.[78]

Two species of cat's claw, *Uncaria guianesis* and *U. tomentosa*, have been used medicinally by Peruvian Indians for over 2000 years. These plants are now attracting much attention in the West because of their immunostimulant properties and potential to help fight AIDS and leukemia. European researchers have suggested that the enhancement of immune function is due to various flavonoids, triterpenes, or alkaloids found in the root and stalk bark.[79,80] Extracts of cat's claw are reported to stimulate T cells, macrophages, and other components of the immune system. An extract of astragalus root (*Astragalus membranaceus*) can stimulate phagocytic activity, interleukin-2 production, and immunoglobulin synthesis. Saponins from astragalus are known to stimulate natural killer cell activity and improve the vitamin C level in the adrenal glands, the production site of cortisol.[81] Chinese clinical studies have shown that astragalus can reduce the incidence and shorten the course of the common cold.[82]

Garlic preparations have also been reported to improve the immune system of patients with AIDS.[83] St. John's Wort (*Hypericum perforatum* L.) possesses antiretroviral activity, and may be useful for treatment of HIV-infected patients.[1] Various researchers have identified tannins, carreic acid, and a polysaccharide in extracts of hyssop (*Hyssopus officinalis*) as having strong anti-HIV activity, without showing significant toxicity to lymphocyte function or T-cell counts.[84,85]

12.7 HERBS WITH ANTI-CANCER ACTIVITY

A number of commonly used herbs have been identified as possessing cancer-protective properties. These herbs include members of the *Allium* sp. (garlic, onions, chives); members of the Labiatae (mint) family (basil, mint, oregano, rosemary, sage, sweet savory, thyme); members of the Zingiberaceae family (turmeric, ginger); licorice root, green tea, flax; members of the *Umbelliferae* (carrot) family (anise, caraway, celery, chervil, cilantro, coriander, cumin, dill, fennel, parsley); and tarragon.[86]

Researchers have identified a host of cancer chemoprotective phytochemicals in these herbs (see Table 12.2). In addition, many herbs contain a variety of phytosterols, terpenes, flavonoids, saponins, and carotenoids, which have been shown from studies on legumes, fruits, and vegetables to be cancer chemoprotective.[96] These beneficial substances act as antioxidants, stimulate the immune system, inhibit nitrosation, inhibit the formation of DNA adducts with carcinogens, and inhibit hormonal actions and metabolic pathways associated with the development of cancer.[66,86-89,93-100] A number of phytochemicals inhibit tumor formation by stimulating the protective phase II enzyme glutathione *S*-transferase (GST). Examples of phytochemicals that stimulate GST activity include the phthalides in the umbelliferous herbs, the sulfides in garlic and onions, curcumin in turmeric and ginger, and terpenoids such as limonene, geraniol, carvone, and perillyl alcohol found in commonly used herbs.[88,96,98]

TABLE 12.2
Active Cancer-Protective Phytochemicals Found in Herbs

Herbal Source	Active Phytochemicals in the Herbs
Allium sp. (garlic, onions, leeks, chives)	Diallyl sulfide, diallyldisulfide, diallyl trisulfide, other disulfides and trisulfides[6,88]
Flaxseed	Lignans[6]
Ginger	Curcumin, gingerols, diarylheptanoids[89]
Ginseng	Ginsenosides[2]
Green tea	Epigallocatechin gallate, and other catechins[90,91]
Labiatae herbs (basil, oregano, rosemary, sage, thyme)	Monoterpenes, sesquiterpenes, flavonoids[1,6,88,92]
Licorice root	Glycyrrhizin, chalcones[78]
Rosemary, sage	Diterpenoids (rosmanol, carnosol, carnosic acid, rosmarinic acid, epirosmanol, isorosmanol), ursolic acid[93,94]
Turmeric	Curcuminoids[8]
Umbelliferous herbs (anise, caraway, celery seed, coriander, cumin, dill, fennel, parsley)	Coumarins, phthalides, polyacetylenes, terpenoids, flavonoids[2,6,95]

Terpenoids in plants are reported to increase tumor latency and decrease tumor multiplicity.[49,101-106] These terpenoids, which are responsible for the unique flavors of the herbs in the Labiatae and Umbelliferеae families, possess strong antioxidative activity[92] and can suppress tumor growth by inhibiting HMG-CoA reductase[101,104,106-108] (see Table 12.3). Elson has shown that the isoprenoids inhibit tumor growth in direct proportion to their ability to inhibit the activity of HMG-CoA reductase.[49] The carotenoid pigments, such as found in rose hips and paprika, are effective antioxidants that quench free radicals, provide protection against oxidative damage to cells, and also stimulate immune function. Persons with high levels of serum carotenoids have a reduced risk of cancer.[110]

A wide variety of organic sulfides and polysulfides provides garlic (*Allium sativum*) with anti-tumor properties. Garlic enhances the activity of the lymphocytes and macrophages to destroy cancer cells, and can also inhibit tumor cell metabolism, especially when the tumor size is small.[41,111] Garlic can inhibit the formation of nitrosamines, and also inhibit the formation of adducts with DNA.[112] A prospective study of 42,000 women living in Iowa revealed that risk of colon cancer was 32% less in those in the highest quartile of garlic consumption compared with those in the lowest quartile.[113] In China, those in the highest quartile of intake of garlic, onions, and other *Allium* herbs had a risk of stomach cancer 40% less than those in the lowest quartile of intake.[114] Case-control studies in Greece have shown a high consumption of onions, garlic, and other alliums to be protective against stomach cancer.[96] A Dutch study revealed that cancer in the noncardia section of the stomach for men and women consuming at least one-half an onion a day was about 50% lower than that in persons consuming no onions at all.[115]

TABLE 12.3
Terpenoids that Inhibit Tumors[1,49,99-104,109]

Terpenoid	Herbs that Contain the Terpenoid
Carvacrol	Thyme, marjoram, mint, dill
Farnesol	Lemongrass, chamomile, lavender
Geraniol	Lemongrass, coriander, melissa, basil, rosemary
β-Ionone	Alfalfa, green tea, black tea, passionflower
Limonene	Caraway, mints, cardamom, dill, celery seed, coriander, fennel
Menthol	Peppermint
Perillyl alcohol	Mint, lavender, sage
Perillaldehyde	Basil, rosemary
Thymol	Thyme, oregano

Flaxseed (*Linum usitatissimum*) contains a very rich supply of lignans, which are converted to enterolactone and enterodiol by bacterial fermentation in the colon.[116] These lignan metabolites can act as phytoestrogens, by binding to estrogen receptors and inhibiting the growth of estrogen-stimulated breast cancer.[117,118] The phenolic constituents of turmeric (*Curcuma domestica*) inhibit cancer as well as having antimutagenic activity. The major active component of turmeric is curcumin, an antioxidant, cancer-preventive and anti-inflammatory agent.[8,119] The rhizome of ginger also contains curcumin in addition to the phenolic compounds, gingerols and diarylheptanoids, which have a high antioxidant activity.[89]

Polyphenolics in green tea (*Camellia sinensis*) possess antimutagenic and anticancer activity. Evidence suggests a possible protective effect of tea against stomach and colon cancer.[72] Animal studies also point to a reduction in the risk of cancer in several organs resulting from the consumption of green and black tea or their principal catechins.[72] Tumor incidence and average tumor yield in rats with chemically induced colon carcinogenesis was significantly reduced when the rats received (-)-epigallocatechin gallate, a major polyphenolic constituent of green tea.[91] In another study, extracts of both black and green tea significantly inhibited leukemia and liver tumor cells.[120]

Korean studies suggest that ginseng (*Panax ginseng*) may lower the risk of human cancer.[121] Ginseng extract and powder have been found to be more effective than fresh sliced ginseng, the juice, or a ginseng tea, in reducing the risk of cancer.[122] In a large case-control study, those who had taken ginseng for 1 year had 36% less cancer than nonusers, while those who used ginseng for 5 years or more had 69% less cancer. In addition, those who had used ginseng less than 50 times during their life had 45% less cancer, while those who used ginseng more than 500 times in their life had 72% less cancer.[123] Ginseng seemed to be most protective against cancer of the ovaries, larynx, pancreas, esophagus, and stomach and less effective against breast, cervical, and bladder cancer. The ginsenosides, a family of triterpene saponins, are considered the main active ingredients of ginseng root.[1] Other cancer-protective constituents possibly include flavonoids, polysaccharides, and polyacetylenes.[121]

12.8 HERBS THAT PROMOTE MENTAL HEALTH

All too frequently, Americans experience various degrees of anxiety and depression. The hectic pace of life can put people under great stress. This can lead to headaches, sleep disorders, restlessness, and other health conditions. A variety of herbal medications are available for the relief of these conditions. In addition, regular exercise, good relationships and a sense of community, good time management, and helpfulness to others are all-important components of a healthy lifestyle that help promote positive mental health.

12.8.1 Gentle Sedation

There are a number of herbs which provide sedative effects safely without the side effects of conventional tranquilizers. Valerian, hops, lemon balm, passionflower, and kava-kava all possess sedative properties to some degree and find common use as sleep aids. The dried rhizome and roots of valerian (*Valeriana officinalis*) are quite effective for the treatment of anxiety and sleep disturbances caused by anxiety and have been used as a mild tranquilizer and sleep aid for many years.[4] Valerian reduces sleep latency, and produces a better quality of sleep including a reduced number and length of nighttime awakenings, all without a sleep hangover.[124] Women with sleep disorders derived benefit from a valerian-lemon balm mixture taken twice daily. The continuity and quality of sleep was superior to that of placebo.[125] The effect of the valerian-lemon balm treatment continued for one week after treatment was discontinued. The activity of valerian is not fully understood but the compounds believed to be responsible for its sedative and anxiety-reducing properties are a variety of monoterpenes in the volatile oil, the iridoids (valepotriates), and the flavonoids.[1]

Lemon Balm (*Melissa officinalis*) has pleasant-tasting citrus-scented leaves which can be brewed into a delicious tea. Melissa oil is used as a sedative to treat insomnia caused by nervous conditions, as well as being used as an antispasmodic and antibacterial agent.[2] The active principles of melissa are found in the terpenoid-rich essential oil of the leaves — citronellal, geraniol, linalool, citral, limonene, caryophyllene, and eugenol.[2,12] Hops are derived from the fruit of the vine, *Humulus lupulus*. Hop teas are commonly used for insomnia, restlessness, nervous tension, sleep disturbances, and other nervous conditions. The active principles of hops includes the essential oil components (which includes humulene, myrcene, beta-caryophyllene, and farnesene), flavonoids, and the resinous bitter principles, including humulone and lupulone. During storage the latter two compounds degrade to 2-methyl-3-buten-2-ol, which has central nervous system depressant activity.[4,6] The German Commission E notes that the effectiveness of hops is enhanced when used with other sedatives, such as valerian root, lemon balm, and passionflower.

Due to its mild sedative action, passionflower (*Passiflora incarnata*) is widely used in Europe to treat nervous anxiety and sleep disturbances. Pharmacological studies have shown that passionflower depresses the central nervous system. Its sedative and anxiety-relieving activity is possibly due to several substances that may act synergistically.[2,4,126] Kava-kava (*Piper methysticum*) is made from the dried rhizomes and roots of a shrub that grows throughout the South Pacific Islands and Hawaii. Polynesians take modest amounts of kava beverage to achieve a state of tranquility and contentment without the hangover and boisterous behavior associated with the use of alcohol. In the U.S. today, kava-kava is becoming widely used to treat stress, nervous anxiety, and insomnia. In a placebo-controlled, double-blind study, a significant reduction in anxiety and tension was observed after only 1 to 2 weeks in those patients taking 100 mg of kava-kava extract three times a day. The clinical picture continued to improve during the 4 weeks of the study.[127] The sedative activity of kava-kava derives from the presence of kava lactones, such as kavain, dihydrokavain, and methysticin, which relax skeletal muscles.[2] No side effects are seen with the use of small amounts of kava. However, with long-term heavy use, visual disturbances may occur along with itching and yellow discoloration of the skin. Overdosage can result in disorders of movement, and tendency to sleep. Kava-kava is contraindicated during pregnancy, lactation, or depression. Kava-kava appears to be safe and effective and nonaddictive if used carefully and in modest amounts. However, kava-kava can potentiate the effectiveness of alcohol and barbiturates.[2]

A tea prepared from the leaves and flowering tops of St. John's wort (*Hypericum perforatum*) is a popular herbal remedy for anxiety and depression. In Europe it is widely used as an effective treatment for nervousness, sleep disturbances, anxiety, and depression without the side effects commonly seen with chemical psychiatric medications.[2,4] Clinical trials have demonstrated the effectiveness of St. John's wort in treatment mild to moderate depression. After 4 weeks, 66% of the patients with depressive symptoms responded positively to taking 300 mg of St. John's wort extract three times a day, compared with a 28% response in the placebo group. Recent studies suggest that the antidepressant activity of St. John's wort may be largely due to the ability of the herb to inhibit the uptake of serotonin.[2] Active compounds include hypericin (a photosensitizing agent), pseudohypericin, terpenoids, and phenolic acids. While St. John's wort is a safe antidepressant, it may not be suited for the treatment of serious depressions.[128]

Recently, Brazilian researchers observed that the monoterpene linalool provided significant sedative effects in experimental animals. Linalool showed dose-dependent sedative effects at the central nervous system, including hypnotic and anticonvulsant properties.[129] Linalool occurs in rich amounts in lavender and coriander seed, and in lesser amounts in the essential oil of lemongrass, lemon balm, basil, feverfew, rosemary, sage, thyme, and other aromatic herbs.[6] Preliminary research suggests that certain fragrances such as vanilla may reduce stress and help provide some pain relief.

12.8.2 Headache Relief

Headache is a common discomfort experienced by many Americans while migraines afflict fewer people. Feverfew (*Tanacetum parthenium*) is valued for its ability to reduce the frequency and severity of migraines.[130] In addition, it is used for the treatment of arthritis and rheumatic diseases.[2] Feverfew may also reduce the discomfort of nausea and vomiting often associated with the migraine. The active components of feverfew are parthenolide and related sesquiterpenoids. These act as serotonin antagonists, and inhibit its release from platelets. Serotonin is a very important vasoactive substance mediating vascular headaches.[4] Feverfew also impedes prostaglandin synthesis and the release of histamines.[2]

External applications of mixed essential oils have been used for relieving stress and headaches. The oils are normally rubbed on the forehead or temples to relieve headache pain. A double-blind clinical trial conducted on healthy subjects in Germany found that peppermint oil, but not eucalyptus oil, was effective in relieving headaches.[131] Lavender (*Lavandula angustifolia*) has also been used to relieve headaches. Lavender can reduce muscle spasms, which may cause some tension headaches. Lavender is recognized as a mild sedative and finds use for mood disturbances such as restlessness or insomnia in addition to nervous intestinal discomfort.[2] Up to 50% of the volatile oil of lavender is linalool, a known sedative.

12.8.3 Ginseng

There are several commercial varieties of ginseng (*Panax* sp.), including Chinese, Korean, and American ginseng. The name *Panax* is derived from the Greek *pan* ("all") and *akos* ("remedy"), clearly reflecting the root's reputation as a panacea or cure-all. Asian ginseng (*Panax ginseng*) is used as a general tonic to combat feelings of debility and fatigue, an inability to concentrate, and to increase stamina, work efficiency, and endurance. Ginseng has been considered an adaptogen to enhance adaptation to stress.[6] Ginseng extracts can also enhance RNA and protein synthesis.[6]

It is suggested that for effectiveness, ginseng be used no longer than 2 to 3 months, and then discontinued for one month. The main active ingredients of ginseng root are believed to be a family of triterpene saponins, called ginsenosides. A major problem with ginseng has been its frequent contamination with other products and the lack of standardization of its active principles. When *Consumer Reports* analyzed 10 different brands of ginseng on the market they found a wide variation in the content of ginsenosides, ranging from 0.4 mg per capsule in one brand to 23.2 mg per capsule in another brand.[132] Such a lack in the standardization of herbal products makes it difficult for the consumer to obtain a reliable therapeutic product.

12.9 HERBAL MEDICINE FOR MENOPAUSE

Menopausal symptoms such as hot flashes, insomnia, depression, and emotional lability commonly strike women in their forties and early fifties. While some postmenopausal women take estrogen to help reduce such symptoms, most do not take hormone replacement therapy due to negative side effects and the fear of breast and uterine cancer. A number of herbs have been recommended for the relief of menopausal symptoms. These include black cohosh, chaste tree, and red clover.

Clinical studies over the past 40 years have confirmed that the rhizome and roots of black cohosh (*Cimicifuga racemosa*) are a safe and effective alternative for hormone replacement therapy in the treatment of menopausal symptoms. Experiments have shown that women taking black cohosh experienced a marked reduction in menopausal symptoms (hot flashes, mood swings, depression, headache, and nervousness) as well as menstrual difficulties. Young women suffering from dysmenorrhea, premenstrual syndrome (PMS), and other related conditions have also derived benefit from using black cohosh preparations.[133] In a double-blind study Stoll found that, compared with placebo, neurovegetative symptoms such as hot flashes, profuse perspiration, headache, vertigo, and heart palpitation, and psychiatric symptoms such as nervousness, irritability, sleep disturbances, and depressive moods were significantly improved when black cohosh extract (Remifemin) was consumed.[133] A clinical study of 60 women under 40 years of age, all of whom had at least one ovary removed, found that the use of black cohosh extract was equally as effective as estrogen hormone therapy for the relief of hot flashes, sweating, sleep disturbances, depressive moods, and other related menopausal symptoms.[134] The active principles in black cohosh root are reported to be triterpene glycosides. Recently, experimental data revealed that black cohosh does not suppress luteinizing hormone, nor does it have an estrogenic effect as earlier believed.[2]

Extracts of the ripe, dried fruits of the chaste tree (*Vitex agnus castus*) have been used for treatment of premenstrual complaints and irregularities of the menstrual cycle. The oils from evening primrose (*Oenothera biennis*) and black currant (*Ribes nigrum* L.) have been used for treatment of PMS. The reported effectiveness of these oils is believed to result from their substantial levels of gamma-linolenic acid, an important precursor of prostaglandins.[2,4] Since red clover (*Trifolium pratense*) is rich in the phytoestrogens (isoflavones) similar to those found in soy, it comes as no surprise that red clover has physiological effects similar to soy.[135] Red clover is currently being utilized as an alternative to hormone replacement therapy for menopausal women in a fashion similar to soy.

12.10 CONCLUSION

A variety of herbs containing different phytochemicals are available to provide different therapeutic functions. Many herbs possess potent antioxidant compounds that provide significant protection against chronic diseases. A number of herbs are known to provide help for cardiovascular problems; provide relief for problems of the gastrointestinal and urogenital tracts; provide protection against cancer and immune deficiencies; are useful adjuncts for the control of elevated blood sugar; and provide help for a variety of other health problems. A diet in which culinary herbs are generously used to flavor food will also provide a variety of phytochemicals that promote health and protect against chronic diseases. While the discriminate use of many herbal products is safe and, in some cases, of therapeutic value, the indiscriminate or excessive use of herbs can be unsafe and may even be toxic.[4]

REFERENCES

1. Bruneton, J., *Pharmacognosy, Phytochemistry, Medicinal Plants*, Lavoisier, Paris, 1995.
2. *Physician's Desk Reference for Herbal Medicines*, Medical Economic, Montvale, NJ, 1998.

3. Kawai, T., Kinoshita, K., and Takahashi, K., Anti-emetic principles of *Magnolia obovata* bark and *Zingiber officinale* rhizome, *Planta Med.*, 60, 17, 1994.
4. Tyler, V., *Herbs of Choice. The Therapeutic Use of Phytomedicinals*, Pharmaceutical Products Press, New York, 1994.
5. Dew, M.J., Evans, B.K., and Rhodes, J., Peppermint oil for the irritable bowel syndrome: a multicentre trial, *Br. J. Clin. Pract.*, 38, 394, 1984.
6. Bisset, N.G., Ed., *Herbal Drugs and Phytopharmaceuticals. A Handbook for Practice on a Scientific Basis*, Medpharm Scientific Publishers, Stuttgart, Germany, 1994.
7. Foster, S., *Herbal Renaissance. Growing, Using and Understanding Herbs in the Modern World*, Gibbs Smith, Layton, UT, 1993.
8. Nagabhushan, M. and Bhide, S.V., Curcumin as an inhibitor of cancer, *J. Am. Coll. Nutr.,* 11, 192, 1992.
9. Turnbull, W.H. and Thomas, H.G., The effect of a *Plantago ovata* seed containing preparation on appetite variables, nutrient and energy intake, *Int. J. Obesity,* 19, 338, 1995.
10. Foster, S., Laxatives. Plants Can Offer Gentle Relief, *The Herb Companion*, Aug/Sept, 67, 1996.
11. Foster, S. and Tyler, V.E., *Tyler's Honest Herbal. A Sensible Guide to the Use of Herbs and Related Remedies*, 4th ed., Haworth Press, Binghamton, NY, 1999.
12. Tyler, V.E., Phytomedicines in Western Europe: Their potential impact on herbal medicine in the United States, *Herb. Gram.,* 30, 24, 1994.
13. Avorn, J., Monane, M., Gurwitz, J. H., Glynn, R.J., Choodnovskiy, I., Lipsitz, L.A., et al., Reduction of bacteriuria and pyuria after ingestion of cranberry juice, *J. Am. Med. Assoc.,* 271, 751, 1994.
14. Braeckman, J., The extract of *Serenoa repens* in the treatment of benign prostatic hyperplasia: A multicenter open study, *Curr. Ther. Res.,* 55, 776, 1994.
15. Belaiche, P. and Lievoux, O., Clinical studies on the palliative treatment of prostatic adenoma with extract of Urtica root, *Phytother. Res.,* 5, 267, 1991.
16. Hirano, T., Homma, M., and Oka, K., Effects of stinging nettle root extracts and their steroidal components on the Na+,K+- ATPase of the benign prostatic hyperplasia, *Planta Med.,* 60, 30, 1994.
17. Gansser, D. and Spiteller, G., Aromatase inhibitors from *Urtica dioica* roots, *Planta Med.,* 61, 138, 1995.
18. Breza. J., Dzurny, O., Borowka, A., Hanus, T., Petrik, R., Blane, G., and Chadha-Boreham, H., Efficacy and acceptability of tadenan (*Pygeum africanum* extract) in the treatment of benign prostate hyperplasia: a multicenter trial in central Europe, *Curr. Med. Res. Opin.,* 14, 127, 1998.
19. Welihinda, J., Karunanayake, E.H., Sheriff, M.H.R., and Jayasinghe, K.S.A., Effect of *Momardica charantia* on the glucose tolerance in maturity onset diabetes, *J. Ethnopharmacol.,* 17, 277, 1986.
20. Srivastava,Y., Venkatakrishna-Bhatt, H., Verma, Y., Venkaiah, K., and Raval, B.H., Antidiabetic and adaptogenic properties of *Momardica charantia* extract: an experimental and clinical evaluation, *Phytother. Res.* 7, 285, 1993.
21. Marles, R.J. and Farnsworth, N.R., Antidiabetic drugs and their active constituents, *Phytomedicine,* 2, 137, 1995.
22. Sharma, R.D. and Raghuram, T.C., Hypoglycaemic effect of fenugreek seeds in non-insulin, dependant diabetic subjects, *Nutr., Res.,* 10, 731, 1990.
23. Ribes, G., Sauvaire, Y., Da Costa, C., Baccou, J.C., and Loubatieres-Mariani, M.M., Antidiabetic effects of subfractions from fenugreek seeds in diabetic dogs, *Proc. Soc. Exp. Biol. Med.,* 182, 159, 1986.

24. Ali, L., Azad Khan, A.K., Hassan, Z., Mosihuzzaman, M., Nahar, N., Nasreen, T., Nur-e-Alam, M., and Rokeya B., Characterization of the hypoglycemic effects of *Trigonella foenum graecum* seed, *Planta Med.,* 61, 358, 1995.
25. Shanmugasundaram, E.R.B., Rajeswari, G., Baskaran, K., Kumar, B.R.R., Shanmugasundaram, K.R., and Ahmath, B.K., Use of *Gymnema sylvestre* leaf extract in the control of blood glucose in insulin-dependant diabetes mellitus, *J. Ethnopharmacol.,* 30, 281, 1990.
26. Baskaran, K., Ahamath, B.K., Shanmugasundaram, K.R., and Shanmugasundaram, E.R.B., Antidiabetic effect of a leaf extract from *Gymnema sylvestre* in non-insulin dependent diabetes mellitus patients, *J. Ethnopharmacol.,* 30, 295, 1990.
27. Cunnane, S.C., Ganguli, S., Menard, C., Liede, A.C., Hamadeh, M.J., Chen, Z.Y., Wolever, T.M., and Jenkins, D.J., High alpha-linolenic acid flaxseed (*Linum usitatissimum*): some nutritional properties in humans, *Br. J. Nutr.,* 69, 443, 1993.
28. Imparl-Radosevich, J., Deas, S., Polansky, M.M., Baedke, D.A., Ingebritsen, T.S., Anderson, R.A., and Graves, D.J., Regulation of PTP-1 and insulin receptor kinase by fractions from cinnamon: implications for cinnamon regulation of insulin signalling, *Horm. Res*., 50, 177, 1998.
29. Sotaniemi, E.A., Haapakoski, E., and Rautio, A., Ginseng therapy in non-insulin-dependent diabetic patients, *Diabetes Care,* 118, 1373, 1995.
30. Sheela, C.G. and Augusti, K.T., Antidiabetic effects of S-allyl cysteine sulphoxide isolated from garlic (*Alium sativum* L.), *Indian J. Exp. Biol.,* 30, 523, 1992.
31. Sharma, K.K., Gupta, R.K., Gupta, S., and Samuel, K.C., Antihyperglycemic effect of onion: effect on fasting blood sugar and induced hyperglycemia in man, *Indian J. Med. Res.,* 65, 422, 1977.
32. Broadhurst, C.L., Keeping diabetes in check, *Herbs for Health,* 14, 30, 1997.
33. Khan, A., Bryden, N.A., Polansky, M.M., and Anderson, R.A., Insulin potentiating factor and chromium content of selected foods and spices, *Biol. Trace Elem. Res.,* 24, 183, 1990.
34. Warshafsky, S., Kramer, R.S., and Sivak, S.L., Effect of garlic on total serum cholesterol: a meta-analysis, *Ann. Intern. Med.,* 119, 599, 1993.
35. Kleijnen, J., Knipschild, P., and Riet, G.T., Garlic, onions and cardiovascular risk factors. A review of the evidence from human experiments with emphasis on commercially available preparations, *Br. J. Clin. Pharm.,* 28, 535, 1989.
36. Kendler, B.S., Garlic (*Allium sativum*) and onion (*Allium cepa*): A review of their relationship to cardiovascular disease, *Prev. Med.,* 16, 670, 1987.
37. Nishimura, H. and Ariga, T., Vinyldithiins in garlic and Japanese domestic allium (*A. victorialis*), in *Food Phytochemicals for Cancer Prevention. Fruits and Vegetables,* Huang, M.T., Osawa, T., Ho, C.T., Rosen, R.T., Eds., American Chemical Society, Washington, D.C., 1994, 128.
38. Bordia, A., Verma, S.K., and Srivastava, K.C., Effect of garlic (*Allium sativum*) on blood lipids, blood sugar, fibrinogen and fibrinolytic activity in patients with coronary artery disease, *Prostaglandins Leukot. Essent. Fatty Acids,* 58, 257, 1998.
39. Ali, M. and Thomson, M., Consumption of a garlic clove a day could be beneficial in preventing thrombosis, *Prostaglandins, Leukot. Essent. Fatty Acids,* 53, 211, 1995.
40. Silagy, C.A. and Neil, H.A., A meta-analysis of the effect of garlic on blood pressure, *J. Hypertens.,* 12, 463, 1994.
41. Dauusch, J.G. and Nixon, D.W., Garlic: A review of its relationship to malignant disease, *Prev. Med.,* 19, 346, 1990.
42. Berthold, H.K., Sudhop, T., and von Bergmann, K., Effect of a garlic oil preparation on serum lipoproteins and cholesterol metabolism: a randomized controlled trial, *J.*

43. Kawakishi, S. and Morimitsu, Y., Sulfur chemistry of onions and inhibitory factors of the arachidonic acid cascade, in *Food Phytochemicals for Cancer Prevention I. Fruits and Vegetables*, Huang, M.T., Osawa, T., Ho, C.T., and Rosen, R.T., Eds., American Chemical Society, Washington, D.C., 1994, 120.
44. Sprecher, D.L., Harris, B.V., Goldberg, A.C., Anderson, E.C., Bayuk, L.M., Russell, B.S., Crone, D.S., Quinn, C., Bateman, J., and Kuzmak, B.R., Efficacy of psyllium in reducing serum cholesterol levels in hypercholesterolemic patients on high- or low-fat diets, *Ann. Intern. Med.,* 119, 545, 1993.
45. Bierenbaum, M.L., Reichstein, R., and Walkins, T., Reducing atherogenic risk in hyperlipemic humans with flax seed supplementation: a preliminary report, *J. Am. Coll. Nutr.,* 12, 501, 1993.
46. Nityanand, S., Srivastava, J.S., and Asthana, O.P., Clinical trials with gugulipid, a new hypolipidaemic agent, *J. Assoc. Phys. India,* 37, 321, 1989.
47. Dalvi, S.S., Nayak, V.K., Pohujani, S.M., Desai, N.K., Kshirsagar, N.A., and Gupta, K.C., Effect of gugulipid on bioavailability of diltiazem and propranolol, *J. Assoc. Phys. India*, 42, 454, 1994.
48. Case, G.L., He, L., Mo, H., and Elson, C.E., Induction of geranyl pyrophosphate pyrophosphatase activity by cholesterol-suppressive isoprenoids, *Lipids,* 30, 357, 1995.
49. Elson, C.E., Suppression of mevalonate pathway activities by dietary isoprenoids: protective roles in cancer and cardiovascular disease, *J. Nutr.,* 125, 1666S, 1995.
50. Elson, C.E., Underbakke, G.L., Hanson, P., Shrago, E., Wainberg, R.H., and Qureshi, A.A., Impact of lemongrass oil, an essential oil, on serum cholesterol, *Lipids,* 24, 677, 1989.
51. Sharma, R.D. and Raghuram, T.C., Hypoglycaemic effect of fenugreek seeds in non-insulin dependant diabetic subjects, *Nutr. Res.,* 10, 731, 1990.
52. Sharma, R.D., Raghuram, T.C., and Rao, V.D., Hypolipidaemic effect of fenugreek seeds. A clinical study, *Phytother. Res.* 5, 145, 1991.
53. Park, H.J., Rhee, M.H., Park, K.M., Nam, K.Y., and Park, K.H., Effect of non-saponin fraction from *Panax ginseng* on cGMP and thromboxane A2 in human platelet aggregation, *J. Ethnopharmacol.,* 49, 157, 1995.
54. Renaud, S., McGregor, L., Morazain, R., Thevenon, C., Benoit, C., Dumont, E., and Mendy, F.B., Comparative beneficial effects on platelet functions and atherosclerosis of dietary linoleic and gamma-linolenic acids in the rabbit, *Atherosclerosis,* 45, 43, 1982.
55. Ishikawa, T., Fujiyama, Y., Igarashi, O., Morino, M., Tada, N., Kagami, A., Sakamoto, T., Nagano, M., and Nakamura, H., Effects of gammalinolenic acid on plasma lipoproteins and apolipoproteins, *Atherosclerosis,* 75, 95, 1989.
56. Kawakishi, S., Morimitsu, Y., and Osawa, T., Chemistry of ginger components and inhibitory factors of the arachidonic acid cascade, in *Food Phytochemicals for Cancer Prevention. II. Teas, Spices and Herbs,* Huang, M.T., Osawa, T., Ho, C.T., and Rosen, R.T., Eds., American Chemical Society, Washington, D.C., 1994, 244.
57. Nuttall, S.L., Kendall, M.J., Bombardelli, E., and Morazzoni, P., An evaluation of the antioxidant activity of a standardized grape seed extract, Leucoselect., *J. Clin. Pharm. Ther.,* 23, 385, 1998.
58. Pittler, M.H. and Ernst, E., Horse-chestnut seed extract for chronic venous insufficiency. A criteria-based systematic review, *Arch. Dermatol.,* 134, 1356, 1998.
59. Curtis-Prior, P., Vere, D., and Fray, P., Therapeutic value of *Ginkgo biloba* in reducing symptoms of decline in mental function, *J. Pharm. Pharmacol.,* 51, 535, 1999.
60. Kleijnen, J. and Knipschild, P., Gingko biloba for cerebral insufficiency, *Br. J. Clin. Pharmacol.,* 34, 352, 1992.

61. Kleijnen, J. and Knipschild, P., Gingko biloba, *Lancet,* 340, 1136, 1992.
62. Vibes, J., Lasserre, B., Gleye, J., and Declume, C., Inhibition of thromboxane A2 biosynthesis in vitro by the main components of Crataegus oxyacantha (*Hawthorn*) flower heads, *Prostaglandins Leukot. Essent. Fatty Acids,* 50, 173, 1994.
63. Schmidt, U., Kuhn, U., Ploch, M., and Hubner, W.D., Efficacy of the Hawthorn (*Crataegus*) preparation LI 132 in 78 patients with chronic congestive heart failure defined as NYHA functional class II, *Phytomedicine,* 1:17, 1994.
64. Cook, N.C. and Samman, S., Flavonoids — chemistry, metabolism, cardioprotective effects, and dietary sources, *J. Nutr. Biochem.*, 7, 66, 1996.
65. Manach, C., Regerat, F., Texier, O., Agullo, G., Demigne, C., and Remesy, C., Bioavailability, metabolism and physiological impact of 4-oxo-flavonoids, *Nutr. Res.*, 16, 517, 1996.
66. Smith, T.J. and Yang, C.S., *Effects of food phytochemicals or xenobiotic metabolism, in Food Phytochemicals for Cancer Prevention. I. Fruits and Vegetables,* Huang, M.T., Osawa, T., Ho, C.T., Rosen, R.T., Eds., American Chemical Society, Washington, D.C., 1994, 17.
67. Hertog, M.G.L., Feskens, E.J.M., Hollman, P.C., Katan, M.B., and Kromhout, D., Dietary antioxidant flavonoids and risk of coronary heart disease, *Lancet*, 342, 1007, 1993.
68. Keli, S.O., Hertog, M.G., Feskins, E.J., and Kromhout, D., Dietary flavonoids, anti-oxidant vitamins, and incidence of stroke: the Zutphen study, *Arch. Intern. Med.,* 156, 637, 1996.
69. Hertog, M.G.L., Kromhout, D., Aravanis, C., Blackburn, H., Buzina, R., Fidanza, F., Giampaoli, S., Jansen, A., Menotti, A., Nedeljkovic, S., Pekkarinen, M., Simic, B.S., Toshima, H., Feskens, E.J.M., Hollman, C.H., and Katan, M.B., Flavonoid intake and long-term risk of coronary heart disease and cancer in the Seven Countries Country, *Arch. Intern. Med.,* 155, 381 1995.
70. Decker, E.A., The role of phenolics, conjugated linoleic acid, carnosine, and pyrrolo-quinoline quinone as nonessential dietary antioxidants, *Nutr. Rev.,* 53, 49, 1995.
71. Fuhrman, B., Buch, S., Vaya, J., Belinky, P.A., Coleman, R., Hayek, T., and Aviram, M., Licorice extract and its major polyphenol glabridin protect low-density lipoprotein against lipid peroxidation: *in vitro* and *ex vivo* studies in humans and in atherosclerotic apolipoprotein E-deficient mice, *Am. J. Clin. Nutr.*, 66, 267, 1997.
72. Dreosti, E., Bioactive ingredients: antioxidants and polyphenols in tea, *Nutr. Rev.,* 54(11), S51, 1996.
73. Ishikawa, T., Suzukawa, M., Ito, T., Yoshida, H., Ayaori, M., Nishiwaki, M., Yonemura, A., Hara, Y., and Nakamura, H., Effect of tea flavonoid supplementation on the susceptibility of low-density lipoprotein to oxidative modification, *Am. J. Clin. Nutr.,* 66, 261, 1997.
74. Schoneberger, D., The influence of immune-stimulating effects of pressed juice from *Echinacea purpurea* on the course and severity of colds, *Forum Immunol.,* 8, 2, 1992.
75. Schulz, V., Hansel, R., and Tyler, V.E., *Rational Phytotherapy. A Physicians' Guide to Herbal Medicine,* 3rd ed., Springer-Verlag, Berlin, 1998.
76. Mori, K., Sakai, H., Suzuki, S., Akutsu, Y., Ishikawa, M., Aihara, M., Yokoyama, M., Sato, Y., Okaniwa, S., and Endo, Y., The present status in prophylaxis and treatment of HIV infected patients with hemophilia in Japan, *Rinsho Byhori,* 37, 1200, 1989.
77. Abe, N., Ebina, T., and Ishida, N., Interferon induction by glycyrrhizin and glycyrrhetinic acid in mice, *Microb. Immunol.,* 26, 535, 1982.
78. Shibata, S., Antitumor-promoting and anti-inflammatory activities of licorice principles and their modified compounds, in *Food Phytochemicals for Cancer Prevention. II. Teas, Spices and Herbs,* Huang, M.T., Osawa, T., Ho, C.T., Rosen, R.T., Eds., American Chemical Society, Washington, D.C., 308, 1994.

79. Aquino, R., De Feo, V., De Simone, F., Pizza, C., and Cirino, G., Plant metabolites. New compounds and anti-inflammatory activity of *Uncaria tomentosa*, *J. Nat. Prod.*, 54, 453, 1991.
80. Wagner, H., Kreutzkamp, B., and Jurcic, K., The alkaloids of Uncaria tomentosa and their phagocytosis-stimulating action, *Planta Med.*, 51, 419, 1985.
81. Zhang, Y., Xu, Q., and Liu, X., The anti-leukocytopenic and anti-stress effects of Astragalus saponins on mice, *Nanjing Yixueyuan,* 12, 244, 1992.
82. Chang, H.M. and But, P.P.H., *Pharmacology and Applications of Chinese Materia Medica,* Vol. 2., World Scientific, Teaneck, NJ, 1987, 1041.
83. Abdullah, T.H., Kirkpatrick, D.V., and Carter, J., Enhancement of natural killer cell activity in AIDS with garlic, *Dtsch. Z. Onkol.,* 21, 52, 1989.
84. Kreis, W., Kaplan, M.H., Freeman, J., Sun, D.K., and Sarin, P.S., Inhibition of HIV replication by *Hyssopus officinalis* extracts, *Antiviral Res.,* 14, 323, 1990.
85. Gollapudi, S., Sharma, H.A., Aggarwal, S., Byers, L.D., Ensley, H.E., and Gupta, S., Isolation of a previously unidentified polysaccharide (MAR-10) from *Hyssopus officinalis* that exhibits strong activity against human immunodeficiency virus type 1, *Biochem. Biophys. Res. Commun.,* 210, 145, 1995.
86. Caragay, A.B., Cancer-preventative foods and ingredients, *Food Technol.,* 46(4), 65, 1992.
87. Craig, W.J., Health-promoting properties of common herbs, *Am. J. Clin. Nutr.,* 70, 491S, 1999.
88. Huang, M.T., Ferraro, T., and Ho, C.T., Cancer chemoprevention by phytochemicals in fruits and vegetables. An overview, in *Food Phytochemicals for Cancer Prevention. I. Fruits and Vegetables,* Huang, M.T., Osawa, T., Ho, C.T., and Rosen, R.T., Eds., American Chemical Society, Washington, D.C., 1994, 2.
89. Kikuzaki, H. and Nakatani, N., Antioxidant effects of some ginger constituents, *J. Food Sci.*, 58, 1407, 1993.
90. Hara, Y., Prophylactic functions of tea polyphenols, in *Food Phytochemicals for Cancer Prevention. II. Teas, Spices and Herbs,* Huang, M.T., Osawa, T., Ho, C.T., and Rosen, R.T., Eds., American Chemical Society, Washington, D.C., 1994, 34.
91. Kim, M., Hagiwara, N., Smith, S.J., Yamamoto, T., Yamane, T., and Takahashi, T., Preventive effect of green tea polyphenols on colon carcinogenesis, in *Food Phytochemicals for Cancer Prevention. II. Teas, Spices and Herbs,* Huang, M.T., Osawa, T., Ho, C.T., and Rosen, R.T., Eds., American Chemical Society, Washington, D.C., 1994, 51.
92. Nakatani, N., Chemistry of antioxidants from Labiatae herbs, in *Food Phytochemicals for Cancer Prevention. II. Teas, Spices and Herbs,* Huang, M.T., Osawa, T., Ho, C.T., and Rosen, R.T., Eds., American Chemical Society, Washington, D.C., 1994, 44.
93. Cuvelier, M.E., Berset, C., and Richard, H., Antioxidant constituents in sage (*Salvia officinalis*), *J. Agric. Food Chem.*, 42, 665, 1994.
94. Ho, C.T., Ferraro, T., Chen, Q., Rosen, R.T., and Huang, M.T., Phytochemicals in teas and rosemary and their cancer-preventive properties, in *Food Phytochemicals for Cancer Prevention. II. Teas, Spices and Herbs,* Huang, M.T., Osawa, T., Ho, C.T., and Rosen, R.T., Eds., American Chemical Society, Washington, D.C., 1994, 2.
95. Sauberlich, H.E., Weinberg, D.S., Freeburg, L.E., Juan, W., Sullivan, T.R., Tamura, T., and Craig, C.B., Effects of consumption of an Umbelliferous vegetable beverage on constituents in human sera, in *Food Phytochemicals for Cancer Prevention. I. Fruits and Vegetables,* Huang, M.T., Osawa, T., Ho, C.T., Rosen, R.T., Eds., American Chemical Society, Washington, D.C., 1994, 258.
96. Steinmetz, K.A. and Potter, J.D., Vegetables, fruit, and cancer, II. Mechanisms, *Cancer Causes Control,* 2, 427, 1991.

97. Haraguchi, H., Saito, T., Okamura, N., and Yagi, A., Inhibition of lipid peroxidation and superoxide generation by diterpenoids from *Rosmarinus officinalis*, *Planta Med.*, 61, 333, 1995.
98. Zheng, G.Q., Zhang, J., Kenney, P.M., and Lam, L.K.T., Stimulation of glutathione S-transferase and inhibition of carcinogenesis in mice by celery seed oil constituents, in *Food Phytochemicals for Cancer Prevention. I. Fruits and Vegetables,* Huang, M.T., Osawa, T., Ho, C.T., and Rosen, R.T., Eds., American Chemical Society, Washington, D.C., 1994, 230.
99. *d*-Limonene, an anticarcinogenic terpene, *Nutr. Rev.,* 46, 363, 1988.
100. Robbers, J.E., Speedie, M.K., and Tyler, V.E., *Pharmacognosy and Pharmacobiotechnology*, Williams & Wilkins, Baltimore, MD, 1994.
101. Elson, C.E. and Yu, S.G., The chemoprevention of cancer by mevalonate-derived constituents of fruits and vegetables, *J. Nutr.,* 124, 607, 1994.
102. Zheng, G.Q., Kenney, P.M., and Lam, L.K.T., Potential anticarcinogenic natural products isolated from lemongrass oil and galanga root oil, *J. Agric. Food Chem.*, 41, 153, 1993.
103. Zheng, G.Q., Kenney, P.M., and Lam, L.K.T., Anethofuran, carvone, and limonene: potential cancer chemopreventive agents from dill weed oil and caraway oil, *Planta Med.*, 58, 338, 1992.
104. Zheng, G.Q., Kenney, P.M., and Lam, L.K.T., Sesquiterpenes from clove (*Eugenia caryophyllata*) as potential anticarcinogenic agents, *J. Nat. Prod.,* 55, 999, 1992.
105. Burke, Y.D., Stark, M.J., Roach, S.L., Sen, S.E., and Crowell, P.L., Inhibition of pancreatic cancer growth by the dietary isoprenoids farnesol and geraniol, *Lipids,* 32, 151, 1997.
106. Yu, S.G., Anderson, P.J., and Elson, C.E., Efficacy of β-ionone in the chemoprevention of rat mammary carcinogenesis, *J. Agric. Food Chem.,* 43, 2144, 1995.
107. Yu, S.G., Abuirmeilah, N.M., Quershi, A.A., and Elson, C.E., Dietary beta ionone suppresses hepatic 3-hydroxy-3-methylglutaryl coenzyme A reductase activity, *J. Agric. Food Chem.,* 42, 1493, 1994.
108. Quershi, A.A., Mangels, W.R., Din, Z.Z., and Elson, C.E., Inhibition of hepatic mevalonate biosynthesis by the monoterpene, *d*-limonene, *J. Agric. Food Chem.,* 36, 1220, 1988.
109. He, L., Mo, H., Hadisusilo, S., Qureshi, A.A., and Elson, C.E., Isoprenoids suppress the growth of murine B16 melanoma *in vitro* and *in vivo, J. Nutr.,* 127, 668, 1997.
110. van Poppel, G. and Goldbohm, R.A., Epidemiologic evidence for beta-carotene and cancer prevention, *Am. J. Clin. Nutr.,* 62, 1393S, 1995.
111. Lau, B.H.S., Tadi, P.P., and Tosk, J.M., *Allium sativum* garlic and cancer prevention, *Nutr. Res.,* 10, 937, 1990.
112. Milner, J.A., Garlic: its anticarcinogenic and antitumorigenic properties, *Nutr. Rev.,* 54(11), S82, 1996.
113. Steinmetz, K.A., Kushi, L.H., Bostick, R.M., Folsom, A.R., and Potter, J.D., Vegetable, fruit, and colon cancer in the Iowa women's health study, *Am. J. Epidemiol.* 139, 1, 1994.
114. You, W.C., Blott, W.J., Chang, Y.S., Ershow, A., Yang, Z.T., An, Q., Henderson, B.E., Fraumeni J.F., Jr., and Wang T.G., Allium vegetables and reduced risk of stomach cancer, *J. Natl. Cancer Inst*., 81, 162, 1989.
115. Dorant, E., van den Brandt, P.A., Goldbohm, R.A., and Sturmans, F., Consumption of onions and a reduced risk of stomach carcinoma, *Gastroenterology*, 110, 12, 1996.
116. Thompson, L.U., Robb, P., Serraino, M., and Cheung, F., Mammalian lignan production from various foods, *Nutr. Cancer,* 16, 43, 1991.

117. Serraino, M. and Thompson, L.U., The effect of flaxseed supplementation on the initiation and promotional stages of mammary tumorigenesis, *Nutr. Cancer,* 17, 153, 1992.
118. Hirano, T., Fukuoka, K., Oka, K., Naito, T., Hosaka, K., Mitsuhashi, H., and Matsumoto, Y., Antiproliferative activity of mammalian lignan derivatives against the human breast carcinoma cell line, ZR-75-1, *Cancer Invest.*, 8, 595, 1990.
119. Chan, M.M. and Fong, D., Anti-inflammatory and cancer-preventive immunomodulation through diet: effects of curcumin on T-lymphocytes, in *Food Phytochemicals for Cancer Prevention. II. Teas, Spices and Herbs,* Huang, M.T., Osawa, T., Ho, C.T., and Rosen, R.T., Eds., American Chemical Society, Washington, D.C., 1994, 222.
120. Lea, M.A., Xiao, Q., Sadhukhan, A.K., Cottle, S., Wang, Z,Y., and Yang, C.S., Inhibitory effects of tea extracts and (-)-epigallocatechin gallate on DNA synthesis and proliferation of hepatoma and erythroleukemia cells, *Cancer Lett.,* 68, 231, 1993.
121. Yun, T.K., Experimental and epidemiological evidence of the cancer-preventive effects of *Panax ginseng, Nutr. Rev.,* 54(11), S71, 1996.
122. Yun, T.K. and Choi, S.Y., A case-control study of ginseng intake and cancer, *Int. J. Epidemiol.,* 19, 871, 1990.
123. Yun, T.K. and Choi, S.Y., Preventive effect of ginseng intake against various human cancers: a case-control study on 1987 pairs, *Cancer Epidemiol., Biomarkers Prev.,* 4, 401, 1995.
124. Balderer, G. and Borbely, A.A., Effect of valerian on human sleep, *Psychopharmacology,* 87, 406, 1985.
125. Dressing, H., Kohler, S., and Muller, W.E., Improvement in sleep quality with a high dose valerian-melissa preparation, *Psychopharmacotherapie,* 3, 123, 1996.
126. Speroni, E. and Minghetti, A., Neuropharmacological activity of extracts from Passiflora incarnata, *Planta Med.,* 54, 488, 1988.
127. Lehmann, E., Kinzler, E., and Friedemann, J., Efficacy of a special Kava extract (*Piper methysticum*) in patients with states of anxiety, tension and excitedness of non-mental origin — a double-blind, placebo-controlled study of four weeks treatment, *Phytomedicine,* 3, 113, 1996.
128. Harrer, G. and Sommer, H., Treatment of mild/moderate depression with Hypericum, *Phytomedicine,* 1, 3, 1994.
129. Elisabethsky, E., Marschner, J., and Souza, D.O., Effects of linalool on glutamatergic system in the rat cerebral cortex, *Neurochem. Res.,* 20, 461, 1995.
130. Johnson, E.S., Kadam, N.P., Hylands, D.M., and Hylands, P.J., Efficacy of feverfew as prophylactic treatment of migraine, *Br. Med. J.,* 291, 569, 1985.
131. Gobel, H., Schmidt, G., and Soyka, D., Effect of peppermint and eucalyptus oil preparations on neurophysiological and experimental algesimetric headache parameters, *Cephalalgia,* 14, 228, 1994.
132. Ansley, D., Sci. Ed., Ginseng. Much ado about nothing?, *Consumer Reports,* 60(11), 699, 1995.
133. Foster, S., Black Cohosh: *Cimicifuga racemosa*. A literature review, *HerbalGram,* 45, 35, 1999.
134. Lehmann-Willenbrock, E. and Riedel, H.H., Clinical and endocrinological examinations concerning therapy of climacteric symptoms following hysterectomy with remaining ovaries, *Z. Gynakol.*, 110, 611, 1988.
135. Newall, C.A., Anderson, L.A., and Phillipson, J.D., *Herbal Medicines. A Guide for Health-Care Professionals*, Pharmaceutical Press, London, 1996.

13 Garlic and Health

Walt Jones and Richard J. Goebel

CONTENTS

13.1 INTRODUCTION

It has been called "Russian penicillin." Its role in the so-called healthful Mediterranean diet is well known. Its virtues in promoting good health have been part of the folklore in many cultures for generations. It is garlic, a common name for several members of the lily family (Liliaceae) such as cloves or bulbs, whose pungent odor can liven up an otherwise bland dish. It is also a chemically complex herb containing

0-8493-0038-X/97/$0.00+$.50

more than 200 different compounds, 100 of which are sulfur compounds, which confer — at least anecdotally — a number of medicinal benefits.

The chief active ingredient is allicin. Research has suggested that allicin is the component of garlic that is useful in killing bacteria and fungi. Herbalists also contend that garlic preparations help suppress the growth of cancer cells and promote a healthy cardiovascular system. The medical community still looks at such claims with a jaundiced eye, especially since garlic supplements are widely available in a variety of forms and strengths, many of which have been subjected to tests with differing results.

Nevertheless, new studies on the benefits of garlic give food for thought that should not be ignored. As Koch and Lawson note in their book, *Garlic: The Science and Therapeutic Application of Allium sativum L. and Related Species*,

> "In light of the long historical use of garlic for medicinal purposes, it has become very intriguing and important to determine the composition of garlic so that its active compounds might be revealed….Discovery and quantitation of the active ingredients are also important so that we can assess the level and uniformity of the medicinal quality among the many strains of garlic and to determine any adverse effects of agricultural variables, such as soil nutrition, weather, moisture, harvest time, storage conditions and so on."[1]

The authors point out that — unlike other vegetables with known nutritional benefits such as broccoli — garlic is normally consumed in relatively small amounts. Research of the herb's benefits has tended to focus on fresh garlic powders, aged garlic extracts, distilled oils (from steaming), and other forms. The forms and preparations of garlic which are the most efficacious would make for a very interesting study all by itself.

Research studies on garlic discussed here cover a wide topical area, from cardiovascular benefits to garlic's anticarcinogenic properties. Proponents claim that garlic's benefits include the reduction of harmful LDL cholesterol and triglycerides; the prevention of blood clots and blood platelet clumping; the ability to block chemical carcinogens; the stimulation of various immunological factors that may help combat cancer as well as fungal infections; and the protection of cells against various oxidizing agents.

Research on the therapeutic effects of garlic can be grouped into four main areas:

1. Antibacterial/antifungal properties
2. Cardiovascular effects
3. Anticarcinogenic components
4. Other benefits

13.2 ANTIBACTERIAL/ANTIFUNGAL PROPERTIES

Before World War II, garlic was used as a remedy for indigestion and diarrhea, to destroy microorganisms for bacterial, fungal, and viral infections, and to expel intestinal worms and parasites.

Allicin gets the credit for the antibiotic properties of garlic. Many studies both *in vitro* and *in vivo* show that alliin has no activity in this area; 1 mg of allicin is equal to the antibiotic activity of 15 I.U. of penicillin.

Garlic has been used to treat all kinds of illnesses throughout history. From protecting people from infection during the Great Plague in London to its use in World War I by physicians to treat intestinal illnesses, garlic has been used for centuries as a remedy both internally and externally.

Through research and testing, garlic has shown to be an antibiotic against both Gram-positive and Gram-negative bacteria. In 1966, Jezowa and colleagues compared garlic to modern antibiotics.[2] Not only was it effective in all cases, but garlic also worked against strains that were resistant to antibiotics.

A study conducted in 1998 in India demonstrated the inhibitory activity of garlic against a variety of food pathogens, most notably *Staphylococcus aureus, Salmonella typhi, Escherichia coli*, and *Listeria monocytogenes*. The results revealed that all bacterial pathogen strains tested were inhibited by garlic, with *Escherichia coli* being the most sensitive.[3]

13.2.1 Antifungal Effects

Garlic has been used in folk medicine for years to treat fungal and yeast infections. Several studies indicate allicin is the active compound in fighting fungal infections and preventing further growth. American researchers tested 139 different types of fungi and yeasts for sensitivity. After 21 days, some microorganisms grew while some showed no growth at all. These results indicate that the use of garlic in treating infections is very specific. The use of aged garlic extract (containing no allicin or allicin-derived compounds) was ineffectual in treating fungal and yeast infections.

13.2.2 Antiprotozoal Effects

In the late 1920s, Russian researchers observed that the volatile constituents of fresh garlic and onion strongly inhibit and even kill various microorganisms. Ensuing experiments with ingredients of these plants, and later of other plants, were mainly performed in protozoa, especially *Paramecium caudatum*, and with eggs and larvae of mollusks and frogs. The favorable results prompted some to coin the descriptive word "phytoncides" for the antibiotically active components of higher plants.[4]

13.2.3 Antiviral Effects

Although there is not much research dealing with garlic as a treatment against viruses, it has been used in China and India as a cheaper alternative to expensive Western medication. In Russia, the use of garlic is so widespread that it is known as "Russian penicillin." During one acute influenza epidemic in Russia, the Soviet Union imported 500 tons of garlic cloves to treat it. In a patent filed in 1992, it is claimed that an allicin-urotropin treatment can be used against viral infections, including AIDS.

13.3 CARDIOVASCULAR BENEFITS

With the appropriate dosage, garlic may protect blood vessels from the negative effects of free radicals, may have a positive influence on blood lipids, increase capillary flow, and decrease elevated blood pressure levels. The combined result is that garlic can prevent arteriosclerosis or ameliorate an existing condition.

Garlic's cardiovascular effects were rediscovered in the late 1960s by Western scientists, but it has been used in Asian folk medicine for heart problems for years. Garlic has also been used in Europe for some time.

Studies have repeatedly shown that garlic strengthens the heart and stimulates well being. Advocates' claims that garlic prevents arteriosclerosis are based on studies conducted on thrombocyte adhesiveness and aggregation, which is reportedly decreased significantly by the effective constituents of garlic. At the same time, the dissolution of coagulated blood, plaques, and clots is enhanced. Garlic decreases the lipoproteins circulating in the blood as LDL (low-density lipoprotein). This occurs through the increased production of HDL (high-density lipoprotein) at the expense of LDL.

13.3.1 Cholesterol and Lipid-Lowering Effects

Several studies conducted primarily on rats but also on rabbits, chickens, dogs, and cats, have shown that garlic, in the form of fresh pressed juice, powder, and oils, caused the thickening of the blood vessel walls to disappear partially or completely. A study in 1982 conducted on rats showed levels of cholesterol, triglyceride, and very low-density lipoprotein (VLDL) fell significantly, while the HDL levels increased after having been fed garlic.[5] However, animals given the residue of distilled garlic oil showed no noticeable changes. It is assumed that the active component in the lipid-lowering effect is allicin.

A study on male albino rats conducted in 1985 compared the effects of garlic to onions. After being fed meals of 20% onion or garlic for 12 weeks, the subjects showed significantly lower serum and liver cholesterol values than at the beginning of the experiment. Garlic was shown to be clearly more effective than onion.[6]

Similar results are seen in studies involving humans, both in healthy people, as well as patients with hyperlipidemia (elevated levels of any or all lipids in the plasma) and hypercholesterolemia (abnormally high concentrations of cholesterol present in the bloodstream).

A study conducted in India demonstrated that garlic, when administered in a daily dose of two capsules twice a day (each capsule containing ethyl acetate extract from 1 g peeled and crushed raw garlic), significantly reduced total serum cholesterol and triglycerides, and significantly increased HDL-cholesterol and fibrinolytic activity.[7]

Russian researchers also reported on the cholesterol-reducing benefits of garlic in a 1997 study. They noted that garlic indirectly affects artherosclerosis by reducing hyperlipidemia, hypertension, and likely, diabetes mellitus, and prevents thrombosis formation. They deduce that its effects are the result of garlic's capacity to reduce lipid content in arterial cells and prevent intracellular lipid accumulation.[8]

The results from a collection of 40 studies with 43 groups of patients and volunteers show a mean decrease in serum cholesterol levels of 10.6%. The forms of garlic used in the studies were fresh garlic, garlic powder tablets, oils (predominantly ether-extracted garlic), and steam-distilled oils. They showed decreases ranging from 4 to 16%. The steam-distilled oils had the lowest decrease, although the amounts used varied considerably, and the effect increased as the dose increased. The lipid-lowering effect is attributed to the active compound allicin.

Additionally, 33 human studies were conducted using garlic cloves and garlic powder tablets. Three of those studies showed no effect on lipid lowering, and the reason given is that the study used tablets that contained either no allicin potential (spray-dried)[9] or low allicin potential.[10] (There was one additional negative study, but its results could not be duplicated in subsequent studies.)

Clinical trials with garlic oils which contain only allicin-derived garlic compounds plus added vegetable oils have lowered serum lipids.

13.3.2 Effects on Blood Pressure and Vascular Resistance

In 1921, Loeper et al. noticed the effect of wild garlic on the circulatory systems of dogs.[11,12] In 1969, tests conducted by Erken revealed that patients treated with a commercial preparation containing oil macerates of garlic experienced a normalization of serum cholesterol and blood pressure levels as well as a reduction of symptoms such as headache, buzzing in the ears, and the sensation of pressure and dizziness.[13]

In 1984, Lutomski noted a significant improvement in the secondary symptoms of patients with arteriosclerosis, such as headache, dizziness, insomnia, and indigestion. He also noticed an improvement in their general sense of well-being.[14]

Although it has not been determined exactly which compound in garlic positively influences blood pressure, it appears that allicin is not responsible. The current theory is that garlic contains two effective compounds: a chloroform-soluble compound which is able to slightly lower blood pressure and exert a tonic action on the heart, and at least one chloroform-insoluble compound which has a strong ability to lower blood pressure and also has a tonic effect on the intestines.

The compound present in garlic that likely does this is adenosine. In order for adenosine to be absorbed properly and thus be effective, the compounds allicin and alliin must be present. (However, the alkaloids present in coffee and tea, caffeine and theophylline, can block the adenosine receptors and trigger an increase in blood pressure.)

Finally, a German study concluded that garlic intake can increase the elastic vascular resistance of the aorta in the elderly.[15]

13.3.3 Effects on Blood Coagulation, Fibrinolysis, and Blood Flow

Generally, arteriosclerosis is partnered with the inability of the blood coagulation system to break down blood clots after coagulation. This process is known as fibrinolysis. To restore balance, drug therapy is used to return fibrinolysis to a normal level. As a replacement for drug therapy, studies in both animals and humans were conducted to ascertain garlic's ability to do the same thing.

The results of 11 clinical studies using 14 groups of subjects reported that small doses of garlic can rapidly activate fibrinolysis. The average in these studies was a 56% fibrinolytic activity increase when compared to the pretreatment condition.

13.3.4 Antithrombotic (Platelet Antiaggregatory) Effects

Blood platelets (thrombocytes) adhere to vessel walls. With the added presence of cholesterol, an aggregation, or clumping, of platelets will occur. If this aggregation continues, it may lead to the occlusion of a vessel which may cause stroke, myocardial infarction, or occlusive arterial disease.

In vitro studies in 1972 by Weissenberger and colleagues showed that platelet aggregation in platelet-rich plasma can be inhibited by an onion extract. The authors believe adenosine to be the inhibiting factor.[16]

> Adenosine acts by competitive blocking of the binding side for ADP (adenosine diphosphate) at the platelet membrane. Adenosine has multiple biological functions, among them vasodilative, antihypertensive and spasmolytic actions, which are especially significant. These effects are explained by the vascular smooth-muscle-relaxing influence of adenosine. In addition, adenosine inhibits lipolysis in fat cells, promotes glucose oxidation and increases the release of the hormone glucagon from the pancreas. The antidiuretic effect can be explained by vasoconstriction in the kidney. Adenosine also stimulates the synthesis of steroid hormones in the adrenal glands. Finally, as already mentioned, it inhibits or prevents the aggregation of platelets.[17]

Allicin (natural and synthetic) has also been shown in recent studies to be effective as an aggregation-inhibiting substance *in vitro*. A product of allicin, ajoene, is also receiving attention for its antiaggregatory ability.

13.3.5 Antioxidant Effects

Garlic's antioxidant effect is primarily of interest in the treatment of arteriosclerosis. In general, it is accepted that free radicals play a vital role in depositing cholesterol on vessel walls. Garlic constituents are able to inhibit the formation of free radicals, promote the radical scavenger process, and protect LDL against oxidation by free radicals.

Once again, allicin and allicin-derived allyl sulfides are believed to be the responsible compounds in garlic's antioxidant activity. "Both allicin and allyl sulfides are metabolized in blood and liver to the same metabolite, allyl mercaptan, which is a strong antioxidant."[18]

13.4 ANTICARCINOGENIC EFFECTS

For decades, garlic has been touted as very effective against various forms of cancer. A study conducted 60 years ago concluded that the occurrence of cancer is lower in countries that have high garlic and onion consumption. The general belief is that garlic is effective as a cancer-inhibitor due to its ability to prevent putrification of the intestines and activate secretions, leading to an increase in the body's resistance.

Garlic's ability to activate gastric secretions makes it a possible agent for preventing gastrointestinal cancer.

Only one study of garlic in the treatment of cancer has been documented. In 1962, Spivak gave a garlic juice preparation to 35 patients with different types of cancer. Of those 35, 26 showed positive results of differing degrees, although no one was cured with the treatment.[19]

13.4.1 Epidemiological Studies

Epidemiological studies comparing cancer incidence with consumption levels of individual or grouped foods are currently the most important evidence that garlic may significantly reduce the risk of cancer, especially cancers of the gastrointestinal tract. The most favorable effect of garlic was seen in stomach cancer patients who were given both raw and cooked garlic.

13.4.2 Animal and *In Vitro* Studies

In 1936, Caspari showed the effectiveness of garlic as a tumor inhibitor by feeding mice garlic and then injecting them with tumor cells. By doing so, he brought about an increase in immunity in his test animals.[20]

In 1973, Nakata reported that tumors incubated with fresh garlic extract for an hour and then injected into animals were no longer lethal to the animals. However, he did not get the same result with tumors incubated with an extract of boiled garlic. The results of this experiment showed that fresh garlic juice (containing allicin) was much more effective as a tumor-inhibiting agent than garlic with the allicin extracted from it.[21] Allicin's enzyme-inhibiting ability may be responsible for its tumor-inhibiting effect.

Another way garlic may inhibit tumor growth is by stimulating and elevating the natural and antioxidative functions within the organism. As long as the garlic was used as a preventative, it was able to prevent mutations of cancer cells, studies revealed.

> People who eat garlic regularly have a low pH and low concentrations of nitrite in their gastric fluid. In addition, fewer nitrate-reducing bacteria are found in their stomach than in people who rarely or never consume any garlic. This is taken as proof for the well-known fact that garlic eaters rarely develop cancer of the stomach.[22]

A possible explanation for this is that the sulfur compounds in garlic act as radical scavengers. The compounds selenium and germanium may also be agents in garlic's cancer-inhibiting effect.

One study involving rats concluded that garlic and associated allyl sulfur components, SAC and DADs, are effective inhibitors of MNU-induced mammary carcinogenesis.[23] Other studies link the cancer-fighting characteristics of other elements and compounds, most notably selenium, with garlic's therapeutic benefits. Schaffer et al. concluded that garlic powder enhanced the selenite inhibition of mammary DNA adducts. They noted that present studies provide evidence that synergistic protection against the initiation of dimethylbenz[a]anthracene-induced (DMBA) carcinogenesis occurs when selenite is supplemented in conjunction with garlic or its allyl sulfur compounds.[24]

Milner also notes that research from several sources shows that garlic and its organic allyl sulfur compounds inhibit the cancer process. These benefits, the researcher adds, are not limited to a specific species, a particular tissue, or a specific carcinogen. However, the report concludes, additional evidence is needed to determine the quantity needed by humans to minimize cancer risk.[25]

The cancer-inhibiting effect of garlic is most likely attributed to allicin and allicin-derived compounds, along with a few unknown compounds unrelated to allicin. It is important to understand the significance of studies using fresh garlic extract because of the allicin and allicin-derived compounds found in fresh garlic.

13.5 OTHER BENEFITS

13.5.1 Immunomodulatory Effects

Although only a few human studies have been conducted, *in vitro* and animal studies suggest that garlic may play an important role in enhancing the immune system. The human studies are encouraging, because they show a positive link between garlic and enhanced immunoreactions and phagocytosis.

A study conducted on rats revealed garlic's antiarthritic effect when used in the form of commercial steam-distilled garlic oil. The effect of garlic was synergistically increased when boron was added to the diet.

Further studies showed garlic extract's necrosis-inhibiting effect along with the compounds of allicin and diallyl disulfide.

13.5.2 Hypoglycemic Effects

Studies conducted from the 1920s to the 1970s show that the consumption of onions and garlic can lower elevated blood glucose concentrations. In 1924, a study by Mahler and Pasterny gave two diabetic patients 10-15 g of fresh garlic sliced and distributed to them throughout the day in three portions. Blood sugar decreased and the urine sugar excretion in one patient was reduced from 3.2 to 1%, and from 3.8% to zero in the second patient.[26]

"Garlic oil was also found to increase insulin and urea levels and to change the activities of key liver enzymes in ethanol-fed rats."[27] The results of another study showed that the glucose level in the blood was lowered by garlic, while the concentrations of glycogen level in the liver and insulin in the blood increased. In a study with diabetic rats, the compound allicin was shown to exert significant antidiabetic effects.

13.5.3 Hormone-Like Effects

In older medical literature, garlic is mentioned to confer hormone-like effects. Aphrodisiac properties are linked with garlic because of the belief that it stimulates male and female sex hormones.

Garlic is also assumed to stimulate the pituitary gland, which in turn influences other glands and has an effect on fat and carbohydrate metabolism.

13.5.4 Enhancement of Thiamin Absorption

In 1924, the Medical Academy in Paris confirmed garlic's effectiveness for scurvy. In the 1800s, the Japanese established garlic's effectiveness for beriberi.

13.5.5 Effects on Organic and Metabolic Disturbances

Garlic is ideal for self-medication. In the 1980s, researchers noticed that people in their mid-40s started using garlic as a preventive tool in strengthening their defense mechanisms.

Garlic contains many unknown factors that block enzymes and modify the functions of biological membranes. Most studies conducted on garlic to determine these compounds and their effectiveness were conducted *in vitro* and must be viewed with caution. Allicin is known to be metabolized very rapidly in blood to allyl mercaptan.

13.5.6 Antihepatotoxic Effects

Studies on rats showed that several known compounds in garlic were able to provide adequate liver protection. In livers with high amounts of lipid peroxides and accumulation of triglycerides, levels were significantly decreased in the animals treated with garlic extract. Vitamin E inhibited lipid peroxidation but not fat deposition.

An aged garlic extract proved to be effective in controlling hepatopathy and liver damage induced by hepatoxins during acute hepatitis.

13.5.7 Dyspepsia and Indigestion

Throughout the ages, garlic has been used in the treatment of stomach and intestinal troubles. The resistance of the people in the Balkans to all kinds of intestinal diseases is credited to their high consumption of garlic.

Garlic oil activates higher secretions of hydrochloric acid and digestive enzymes in the stomach because of its stimulating effect on the mucous membrane of the stomach.

Damrau and Ferguson investigated the effect of dried garlic on gastrointestinal motility by means of roentgenography, and they demonstrated the elimination of flatulence and meteorism, gaseous colic, and nausea, in clinical experiments.[27]

13.5.8 Respiratory Diseases

Recent reports indicate that garlic may help people with respiratory dysfunction, including problems due to high altitude.

Third-World countries have successfully used garlic for years to treat such respiratory ailments as tuberculosis, bronchiectasis, gangrene of the lungs, and whooping cough. The former Soviet Union and Bulgaria also use garlic to treat flu and inflammation of the throat.

13.6 GARLIC — THE WONDER HERB?

Just how wonderful is the wonder herb — this so-called "stinking rose" — and is the research adequate to make any such sweeping, grandiose claims? Koch and Larson[27] point out that garlic contains at least three times more naturally occurring sulfur than any other common fruit or vegetable, including apricots, broccoli, and onions — more than 3 mg/g of fresh weight. The abundance of thiosulfates and other organosulfur compounds gives garlic this natural therapeutic advantage. Research is continuing, as it should, as biochemists, nutritionists, and others add to our body of knowledge about *Allium sativum.*

As one researcher noted, epidemiological, clinical, and laboratory data have proved that garlic contains many biologically and pharmacologically important compounds which are beneficial in the prevention of cardiovascular, neoplastic, and several other diseases. Numerous studies are in progress all over the world to develop effective and odorless garlic preparations, as well as to isolate the active principles that may be therapeutically useful.[28]

Finally, as Milner and others have noted, while garlic's therapeutic benefits have been clearly established, research still is needed to show the dosages, formulas, and preparations that provide the greatest benefits to people.

REFERENCES

1. Koch, H.P. and Lawson, L.D., Eds., (1996) *Garlic: The Science and Therapeutic Application of* Allium sativum L. *and Related Species*, 2nd ed., Williams & Wilkins, Baltimore, 135-212, 172.
2. Jezowa, L., Rafinski, T., and Wrocinski T. (1966) Investigations on the antibiotic activity of *Allium sativum L., Herba (Pol.),* 12:3–13.
3. Kumar, M. and Berwal, J.S., Sensitivity of food pathogens to garlic (1998) *J. Appl. Microbiol.*, 84:213-215.
4. Koch, H.P. and Lawson, L.D., Eds., (1996) *Garlic: The Science and Therapeutic Application of* Allium sativum L. *and Related Species*, 2nd ed., Williams & Wilkins, Baltimore, 135-212, 172.
5. Chi, M.S., Koh, E.T., and Stewart, T.J., (1982) Effects of garlic on lipid metabolism in rats fed cholesterol or lard, *J. Nutr.* 112:241-248; *Chem. Abstr.* 96 (1982) 161 393.
6. Baktsh, R. and Chugtai, M.I.D., (1985) Comparative study of onion and garlic on serum cholesterol, liver cholesterol, prothrombin time, and fecal sterols excretion in male albino rats, *J. Chem. Soc. Pak.* 7:285-288; *Chem. Abstr.* 104 (1986) 108 382.

7. Bordia, A. and Verma S.K., et al., (1998) Effect of garlic on blood lipids, blood sugar, fibrinogen and fibrinolytic activity in patients with coronary heart disease, Dept. of Medicine, RNT Medical College, Udaipur, India, *Prostaglandins Leukot. Essential Fatty Acids*, 58:257-263.
8. Orekhov, A.N. and Grünwald, L., (1997) Effects of garlic on artherosclerosis, *Russ. Acad. Med. Sci. (Moscow).*
9. Sitprija, S., Pengvidhya, C., Kankaya, V., Bhuvapnaich, S., and Tunkayoo, M. (1987) Garlic and diabetes mellitus phase II clinical trial, *J. Med. Assoc. Thailand,* 70:223-227.

9a. Plengvidhya, C., Chinayon, S., Siptprija, S., Pasatrat, S., and Tankeyoon, M. (1988) Effects of spray dried garlic preparation on primary hyperlipoproteinemia, *J. Med. Assoc. Thailand,* 71:248-252.

10. Luley, C., Lehmann-Leo, W., Möller, B., Martin, T., and Schwartzkopff, W. (1986) Lack of efficacy of dried garlic in patients with hyperlipoproteinemia, *Arzneim. Forsch.*, 36:766-768.
11. Loeper, M., Debray, M., and Chailley-Bert, P. (1921) Recherches expérimentales sur l'hypotension par les produits alliaces, *C. R. Séances Soc. Biol.*, Ses Fil.1 85:160-161; *Chem. Zbl.*, 1921, III, 1509.

11a. Loeper, M. and Debray, M. (1921) L'action hypotensive de la teinture d'ail, *Ann. Med. Interne*, 37:1032-1037.

12. Aqel, M.B., Gharaibah, M.N., and Salhab, A.S. (1991) Direct relaxant effects of garlic juice on smooth and cardiac muscles, *J. Ethnopharmacol.*, 33:13-19; *Int. Pharm. Abst.*, 29 (1992) 1705.

12a. Ozturk, Y., Aydin, S., Kosar, M., and Baser, K.H.C. (1994) Endothelium-dependent and independent effects of garlic on rat aorta, *J. Ethnopharmacol.*, 44:109-116.

13. Erken, D. (1969) Schonende Blutdrucksenkung durch Pflanzenstoffe. Über die klinische Prüfung eines Phytotherapeutikums, *Dtsch. Apotheker*, 21:22-24.
14. Lutomski, J. (1984) Klinische Untersuchungen zur therapeutischen Wirksamkeit von Ilja Rogoff Knoblauchpillen mit Rutin, *Z. Phytother.* 5:938-942.
15. Breithhaupt-Grögler, K., Ling, M., Boudoulas, H., and Belz, G.G. (Oct. 1997) Protective effect of chronic garlic intake on elastic properties of aorta in the elderly, *Circulation*, 96:2649-55.
16. Weisenberger, H., Grube, H., Koenig, E., and Pelzer, H. (1972) Isolation and identification of the platelet aggregation inhibitor present in the onion. Allium cepa, *FEBS Lett.*, 26:105-108. *Chem. Abstr.* 77 (1972) 162 867.
17. Koch, H.P. and Lawson, L.D., Eds., (1996) *Garlic: The Science and Therapeutic Application of* Allium sativum L. *and Related Species*, 2nd ed., Williams & Wilkins, Baltimore, 135-212, 172.
18. Koch, H.P. and Lawson, L.D., Eds., (1996) *Garlic: The Science and Therapeutic Application of* Allium sativum L. *and Related Species*, 2nd ed., Williams & Wilkins, Baltimore, 135-212, 172.
19. Spivak, M.Y. (1962) On the use of phytonacides of garlic and onion for the treatment of tumorous patients, *Vopr. Onkol.* (Problems in Oncology), 8:93-96 (Russian).
20. Caspari, W. (1936) Über den Einflub der Kost auf das Wachstum von Impfgeschwülsten, *Z. Krebsforsch.* 43:255-263.
21. Nakata, T. (1973) Effect of fresh garlic extract on tumor growth. Nippon Eiseigaku Zasshi, (*Jpn. J. Hyg.*) 27:538-543; *Chem. Absrt.* 79 (1973) 111 680 (Japanese).
22. Koch, H.P. and Lawson, L.D., Eds., (1996) *Garlic: The Science and Therapeutic Application of* Allium sativum L. *and Related Species*, 2nd ed., Williams & Wilkins, Baltimore, 135-212, 172.

23. Schaffer, E.M. and Liu, J.Z., et al., Garlic and associated allyl sulfur components inhibit N-methyl-N-nitrosource induced rate mammary carcinogenesis (1996), *Cancer Lett.*, 102: 199-204.
24. Schaffer, E.M., Liu, J.Z., and Milner, J.A., Garlic powder and allyl sulfur compounds enhance the ability of dietary selenite to inhibit 7,12-dimethylbenz[a]anthracene-induced mammary DNA adducts, (1997), *Nutr. Cancer,* 27: 162-168
25. Milner, J.A., Garlic: its anticarcinogenic and antitumorigenic properties (1996) Nov., *Nutr. Review,* 54: S82-6
26. Mahler, P. and Pasterny, K. (1924) Klinische Beobachtung über Insulinwirkung beim Diabetes mellitus, *Med. Klin.*, 11:335-338.
27. Koch, H.P. and Lawson, L.D., Eds., (1996) *Garlic: The Science and Therapeutic Application of* Allium sativum L. *and Related Species*, 2nd ed., Williams & Wilkins, Baltimore, 135-212, 172.
28. Agarwal, K.C., Therapeutic actions of garlic constituents, *Med. Res. Rev.*, 16(1): 111-24, 1996.

14 Some Aspects of the Mediterranean Diet

Iman A. Hakim

CONTENTS

14.1 INTRODUCTION

The Mediterranean region spans 3 continents and more than 15 countries connected by blue seas and magnificent terrain. The Mediterranean area is a world of its own and the Mediterranean lifestyle is a mix of cultures and cuisines. Recent medical research has shown that this cuisine is much better for our health than the typical American diet. While the preparation and seasonings vary from country to country, the people of the Mediterranean region all eat larger amounts of vegetables, fruits, beans, and grains; use olive oil as the main source of fat; and consume moderate amounts of protein, primarily from fish and poultry. By embracing the new trend towards healthier eating, we need to adopt the types of cooking which were developed several decades ago around the Mediterranean Sea.

People have become aware that good health is linked to good diet. The real difficulty has been defining a healthy diet. As we have begun to understand that a healthy diet leads to a healthy lifestyle, the concept of the Mediterranean diet is growing in popularity. The Mediterranean diet, as a model of a healthful diet, has attracted considerable attention because of the low rates of chronic diseases and the high life expectancy noted in countries bordering the Mediterranean Sea. Mediterranean diets are found not only to produce favorable effects on blood lipid profiles,[1] but also protect against oxidative stress and carcinogenesis.[2] The high intake of

0-8493-0038-X/97/$0.00+$.50

antioxidants and fiber helps to scavenge even the small amount of oxidants or oxidized compounds.[3] Epidemiological studies[4-7] show that Mediterranean populations who get more than 30% of their daily calories from fat and rely on olive oil as their principal source of fat have lower rates of cancer, stroke, and heart disease than Americans on a low-fat diet. In addition to the benefits of olive oil, there are many biologically plausible reasons why the increase in consumption of fruits and vegetables found in the Mediterranean diet might slow or prevent the appearance of cancer. These reasons include, but are not limited to, the presence of such readily bioavailable anticarcinogenic agents as vitamins C and E, carotenoids, fiber, selenium, plant sterols, phenols, and *d*-limonene. A recently published study[8] has demonstrated that the high fish, fruit, and vegetable diet characteristic of Mediterranean countries is helpful in preventing heart disease and subsequent heart attack and stroke, and that switching to this diet also protects people who have already had one heart attack from having another.

14.2 MEDITERRANEAN DIET

As well as being the cradle of civilization, the Mediterranean region is also the source of many of the world's delicious cuisines. The term Mediterranean diet was first used by Ancel Keys, an American physiologist, in his book *How to Eat Well and Stay Well: the Mediterranean Way*.[9] In ancient times, the residents of the Italian peninsula learned most of what they knew about food and nutrition from the Greeks who colonized Sicily and the southern part of Italy. In Sicily and the southern provinces, the original Mediterranean diet is still very much the standard with its emphasis on fruits, vegetables, and pasta.[10]

"Mediterranean diet" is an imprecise term because dietary patterns within the various Mediterranean countries vary widely in consumption of specific foods and in nutrient intake.[11] However, a common Mediterranean diet is characterized by abundant plant foods (fruits, vegetables, cereals, bread, beans, nuts, and potatoes), olive oil as the principal source of fat, dairy products, fish, poultry, and meat in low to moderate amounts, fresh fruit as the typical daily dessert, and use of garlic, onions, lemon or lime, and herbs as condiments.[12] This diet, when consumed in sufficient amounts, provides all of the known essential micronutrients, and other plant food substances believed to promote health. Minimal processing, seasonal use, freshness of foods, as well as methods of preparation would be expected to maximize contents of dietary fiber, antioxidants, other micronutrients, and nonnutritive substances found in plant foods.

There is no single typical Mediterranean diet. Defining and understanding the Mediterranean diet is not easy because there are several countries that border the Mediterranean Sea. Although dietary patterns in Mediterranean countries vary widely in consumption of specific foods and in nutrient intake, both European and non-European Mediterranean populations benefit from the protective effect of the so-called Mediterranean diet on health.[4] The abundant fruits, vegetables, and whole grains, and the low to moderate intake of dairy products in traditional Mediterranean diets are likely to have contributed to the low rates of chronic diseases observed in these populations.[13] The Mediterranean diet is rapidly changing, especially in large cities where people are slowly abandoning their traditional diet for a Western-style diet. However, the traditional Mediterranean diet is still consumed in the rural areas of most of the Mediterranean countries.

After thousands of years of defining itself, the Mediterranean cuisine is integrating into our American culture, and for good reasons. Food is fresh and it is high in soluble fiber, antioxidants, and other important nutrient and nonnutrients components. The preference for fresh fruits and vegetables in Mediterranean diets results in a higher consumption of raw plants, a lower production of cooking-related oxidants, and a consequent decreased waste of nutritional and endogenous antioxidants.[3] From the nutritional point of view, this diet is rich in vitamins, minerals, fiber, and minor organic, nonnutritive substances. In addition to the nutrients that are involved in normal metabolic activity, fruits and vegetables contain components that may provide additional health benefits. These food components (generally referred to as phytochemicals) are derived from naturally occurring ingredients and are actively being investigated for their health-promoting potential. The Mediterranean diet is notably low in red meat and saturated fats. Red meat is listed at the top of the Mediterranean diet pyramid,[14] while cheese and yogurt, along with poultry and fish, are the predominant sources of protein. As a result, the Mediterranean diet is low in saturated fat and high in monounsaturated fat, a fact that in part may explain the lower rates of heart disease seen in this part of the world.

14.2.1 Fruits and Vegetables in the Mediterranean Diet

Fresh fruits and vegetables feature strongly in the Mediterranean cuisine. Fresh fruit is often the dessert and is eaten raw. Vegetables are generally eaten raw as a side dish or used for the preparation of rice and pasta dishes, sauces, and vegetable soups. The same vegetable can be prepared with different herbs and spices. The Seven Countries Study[15] probably represents the major investigation contributing to knowledge about the relationship between the Mediterranean diet and coronary heart disease. Kromhout et al.,[16] compared the data of the five Mediterranean cohorts (Italy, Yugoslavia, Corfu, Crete, and Greece) to the three Northern European cohorts (The Netherlands, Eastern and Western Finland) for fruit and vegetable intake. The five Mediterranean cohorts consumed more fruits (222 g/day vs. 51 g/day), more vegetables and legumes (226 g/day vs. 150 g/day), and less pastries and sweets (28 g/day vs. 119 g/day).

Despite relatively high tobacco consumption, lung cancer rates are lower than expected in the Mediterranean region. This may be related to the high intakes of fruits and vegetables.[17] The Mediterranean diet is rich in fruits and vegetables, therefore, it contains a remarkable amount of vitamins. Vitamin C is supplied primarily by consumption of raw fruits, especially citrus fruits, and vegetables. Vegetables such as tomatoes, potatoes, carrots, broccoli, cabbage, and green leafy vegetables, supply vitamin E to the diet. β-Carotene is found predominantly in vegetables such as the carrot, pumpkin, cabbage, and spinach, and in some fruits, especially oranges and apricots. Cooked tomato supplies the diet with notably high quantities of lycopene. Fruit and vegetables are also important sources of fiber that contains mostly pectin and cellulose. A daily intake of 20 g of insoluble fiber from fruits and vegetables[18] plus 15 g from other sources, helps regulate both the metabolism of fat and the intestinal function.

14.2.2 Main Characteristics of the Mediterranean Diet

It is difficult to imagine the Mediterranean cuisine without lemons. Lemons, like oranges, are a quintessential part of Italy and the Mediterranean cuisine. In Ancient Rome and Egypt, stories of the lemon's miraculous power against poison persisted.[10]

The main components of a traditional Mediterranean diet[14] are

- An abundance of plant foods, including fruits and vegetables, potatoes, breads and grains, beans, nuts, and seeds, with emphasis on fresh and minimally processed foods
- Total fat ranging from 25% to 35% of energy, with saturated fat no more than 8% of energy intake
- Olive oil as the principal source of fat
- Fresh fruit representing the classic final course of every meal and often is the dessert
- Daily consumption of low to moderate amounts of cheese and yogurt
- Weekly consumption of low to moderate amounts of fish and poultry
- Red meat and sweets are consumed only a few times per month

14.2.3 Food Pyramids

The Food Guide Pyramid has replaced the basic four food groups as the standard for setting up a healthy diet. The USDA pyramid model retains the idea of food groups, but its shape provides the key for interpreting how to make healthy food choices on a daily basis. The broad base highlight the food groups that should constitute the majority of our daily intake, while the top food group of the pyramid should be consumed as little as possible.

The Mediterranean Diet Pyramid is based on relative frequencies and is therefore intended to provide an overall impression of healthy food choices rather than to specify the number and size of recommended servings of certain foods or proportions of energy obtained from them. In the USDA Pyramid animal and plant protein are presented in the same category with a recommended consumption of two to three servings per day, and all fats and oils are combined together at the top of the pyramid. On the other hand, the Mediterranean Diet Pyramid differentiates between fish, poultry, and red meat intake. Fish and poultry are consumed a few times per week while red meat is consumed a few times per month (Figure 14.1).

14.3 MEDITERRANEAN DIET AND CITRUS CONSUMPTION

From 1950 to 1965 the overall fruit and vegetable consumption increased in Italy. The levels reached at that time were then maintained in the following years. The consumption of fresh fruits and vegetables doubled, while the consumption of citrus

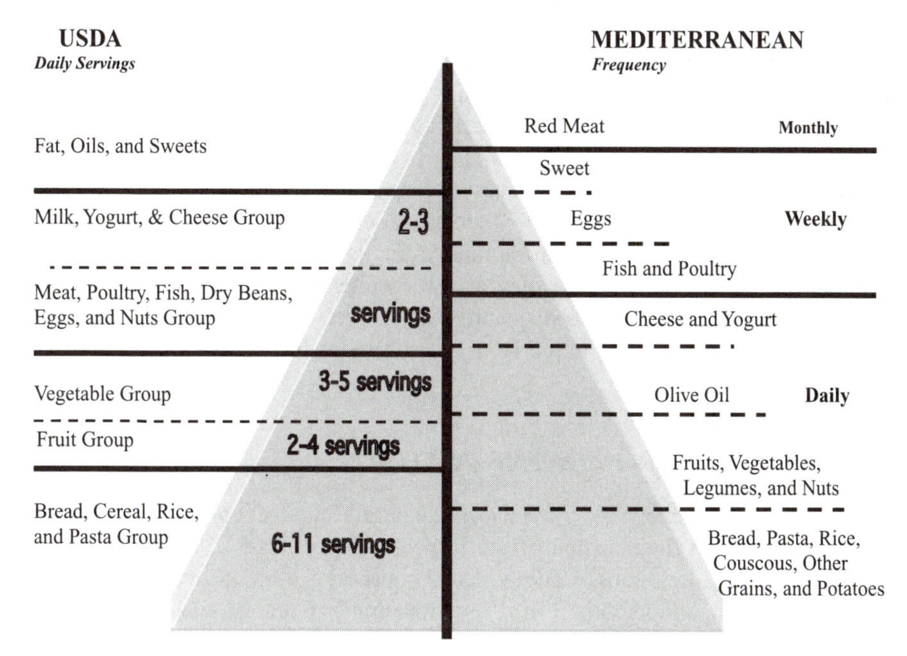

FIGURE 14.1 Food Guide Pyramids.

fruits and tomatoes more than doubled.[19] Citrus fruit is known for its high content of vitamin C, potassium, and *d*-limonene. Vitamin C is an antioxidant that may protect cell membranes and DNA from oxidative damage. Its role in the synthesis of the collagen is crucial; vitamin C deficiency may, therefore, affect the integrity of intercellular matrixes thus promoting tumor growth or hindering tumor encapsulation.[20] Furthermore, there is growing evidence that high-potassium diets may be beneficial in both animal and human genetic hypertension.[21] Citrus fruit also contains *d*-limonene (found specifically in citrus fruit oils), which has been shown to have pronounced chemopreventive and chemotherapeutic activities. Vitamin C and *d*-limonene may contribute to the favorable effects attributable to diets relatively rich in fruits and vegetables, and are associated with a lower incidence of breast, lung, pancreas, colon, rectum, and cervical cancers.

Current amounts of naturally occurring *d*-limonene contained in foods, in portions commonly consumed by the American population, may be inadequate to achieve optimal health benefits. *d*-Limonene is probably present in relatively high levels in the Mediterranean diet compared to U.S. diets, and may be an important component in the putative cancer preventive effect of the Mediterranean diet. The Mediterranean diet includes frequent exposure to citrus oils. Food preparation may play an important role in determining the amount of limonene consumed, since orange zest or parts of the whole lemon fruit are often included during cooking to add a desirable sour taste to the food. Lemon juice (a beverage similar to lemonade) is usually prepared by blending the whole fruit, and thus contains more limonene than American lemonade.

Observational epidemiological data obtained from case-control, cohort, or cross-cultural studies have consistently suggested that those living in the Mediterranean area, who consume large amounts of fruits and vegetables in general, and citrus fruits in particular, have the lowest incidence rates for most tumors associated with diet. Thus, the role of *d*-limonene, a nonnutrient compound of citrus fruit oils, merits careful evaluation as an inhibitor of carcinogenesis. Although dietary factors alone may not fully explain the health of Mediterranean populations, available evidence strongly suggests important contributions from the high consumption of fruits, vegetables, and whole grain. Studies of the Mediterranean diet are of particular interest to better understand and quantify this effect in view of the methods of preparation, frequency, and range of fruit and vegetable consumption by these populations.

14.4 LEVELS OF *d-LIMONENE IN CITRUS*

d-Limonene, a monocyclic monoterpene, is a natural component of a variety of foods and beverages and is found in many fruits (especially citrus fruits), vegetables, meats, spices, and other food items.[22] The principal sources of *d*-limonene are the oils of orange, grapefruit, and lemon.[23,24] It is found naturally in orange juice at an average concentration of 100 ppm. The major use of *d*-limonene is as a lemon fragrance in soap and perfume and as flavoring agent in foods, beverages, and chewing gum. *d*-Limonene (orange oil/essence oil) is used as a flavoring ingredient to impart a citrus flavor in artificial oils and can be found in nonalcoholic beverages (31 ppm), ice cream and ices (68 ppm), candy (49 ppm), baked goods (120 ppm), and gelatins, and puddings (48 to 400 ppm).[25] When citrus juices are packed aseptically into laminated cartons, the *d*-limonene content of the juice is reduced by about 25% within 14 days of storage owing to absorption by the polyethylene.[26] Limonene has been found in packaging material at 25 ppm (25 μg/g).[27] Oxidation is not reported to occur to a significant extent in over four weeks of storage in glass.[28] The effects of packaging materials on *d*-limonene contents in commercially available citrus juices has been clearly demonstrated.[28-31] Our data show that the level of *d*-limonene in orange juice samples varied considerably depending on whether the juice is packaged with or without pulp (8 to 10% less in *d*-limonene content). By comparing orange juice samples in glass and plastic containers, we found a 50 to 58% decrease in *d*-limonene levels based on the type of packaging alone.[29]

Daily U.S. per capita consumption of *d*-limonene, as a result of both its natural occurrence in food and of its presence as a flavoring agent, was estimated to be 0.27 mg/kg body weight per day, or 16.2 mg/day for a 60-kg individual.[32] Intake of *d*-limonene can vary considerably, however, depending on the types of food consumed. Citrus juice products are among the richest sources of *d*-limonene: daily intake owing to consumption of these products may approach 1 mg/kg body weight for adults and 2 mg/kg body weight for young children. Preliminary results from our studies in Arizona suggest, however, that source, preparation practices, and packaging materials have major influences on actual *d*-limonene levels in citrus products. The largest sources of *d*-limonene (averaged concentrations) identified to date are fresh Mediterranean-style lemonade 600 mg/l and limeade 350 mg/l, followed by commercial orange juices. Many commonly produced citrus beverages actually contain no *d*-limonene.

Human exposure to *d*-limonene through the diet or environment is widespread. However, in human populations, the amount of *d*-limonene ingested is determined not only by the frequency and amount of citrus food intake but also by the amount of citrus oil (peel) consumed.[29] Discussions with individual Americans suggest that peel (zest) consumption is not uncommon, and may vary between ethnic groups. Our current work in Arizona suggests that adults with the highest citrus juice intake (two cups per day) were consuming 20 to 50 mg *d*-limonene per day. In the same study, peel consumption was not uncommon, with one-third of the subjects interviewed (163/470) reporting some citrus peel use. Individuals reporting citrus peel use were consuming 90 to 250 mg *d*-limonene per day.

14.5 METABOLISM OF *d*-LIMONENE

In human subjects and several other mammalian species, oral *d*-limonene is completely absorbed and undergoes extensive biotransformation to active metabolites.[33-35] *d*-Limonene metabolites were analyzed in plasma extracts by gas chromatography. Rapid conversion of *d*-limonene into its two major metabolites, perillic acid and dihydroperillic acid, was detected. These metabolites comprised more than 89% of the circulating limonene-derived material at 1 h after administration and thereafter, whereas *d*-limonene itself accounted for only 15%.[36] The most recent human study[37] has shown humans produce all of the same rat plasma metabolites in approximately the same proportions, and the investigators were able to identify two more metabolites in plasma extracts, namely limonene-8,9-diol and an isomer of perillic acid. A comparison of the rat metabolism of orange oil (95% *d*-limonene, from Sunkist) vs. 99% *d*-limonene (Aldrish) indicated that identical metabolites were formed at identical concentrations.[35] In both plasma[36] and urine, [38] limonene is only a minor component of the total limonene-derived material. Metabolites of limonene have been shown to be more potent pharmacological agents than limonene itself in several experimental systems.[39]

Limonene and/or its metabolites distribute throughout the body, showing some preference for fatty tissues.[36,40] No studies have been done to assess the level of *d*-limonene and its metabolites in fatty tissues. In Japan, limonene has been used locally for the purpose of dissolving gallstones in human gallbladders at daily doses of up to 20 g per patient, or approximately 285 mg/kg, with no overt toxicity.[41] It is extensively metabolized by rats, humans, and other species.

14.6 LIMONENE AND TUMOR REGRESSION

The Mediterranean diet was found not only to produce favorable effects on blood lipid profiles, but also found to protect against oxidative stress and carcinogenesis.[14] The chemopreventive efficacy of limonene during both the initiation and promotion stages of carcinogenesis has been demonstrated in chemically induced rodent mammary,[42-44] skin,[45,46] liver,[47] lung and forestomach,[48,49] colon,[50] and gastric[51] tumor model systems. *d*-Limonene inhibits activation of the tobacco-specific carcinogen NNK, and accordingly may have the capacity to diminish carcinogenic response to exposures to tobacco.[52]

It was recently demonstrated that dietary *d*-limonene exhibits therapeutic effects against chemically induced mammary tumors in rats, with a regression of >80% of carcinomas with little host toxicity. Chander et al.[53] found that a 10% limonene dose mixed in the diet caused tumor regression in all animals, while a 5% limonene dose was only able to cause regression in 50% of the rats. The limonene dose-tumor regression response relationship is steep. Significant regressions are not observed at 5% dietary levels, while a majority of tumors completely regress above the 7.5% dietary level. Limonene appears to act in a cytostatic fashion. Its removal from the diet results in a significant number of tumor recurrences.[54] Regressing tumors have a unique histopathological appearance that is not associated with gross cytotoxicity, immune cell involvement, or apoptosis. The postinitiation chemopreventive/tumor suppressive activity may be due in part to the inhibition of isoprenylation of cell growth-associated small G proteins such as p21 ras by limonene and its metabolites.[54,55] Posttranslational isoprenylation is required for functionality of these proteins, e.g., transformation by ras.[56,57] Perillic acid and dihydroperillic acid, the two major metabolites of limonene in the rat and human, are more potent inhibitors of small G-protein isoprenylation than is limonene. Perillic acid is a more potent inhibitor of cell growth than is limonene. These findings coupled with the extensive metabolism of limonene *in vivo*[36,38] raise the possibility that the antitumor effects of limonene *in vivo* may be mediated via perillic acid, and perhaps other metabolites.[36] Since farnesylation of ras protein is critical for its ability to cause oncogenic transformation, inhibition of protein prenylation may be the basis of the antitumor effects of limonene and perillic acid.

A minor metabolite of limonene, perillic acid methyl ester, is a potent inhibitor of the enzyme protein farnesyl transferase. These data suggest that if the inhibition of protein prenylation is a mechanism for limonene's anti-cancer activities, this monoterpene may be a prodrug that is converted into pharmacologically active substances by metabolic modification.[58] *d*-Limonene can also inhibit carcinogen-induced neoplasia when administered at a short time interval prior to carcinogen challenge.[44] The initiation-phase chemopreventive effects of *d*-limonene have been attributed to the induction of phase I[59] and phase II[60] carcinogen-metabolizing enzymes, resulting in carcinogen detoxification.[59]

d-Limonene was recently tested in phase I therapeutic trials.[37,61] A single-center phase I clinical trial was undertaken to determine the toxicity and maximum tolerated dose of orally administered *d*-limonene in patients with advanced solid tumors.[37] One partial response in a breast cancer patient on 8 g/m^2 per day was maintained for 11 months and 3 patients with colorectal carcinoma had prolonged stable disease.

A conceptual limitation that has plagued epidemiological studies has been the approach to analysis. In most studies, food intake data have been converted to summarized nutrients, which have been the focus of the risk analysis. Thus, the limitations of food composition databases have placed important contraints on what could be analyzed. In addition, in studies that have analyzed food intake by food groups as well as by nutrients, food groups have generally been found to have greater relative risks (or relative protection) associated with them than specific nutrients. This may be due both to the presence of important compounds not included in standard food composition databases and to the importance of combinations of factors present in whole foods. The Arizona population offered a unique opportunity to study potential associations between citrus consumption and risk of skin squamous cell carcinoma (SCC). A total of 274 men and 196 women who had participated in the Southeastern Arizona Skin Cancer Study completed a citrus consumption study. Our results show that peel consumption, the major source of dietary *d*-limonene, was not uncommon and may have a potential protective effect in relation to skin SCC. We found no association between the overall consumption of citrus fruits or citrus juices and skin SCC. However, the most striking feature was the protection purported by citrus peel consumption. Moreover, there was a dose-response relationship between higher citrus peel in the diet and degree of risk lowering.[62]

14.7 CONCLUSION

The benefits of phytochemicals have been extensively publicized in the popular press, which has resulted in increased public awareness and interest in consumption of phytochemical-rich foods as a method of enhancing health and well-being. Health benefits of these foods are best obtained through the consumption of a varied diet using our normal food supply. The Mediterranean cuisine is able to offer hundreds of delicious and nutritious recipes and is easily accepted by most people. Therefore, the Mediterranean diet provides the best chance for influencing people to abandon unhealthy foods in favor of fresh vegetables, fruits, grain, and olive oil. It introduces a dietary pattern that is attractive for its delicious palatability as well as for its health benefits. Of course, food alone is not the answer. Mediterranean area inhabitants were and, in many regions, still are more physically active than Americans.

Data from several clinical trials,[63-66] indicate that the beneficial effects associated with a diet high in fruits and vegetables may not be demonstrated when individual nutrients, such as vitamins C and E or beta-carotene, are consumed in supplement form. Neverless, pharmaceutical companies will be motivated to isolate components in foods into pill or supplement form to market the individual components for their health benefit(s). We don't have to wait for more analyses of individual components of the diet when it is clear that the whole diet is important. The public must be convinced that the more appropriate choice would be to increase fruit and vegetable consumption and choose a varied diet based on the principles of the Mediterranean Food Guide Pyramid. However, whether or not the Mediterranean diet is followed, always include regular exercise as a part of a healthy lifestyle. It has become increasingly clear that the Mediterranean Diet is one of the best ways to maintain lifetime wellness and prevention of chronic diseases.

REFERENCES

1. Avellone G., Di Garbo V., Codovaa R., Panno, A.V., Verga, S., and Bompiani, G. Food habits and cardiovascular risk factors in 2 population samples of western Sicily. *Ann. Ital. Med. Int.* 12(4):210-6, 1997.
2. Tavani, A. and LaVecchia, C. Fruit and vegetable consumption and cancer risk in a Mediterranean population. *Am. J. Clin. Nutr.* 61(Suppl. 6):1347s-1377s, 1995.
3. Ghiselli A., D'Amicic, A., and Giacosa, A. The antioxidant potential of the Mediterranean diet. *Eur. J. Cancer Prev.* 6(Suppl. 1):15s-19s, 1997.
4. Khlat, M. Cancer in Mediterranean migrants — based on studies in France and Australia. *Cancer Causes Control.* 6(6):525-31, 1995.
5. LaVecchia, C. and Tavani, A. Fruit and vegetable, and human cancer. *Eur. J. Cancer Prev.* 7(1):3-8, 1998.
6. Macini, M, Parfitt, V.J., and Rubba, P. Antioxidants in the Mediterranean diet. *Can. J. Cardiol.* 11(Suppl. G): 105G-109G, 1995.
7. Renaud, S., de Lorgeril, M., Delave, J., Guidollet, J., Jacquard, F., Mamelle, N., Martin, J.L., Monjaud, I., Salen, P., and Toubol, P. Cretan Mediterranean diet for prevention of coronary heart disease. *Am. J. Clin. Nutr.* 61(Suppl. 6):1360s-1367s, 1995.
8. de Lorgeril, M., Salen, P., Martin, J.L., Monjaud, I., Delaye, J., and Mamelle, N. Mediterranean diet, traditional risk factors, and the rate of cardiovascular complications after myocardial infarction: final report of the Lyon Diet Heart Study. *Circulation.* 99(6): 779-85, 1999.
9. Keys, A. and Keys, M. *How To Eat Well and Stay Well, the Mediterranean Way.* Doubleday, Garden City, NJ, 1975.
10. Braun T., Ancient Mediterranean food. In *The Mediterranean Diets in Health and Disease.* Gene A. Spiller, Ed. Van Nostrand Reinhold, New York, 10-58, 1991.
11. Ferro-Luzzi, A., and Branka, F. Mediterranean diet, Italian style: Prototype of a healthy diet. *Am. J. Clin. Nutr.* 61(Suppl. 6):1338s-1345s, 1995.
12. Trichopoulou, A. and Lagiou, P. Healthy traditional Mediterranean diet: an expression of culture, history, and lifestyle. *Nutr. Rev.* 55(11, Pt. 1):383-9, 1997.
13. Kushi, L.H., Lenart, E.B., and Willet, W.C. Health implications of Mediterranean diets in light of contemporary knowledge. 1. Plant foods and dairy products. *Am. J. Clin. Nutr.* 61(Suppl. 6): 1407s-1415s, 1995.
14. Willet, W.C., Sacks, F., Trichopoulou, A., Drescher, G., Ferro-Luzzi, A., Helsing, E., and Trichopoulos, D. Mediterranean diet pyramid: a cultural model for healthy eating. *Am. J. Clin. Nutr.* 61(Suppl. 6):1402s-1406s, 1995.
15. Keys, A., Aravanis, C., Blackburn, H., Van Buchem, F.S.P., Buzina, R., Djordjevic, B.S., Dontas, A.S., Fidanza, F., Karvonen, M.J., Kimura, N., Lekos, D., Monti, M., Puddu, V., and Taylor, H.L. Epidemiological studies related to coronary heart disease: characteristics of men aged 40-59 in Seven Countries. *Acta. Med. Scand.* 460 (Suppl. 180):1, 1967.
16. Kromhout, D., Keys, A., Arvanis, C., Buzina, R., Fidanza, F., Jensen, A., Menotti, A., Nedeljkovic, S., Pekkarinen, M., Simic, B.S., and Toshima, H. Food consumption patterns on the1960s in Seven Countries. *Am. J. Clin. Nutr.*, 49(5):889-94, May 1989.
17. LeMarchand, L., Yoshizawa, C.N., Kolonel, L.N., Hankin, J.H., and Goodman, M.T. Vegetable consumption and lung cancer risk: a population-based case-control study in Hawaii. *J. Natl. Cancer Inst.* 81:1158-1164, 1989.

18. Lewis, B., Mancini, M., and Puska, P. Dietary measures for control of lipoprotein risk factors. In *Atherosclerosis Biology and Clinical Science*, Olsson, A.G., Ed., pp. 409-417. Churchill Livingstone. New York, 1987.
19. Istituto Centrale di Statistica. 1960-1985. Annuari statistica italiani. Rome. 1960-1985.
20. Cameron, E. and Pauling, L. Cancer and vitamin C. Linus Pauling Institute of Science and Medicine, Palo Alto, CA, 1979.
21. Treasure, J. and Ploth, D. Role of dietary potassium in the treatment of hypertension. *Hypertension*. 5:864, 1983.
22. Marshall, J.R. Editorial: Improving American's Diet-Setting Public Policy with Limited Knowledge. *Am. J. Public Health.* 85:1609-1611, 1995.
23. U.S National Toxicology Program, Research Triangle Park, NC (Jan. 1990). Toxicology and carcinogenesis studies of *d*-limonene in F344/N rats and B6c3F1 Mice. NTTS, p. 12.
24. Kesterson, J.W., Hendrickson, R., and Braddock, R.J. Florida Citrus Oils. Tech. Bull. 749, University of Florida, Gainesville, FL, pp. 3-174, 1971.
25. *D*-Limonene Monograph, Flavor and Extract Manufacturers' Association. Washington, D.C., pp. 1-4, 1991.
26. Marsili, R. Measuring volatiles and limonene-oxidation products in orange juice by capillary GC. *LC-GC.* 4:358-362,1986.
27. Mannheim, C.H., Miltz, J., and Letzter, A. Interaction between polyethylene laminated cartons and aseptically packed citrus juice. *J. Food Sci.* 52:737-740, 1987.
28. Shaw, P.E. Review of quantitative analyses of citrus essential oils. *J. Agric. Food Chem.* 27:246-257, 1979.
29. Hakim, I.A., McClure T., and Liebler, D. Assessing dietary *d*-limonene intake for epidemiological studies. Abstr. Third Int. Food Data Conf., July 1999, Rome, Italy. Accepted in JFCA (in press).
30. Charara, Z.N., Williams, J.W., Schmidt, R.H., and Marshall, M.R. Orange flavor absorption into various polymeric packaging materials. *J. Food Sci.* 57(4):963-967, 1992
31. Sadler, G., Parish, M., Van Clief, D., and Davis, J. The effect of volatile absorption by packaging polymers on flavor, microorganisms and ascorbic acid in reconstituted orange juice. *Lebensm-Wiss u-Technol.* 30 (7):686-690, 1997.
32. Lloyd, R.J. Instrumentation for automated thermal desorption-pyrolysis capillary gas chromatography. *J. Chromatogr.* 284:357-371, 1984.
33. Kodoma, R., Yano, T., Furukawa, K., et al. Studies on the metabolism of *d*-limonene (p-mentha-1,8-diene). IV. Isolation and characterization of new metabolites and species differences in metabolism. *Xenobiotica.* 6:377-389, 1976.
34. Igimi, H., Nishimura, M., Kodoma, R., and Ide, H. Studies on the metabolism of *d*-limonene (p-mentha-1,8-diene). I. The absorption, distribution and excretion of *d*-limonene in rats. *Xenobiotica*. 4:77-84, 1974.
35. Crowell, P.L., Elson, C.E., Bailey, H.H., Elegbede, J.A., Haag, J.D., and Gould, M.N. Human metabolism of the experimental cancer therapeutic agent *d*-limonene. *Cancer Chemother. Pharmacol.* 35:31-37, 1994.
36. Igimi, H., Nishimura, M., Kodoma, R., and Ide, H. Studies on the metabolism of *d*-limonene (p-mentha-1,8-diene). I. The absorption, distribution and excretion of *d*-limonene in rats. *Xenobiotica*. 4:77-84, 1974.
37. Vigushin, D.M., Poon, G.K., Boddy, A., English, J., Halbert, G.W., Pagonis, C., Jarman, M., and Coombes, R.C. Phase I and pharmacokinetic study of *D*-limonene in patients with advanced cancer. *Cancer Chemother. Pharmacol.* 42:111-117, 1998.

38. IARC Monographs on the evaluation of carcinogenic risks to humans. International Agency for Research in Cancer. 56:135-162, 1993.
39. Crowell, P.L., Lin, S., Vedejs, E., and Gould, M.N. Identification of circulating metabolites of the antitumor agent *d*-limonene capable of inhibiting protein isoprenylation and cell growth. *Cancer Chemother. Pharmacol.* 31:205-212, 1992.
40. Kodoma, R., Yano, T., Furukawa, K., et al. Studies on the metabolism of *d*-limonene (p-mentha-1,8-diene). IV. Isolation and characterization of new metabolites and species differences in metabolism. *Xenobiotica*. 6:377-389, 1976.
41. Igimi, H., Tamura, R., Traishi, K., and Tamamoto, F. Medical dissolution of gallstones. Clinical experience of *d*-limonene as a simple, safe, and effective solvent. *Dig. Dis. Sci.* 36:200, 1991.
42. Elson, C.E., Maltzman, T.H., Boston, J.L., et al. Anti-carcinogenic activity of *d*-limonene during the initiation and promotion/progression stages of DMBA-induced rat mammary carcinogenesis. *Carcinogenesis.* 9:331-332, 1988.
43. Maltzman, T.H., Hurt, L.M., Elson, C.E., Tanner, M.A., and Gould, M.N. The prevention of nitosomethylurea-induced mammary tumors by *d*-limonene and orange oil. *Carcinogenesis.* 10:781-783, 1989.
44. Elegbede, J.A., Elson, C.E., Tanner, M.A., Qureshi, A., and Gould, M.N. Inhibition of DMBA-induced mammary cancer by the monoterpene *d*-limonene. New model for the chemoprevention of premalignant and malignant lesions of the breast. *Carcinogenesis*. 5:661, 1984.
45. Van Duuren, B.L. and Goldschmidt, B.M. Cocarcinogenic and tumor-promoting agents in tobacco carcinogenesis. *J. Natl. Cancer Inst*. 56(6):1237-42, 1976.
46. Elegbede, J.A., Maltzman, T.H., Verma, A.K., Tanner, M.A., and Gould, M.N. Mouse skin tumor promoting activity of orange peel oil and *d*-limonene: A reevaluation. *Carcinogenesis*. 7:2047-2049, 1986.
47. Giri, R.K., Parija, T., and Das, B.R. *D*-Limonene chemoprevention of hepatocarcinogenesis in AKR mice: inhibition of c-jun and c-myc. *Oncol. Rep*. 6(5):1123-1127, 1999.
48. Wattenberg, L.W. and Coccia, J.B. Inhibition of 4-(methylnitrosoamino)-1-(3-pyridyl)-1-butanone carcinogenesis in mice by *d*-limonene and citrus fruit oils. *Carcinogenesis*. 12:115-117, 1991.
49. Wattenberg, L.W., Sparnins, V.L., and Barany, G. Inhibition of N-nitrosodiethylamine carcinogenesis in mice by naturally occurring organosulfur compounds and monoterpenes. *Cancer Res*. 49:2689-2692, 1989.
50. Kawamori, T., Tanaka, T., Hirose, M., and Mori, H. Inhibitory effects of *d*-limonene on the development of colonic aberrant crypt foci induced by azoxymethane in F344 rats. *Carcinogenesis*. 17:369-372, 1996.
51. Yano, H., Tatsuta, M., Iishi, H., Baba, M., Sakai, N., and Uedo, N. Attenuation by *d*-limonene of sodium chloride-enhanced gastric carcinogenesis induced by N-methyl-N'-nitro-N-nitrosoguanidine in Wistar rats. *Int. J. Cancer*. 82(5):665-668, 1999.
52. Wattenberg, L.W. Inhibition of carcinogenesis by minor anutrient constituents of the diet. *Proc. Nutr. Soc.* 49:173-183, 1990.
53. Chander, S.K., Lansdown, A.G., Luqmani, Y.A., et al. Effectiveness of combined limonene and 4-hydroxyandrostenedione in the treatment of NMU-induced rat mammary tumours. *Br. J. Cancer.* 69:897-882, 1994.
54. Haag, J.D., Lindstrom, M.J., and Gould, M.N. Limonene-induced regression of mammary carcinomas. *Cancer Res.* 52:4021-4026, 1992.

55. Gould, M.N., Moore, C.J., Zhang, R., et al. Limonene chemoprevention of mammary carcinoma induction following direct in situ transfer of v-ha-ras. *Cancer Res.* 54:3540-3543, 1994.
56. Crowell, P.L. and Gould, M.N. Chemoprevention and therapy of cancer by *d*-limonene. *Crit. Rev. Oncogenesis.* 5:1, 1994.
57. Kato, K., Cox, A.D., Hisaka, M.M., et al. Isoprenoid addition to Ras protein is the critical modification for its membrane association and transforming activity. *Proc. Natl. Acad. Sci. USA* 89:6403, 1992.
58. Gelb, M.H., Tamanoi, F., Yokoyama, K., et al. The inhibition of protein prenyltransferases by oxygenated metabolites of limonene and perillyl alcohol. *Cancer Lett.* 91:169-175, 1995.
59. Maltzman, T.H., Christou, M., Gould, M.N., et al. Effects of monoterpenoids on in vivo DMBA-DNA adduct formation and on phase I hepatic metabolizing enzymes. *Carcinogenesis.* 12:2081, 1991.
60. Elegbede, J.A., Maltzman, T.H., Elson, C.E., et al. Effects of anticarcinogenic monoterpenes on phase II hepatic metabolizing enzymes. *Carcinogenesis.* 14:1221, 1993.
61. McNamee, D., Limonene trial in cancer. *Lancet*, 342:801, 1993.
62. Hakim, I.A., Harris, R. B., and Ritenbaugh, C. Southeastern Arizona Citrus Study (unpublished).
63. Li, J.-Y., Taylor, P.R., Li, B., Dawsey, S., Liu, S.F., Yang, C.S., and Shan, Q. Nutrition intervention trials in Linxian, China: multiple vitamin/mineral supplementation, cancer incidence, and disease-specific mortality among adults with esophageal dysplagia. *J. Natl. Cancer Inst.* 85:1492-1498, 1993.
64. Blot, W.J., Li, J.-Y., Taylor, P.R., Guo, W., Dawsey, S., Wang, G.Q., Yang, C.S., Zheng, J.F., Gail, M., and Li, G.Y. Nutrition intervention trials in Linxian, China: supplementation with specific vitamin/mineral combinations, cancer incidence and disease-specific mortality in the general population. *J. Natl. Cancer Inst.* 85:1483-1492, 1993.
65. Alpha-Tocopherol, Beta Carotene Cancer Prevention Study Group. The effect of vitamin E and beta-carotene on the incidence of lung cancer and other cancers in male smokers. *N. Engl. J. Med.* 330:1029-1035, 1994.
66. Greenberg, E.R., Baron, J.A., Tosteson, T.D., Freeman, D.H., Beck, G.J., Bond, J.H., Colacchio, T.A., Coller, J.A., Frankl, H.D., and Haile, R.W. A clinical trial of antioxidant vitamins to prevent colorectal adenoma. *N. Engl. J. Med.* 331:141-147, 1994.

Section IV

Fruits and Promotion of Health

15 Gastrointestinal Nutritional Problems in the Aged: Role of Vegetable and Fruit Use

B.S. Ramakrishna

CONTENTS

0-8493-0038-X/97/$0.00+$.50

15.1 INTRODUCTION

Aging leads to a decline in the physiological activities of many body organs and systems. The gastrointestinal tract, which is the primary portal for entry of nutrients into the body, is no exception to this. Nutritional changes may arise in the elderly as a consequence of this decline in gastrointestinal function. On the other hand, dysfunction or disease of the gastrointestinal tract may arise as a result of poor nutritional practices and may potentially be prevented or alleviated by appropriate measures. This chapter will consider these two aspects of the interaction between aging, nutrition, and the gastrointestinal tract, and the relevance to these of fruit and vegetable consumption. Alterations in nutrition consequent to disease of the gastrointestinal tract are not unique to the elderly, and will not be considered.

15.2 CHANGES IN GASTROINTESTINAL FUNCTION AND NUTRITION SECONDARY TO AGING

Both aging and the disease concomitants of the aging process impose barriers to adequate nutrition. Decline in smell and taste perception with diminished enjoyment of food and impaired mastication through dental loss may contribute to poor food intake. Diminished physical activity is an important factor leading to suppressed appetite in the elderly. Social and psychological cues to eating are lacking, and depression is common. Nutritional status is a critical determinant of physiological deterioration in the elderly.[1] Malnutrition represents a serious barrier to recovery from illness, and is correlated with the development of infections, muscle wasting, and weakness that prevent ambulation and self-care. Vitamin deficiencies may be subclinical in the elderly, and may be unmasked by stresses from illness or infection, or by the use of medication.

15.2.1 Gastrointestinal Function in the Aged: Potential Effects on Nutrition

A number of changes in gastrointestinal function occur in the aged.[2,3] Alterations in esophageal motor function are common in the elderly, and may be responsible for difficulty in swallowing and choking. Gastric mucosal atrophy occurs in 11–50% of elderly individuals,[3,4] leading to decreased acid secretion and, to a lesser extent, of pepsin and of intrinsic factor. Reduction in the height of small intestinal villi occurs after the age of 60, as also does mucosal atrophy of the colon with inflammatory infiltration.[3] Atrophy of the pancreas is striking morphologically and may lead to reduced secretion of pancreatic enzymes.[5] Liver size decreases accompanied by reductions in bile flow and bile acid secretion.[6] The mucosal immune system shows minor alterations with decreased helper and killer T cells, along with slight changes in B-cell function.[7,8]

These various changes described above contribute to changes in nutrition in the elderly. Difficulty in swallowing and choking, decreased gastric secretion, and altered intestinal motility may all lead to decreased food intake. Malabsorption of nutrients can be caused by a number of factors and may be aggravated by the effects of infection, surgery, or medications. Reduced gastric acid secretion (secondary to gastric atrophy and the use of antisecretory drugs) results in reduced absorption of iron and folic acid. Reduced acid secretion also commonly leads to bacterial colonization of the small intestine in the elderly in the absence of structural alterations. This "simple colonization" of the upper gastrointestinal tract may remain clinically silent in many elderly.[3] In others, it leads to malabsorption of carbohydrate, fat, and vitamin B12.[9] Reduction of intrinsic factor secretion also contributes to poor absorption of vitamin B12. Diminution of small bowel absorptive surface area is not usually of clinical significance, but may impair the capacity to absorb heavy loads of carbohydrate or protein. Reduced secretion of pancreatic enzymes and bile salts may result in diminished absorption of fat-soluble vitamins (A, D, E, and K) and calcium.

15.2.2 Nutritional Status of the Elderly: Role of Vegetable and Fruit Intake

Overt malnutrition among free-living aged people is common only among the poor and sick. Estimates of dietary intake have uniformly shown that total energy intake and intake of protein is usually low in the elderly.[10-12] High prevalences of inadequate intake have been found for various micronutrients including iron, calcium, magnesium, zinc, thiamine, riboflavin, nicotinic acid, pyridoxine, beta-carotene, vitamin A, vitamin D, and vitamin E.[10-16] Assessment of nutritional status by biochemical indices has demonstrated significant prevalences of deficiencies of vitamin B6, C, D, and of zinc, iron, and protein in the elderly, particularly in those who were institutionalized.[10,15] A study of elderly Seventh-Day Adventists suggested that vegetarians had a lesser prevalence of deficiencies (except vitamin B12 and D) than nonvegetarians.[17] Specific nutrient deficiencies in the elderly, in prevention of which fruit and vegetable consumption may be of relevance, are detailed below.

Iron deficiency in the elderly may be aggravated by iron loss from the gastrointestinal tract secondary to the use of nonsteroidal analgesics or from disease in the gastrointestinal tract. While enriched cereals are the best source of this mineral, iron is present in significant amounts in vegetables such as beans, peas, and spinach and in fruit such as strawberries. Zinc status is marginal in the elderly, and may be worsened by a diet high in fiber and calcium, which interferes with absorption of zinc. Zinc is essential for the immune status and wound healing.[18] Significant plant sources of zinc include peanuts and spices, with lesser amounts in whole grains and turnip greens.

Vitamin A and its precursors are required for epithelial differentiation, and have a protective effect against many cancers. They also enhance cellular immune responses, inhibit mutagenesis, and have an antioxidant effect that is significant in many inflammatory diseases. An increase in T-helper cells, without alteration of T-suppressor cells, has been shown in elderly individuals after daily doses of beta-carotene varying from 15–60 mg/day.[19] Absorption of vitamin A decreases in the elderly.[3] Carotenoids, abundant in yellow and dark-green vegetables, are vitamin A precursors that are converted to retinol by molecular cleavage in the intestinal mucosa. Preformed vitamin A, found in animal foods, may be oxidized and lost by exposure to a hot humid environment.[20] Thus there is a basis for recommending an adequate level of intake of vegetable sources of vitamin A. Vitamin K is required for the synthesis of blood clotting factors II, VII, IX, and X. Leafy green vegetables such as spinach, broccoli, and Brussels sprouts are rich in vitamin K. Since vitamin K synthesized by intestinal bacteria meets part of the daily requirement, levels of the vitamin may decrease in the elderly who are taking antibiotics. The use of mineral oil, for constipation, may also interfere with absorption of the vitamin. In the healthy elderly, a varied diet containing green vegetables is recommended to maintain normal levels of the vitamin. Vitamin E is proposed as an antioxidant that can retard or prevent the aging process. There is no definite deficiency disease that can yet be ascribed to vitamin E, nor is there evidence to suggest that vitamin E requirements increase in the elderly. An adequate nutriture can be maintained by intake of vegetable oils, seeds, grains, and nuts which are all good sources of vitamin E.

Thiamine is required as a coenzyme in reactions that are essential to the intermediary metabolism of cells. Those elderly whose food intake is low may have biochemical evidence of thiamine deficiency.[21] Cereals and bran are the major natural source of this vitamin. Studies of independent-living and institutionalized elderly have shown a high prevalence of folate deficiency.[15,22] While low intake and reduced absorption secondary to hypochlorhydria reduce folic acid levels, there may be some compensation by bacterial synthesis of folate by bacteria colonizing the small intestine in the elderly. Clinical deficiency of this vitamin is likely in alcoholics, those with congestive heart failure, and gastrointestinal or liver disease, and those receiving drugs such as phenytoin and barbiturates. Subclinical deficiency leads to accumulation of homocysteine and increases the risk of heart disease. Adequate folic acid nutriture can be maintained in the elderly if they ingest dark-green vegetables and fortified breakfast cereals, which are good sources of folate.

Vitamin C is an antioxidant vitamin, and in addition helps to enhance iron absorption. It may be protective against gastrointestinal cancers, as discussed later. There is no definite change in vitamin C absorption or metabolism with age. In fact, vitamin C requirements may be 20 to 50% lower than the recommended daily allowance (60 mg/day) in the elderly. The most effective way of increasing intake is to encourage consumption of vitamin C-rich foods, such as fruits and vegetables.

15.3 GASTROINTESTINAL DISEASE IN THE AGED: ROLE OF VEGETABLES AND FRUIT IN PREVENTION

Faulty nutritional habits have the potential to affect the aging process, and may be one pathway leading to functional decline in the elderly. The gastrointestinal tract comes into contact with the environment throughout its length, and is directly subject to the influence of luminal factors including ingested food. Specific dietary constituents, or lack of them, can thus be a cause of gastrointestinal functional decline in the elderly. It is likely that such nutritional factors are co-factors or permissive factors that, in conjunction with genetic or other environmental factors, lead to development of gastrointestinal dysfunction or disease. In some instances, gastrointestinal dysfunction is related to recent changes in nutrition. In other instances, as for example diverticular disease, it is likely to be the result of longstanding alterations in dietary patterns. From a nutritional point of view, prevention should be started during youth and middle age to avoid these diseases in the elderly, but constant care is still necessary to obtain better health as well as to prevent disease in the very old.

Belief in the medicinal power of foods has been a part of traditional systems of medicine in many cultures. Compelling evidence to substantiate these medicinal effects is often lacking, but advances in understanding have been made. Vegetables and fruits have several components that are of relevance to the health of the gastrointestinal tract. Prominent among these are dietary fiber, flavonols and other antioxidants, and plant hormones. The following sections will briefly examine these components of plants and vegetables that may have an effect in preventing gastrointestinal disease, and review the evidence relating vegetable and fruit consumption to occurrence of specific gastrointestinal diseases in the elderly.

15.3.1 Carbohydrates in Vegetables and Fruits that Affect Gastrointestinal Function

Consumption of foods high in dietary fiber has been associated with the lower risk of several gastrointestinal diseases. Burkitt et al. comparing Western populations eating a diet rich in refined foods to African populations consuming a traditional diet, suggested that dietary fiber deficiency was responsible for low stool weight and prolonged intestinal transit, in turn leading to various illnesses affecting Western populations.[23,24] Dietary fiber was originally defined as nonabsorbable carbohydrate of plant origin, and its deficiency was postulated to be related to risk of development of colonic disorders such as constipation, diverticular disease, hemorrhoids, and colon cancer. Since the time of the original hypothesis, the plant components concerned have been more clearly identified, their physiological effects defined, and some information regarding their disease associations has been obtained. The term dietary fiber is now all but discarded, in favor of a more chemically descriptive classification. Food carbohydrates that enter the colon are now classified as monosaccharides, polyols, oligosaccharides (fructo- and galacto-oligosaccharides), resistant starch, and nonstarch polysaccharides (including cell wall materials other than lignin, storage polysaccharides, and plant gums, and mucilages).[25,26] The last category, i.e., nonstarch polysaccharides, comprises the bulk of traditionally designated fiber. Lignins, also part of plant cell wall material that are undigested, are a noncarbohydrate component of dietary fiber. The various unabsorbed carbohydrates share overlapping spectra of physiological effects, depending on the extent to which they are soluble and the degree to which they can be fermented. Within the small bowel their effect is largely physical, serving to moderate carbohydrate, and possibly lipid, absorption. Entering the colon, those carbohydrates that are resistant to breakdown serve to increase fecal bulk, decrease the rate of intestinal transit, and are useful in the management of constipation. They may also be useful in binding toxins and bile acids within the lumen of the colon. Carbohydrates that are easily broken down are fermented by anaerobic bacteria in the colon, leading to production of short-chain fatty acids and gases. Short-chain fatty acids exert a variety of effects within the large intestine that may be of relevance to diarrheal disease, inflammatory bowel disease, and colon cancer.[27]

Early experience with fiber led to its classification into soluble and insoluble components, based on fractional extraction by controlling pH.[28] Insoluble fibers included cellulose, certain hemicelluloses, and lignin, which are found in fruits and vegetables. They affect the rate and site of nutrient absorption, and may bind luminal compounds such as bile acids and affect excretion of these compounds. They aid in laxation by increasing fecal bulk, undigested plant residue being the most significant contributor to fecal weight. Insoluble fiber may interfere with absorption of minerals, and possibly vitamins. Soluble fibers such as pectin, gums, and storage polysaccharides found in grains and legumes are easily fermented to short-chain fatty acids by anaerobic bacteria within the colonic lumen. Soluble fibers can increase the stool weight by increasing fecal bacteria and bacterial cell mass, which accounts for the major proportion of fecal solids.[29,30] Resistant starch, which is not digested in the small bowel, is now recognized to form a major proportion of starch in certain foods.[25,31] Resistant starch granules are found in green banana and in raw potato, while retrograded amylose (also resistant to digestion) may be found in boiled and cooled potato, beans, and lentils. The type of processing and preparation of food may affect the digestibility of starch in the small bowel and thus its availability as a substrate for colonic fermentation. Colonic bacteria easily ferment most of the starch entering the colon, but some starches are resistant even to fermentation and may pass in the feces unchanged. Resistant starch that is fermented in the colon increases fecal bacterial cell mass, fecal weight, and fecal short-chain fatty acids, while lowering fecal pH and deoxycholate concentrations.[31]

Inulin and oligofructose are oligosaccharides that have come under the spotlight recently because of their touted ability to modify the colonic bacterial flora.[32] Like other nonabsorbed carbohydrates, they have the potential to increase fecal weight, short-chain fatty acids, and to lower colonic pH, and specifically they promote the growth of bifidobacteria in the colon. They are found naturally in chicory, dandelion greens, garlic, artichokes, and onions, and to a lesser extent in wheat and asparagus.[33]

Fermentation of unabsorbed carbohydrate within the colon leads to production of short-chain fatty acids (SCFA) such as butyrate, acetate, and propionate. These are rapidly absorbed from the colon, to exert effects within the colonic wall as well as systemically.[34] Acetate is carried to the liver and beyond, and is metabolized in muscle, kidney, heart, and brain. Propionate is cleared by the liver, may help in gluconeogenesis, and helps in suppression of cholesterol synthesis. Butyrate produced in the colon has a significant role to play in the health of the large intestinal mucosa.[34,35] It is the major source of energy for the colonic epithelial cell; stimulates sodium and water absorption from the colon; helps in mucosal proliferation; causes cell differentiation; and helps in wound repair processes. Short-chain fatty acids also enhance mesenteric and colonic blood flow, enhance gut hormone production, and stimulate the autonomic nervous system. These various effects have application in inflammatory bowel disease, diarrhea, and prevention of colon cancer, in addition to a number of other gastrointestinal diseases.[27] Fermentation of unabsorbed carbohydrate to short-chain fatty acids and their subsequent utilization, helps in energy conservation. This contributes to about 10% of energy ingested in many populations, and may increase to 20% in populations with a high intake of vegetable and plant foods. The contribution of colonic fermentation to energy conservation has not been specifically estimated in the elderly.

TABLE 15.1

Noncarbohydrate Phytochemicals that Have a Potentially Beneficial Effect on Gastrointestinal Health And Nutrition

Active agent	Fruit and vegetable source
Alpha-tocopherol	Green leafy vegetables, nuts, grains, vegetable oils
Beta-carotene	Yellow fruits, dark green or yellow vegetables
Lycopene	Tomatoes
Ascorbic acid	Fresh fruits and vegetables
Selenium	Nuts, spices, cabbage, carrots, turnips
Allyl sulfur compounds	Garlic, onions, leeks, chives
Flavonoids	Fruits, vegetables, nuts
Indoles and isothiocyanates	Cruciferous vegetables
Inulin/oligofructose	Bananas, garlic, onions
Lignans	Legumes, garlic, asparagus, broccoli, carrot, pears, plums
Isoflavones	Soy beans, legumes
Capsaicin	Chilli peppers
Arachidonate	Banana
Coumarins and glycosides	Cherries, peaches, apricot pits

15.3.2. Noncarbohydrate Components with Significant Effects on the Gastrointestinal Tract

Plants and vegetables contain other bioactive ingredients that may be responsible for effects on gastrointestinal health. Table 15.1 provides a partial list of noncarbohydrate compounds in plants that are thought to have potentially beneficial effects for gastrointestinal health and nutrition. A number of these compounds are known to be antioxidants, while others may have specific effects on cancer prevention. The known effects of these compounds are briefly reviewed here.

15.3.2.1 Antioxidants in Vegetables and Fruits

Reactive forms of oxygen are involved in the pathogenesis of a broad range of diseases. Oxygen free radicals such as superoxide anion, hydroxyl radical, hydrogen peroxide, and singlet oxygen can damage DNA, RNA, proteins, carbohydrates, and unsaturated lipids in cell membranes. The gastrointestinal tract has been described as a free radical time bomb,[36] since reactive oxygen species are generated in significant quantities both within the lumen and the wall of the healthy intestine. It has the highest concentration of xanthine oxidase, a large number of resident phagocytic cells, and a large number of catalase-negative bacteria in the colon capable of producing large amounts of O_2^-.The balance between the oxidants and antioxidant defenses in the wall of the gastrointestinal tract may be upset in a number of gastrointestinal diseases. Examples of such diseases especially prevalent in the elderly include cancer, ischemic bowel disease, and inflammatory bowel disease. A number of enzymatic and nonenzymatic reaction systems comprise the antioxidant defenses of the gastrointestinal mucosa.[37,38] Several of the antioxidant enzymes are metalloenzymes, which contain trace minerals for which vegetables and fruits are significant sources. Superoxide dismutase is a manganese-containing enzyme, while glutathione peroxidase is selenium-containing. Vegetables and fruits are rich sources of manganese, while selenium may be obtained from nuts, spices, whole grains, cabbage, carrots, and turnips.

Antioxidant vitamins, including vitamin A, carotenoids, vitamin C, and vitamin E, potentiate the antioxidant status and reduce lipid oxidation.[39,40] Decreased oxidation of lipids and DNA has been reported in most studies with either individual antioxidant agents or with the intake of vegetables and fruits.[41] In one study, however, plasma protein oxidation was noted to increase, despite decreased lipid oxidation, in subjects drinking large volumes of apple and blackcurrant juice.[42]

Besides the vitamin antioxidants, fruits and vegetables also contain nonnutrient antioxidants such as the flavonoids, polyphenols, and terpenes. Flavonoids such as catechin, chrysin, cyanidin, kaempferol, myricetin, and quercetin are found in fruits, onions, tea, and wines and are assuming importance as dietary antioxidants.[43] In one study, analysis of several common foods revealed that green leafy vegetables had the highest ability to inhibit iron-dependent lipid peroxidation, followed by wheat and rice.[44]

Availability of antioxidants in fruits and vegetables may depend on the food matrix.[38] Beta-carotene is organized in a pigment-protein complex in green vegetables but is in lipid droplets in other vegetables and fruits, and is available much more readily from the latter. Fat-soluble vitamins and carotenoids require sufficient fat in the meal to ensure efficient absorption. Lycopene, an antioxidant available in tomatoes, has a low availability in tomato juice, but cooking tomatoes in an oil-based medium substantially enhances intestinal absorption.[45]

15.3.2.2 Enzyme Modulators

Detoxification enzymes are essential for biotransformation of endogenous compounds and detoxification of many xenobiotics. Modulation of cytochrome P450-dependent monooxygenases and flavin-containing monooxygenases may be important in inactivation of carcinogens. Allium vegetables (onions, garlic, leeks, chives) contain a number of allyl sulfur compounds, which have anticarcinogenic activity. They appear to act at the induction stage of carcinogenesis, by strongly inhibiting alkylating carcinogens.[46] They modify metabolism of carcinogens through cytochrome P450, and also induce glutathione *S*-transferase, an enzyme necessary for detoxification of xenobiotics. Flavonoids, mentioned earlier, and isothiocyanates and indoles found in cruciferous vegetables, also appear to have significant effects on these enzyme systems.[41]

15.3.2.3 Phytoestrogens

Phytoestrogens are a family of plant compounds that bind to estrogen receptors, with resulting partial estrogenic activity. Because of the concentrations obtained in the body relative to endogenous hormones, there is considerable anti-estrogenic activity.[47] They exhibit a variety of actions including effects on protein synthesis, enzymes, cell proliferation and differentiation, angiogenesis, calcium transport, Na-

K-ATPase, vascular smooth muscle, lipid oxidation, and growth factor activity. The two main categories of phytoestrogens are isoflavones and lignans. Isoflavones include genistein, daidzein, and glycetin, and the major sources are soy beans and legumes. Lignans, building blocks for lignin and found in many plants, are found in largest quantities in flaxseed, but also in legumes, soybean, whole grains, and vegetables such as garlic, asparagus, broccoli, carrot, and sweet potato, and in fruits such as pears and plums. Phytoestrogens may have a role to play in the prevention of colon cancer. Due to their effects on small blood vessels, they have a potential, but unexplored, role in degenerative diseases of the vasculature such as angiodysplasia, which is common in the elderly and leads to gastrointestinal bleeding.

15.3.3 Role of Vegetables and Fruits in Prevention of Specific Gastrointestinal Diseases in the Elderly

15.3.3.1 Peptic Ulcer

There is a high prevalence of duodenal and gastric ulcers in the elderly. In community studies, peptic ulcers were detected in more than 12% of men and 8% of women over the age of 60.[48] Particularly in the elderly, peptic ulcers may remain silent until development of a complication such as gastrointestinal bleeding. There is a strong epidemiological association of duodenal ulcer complications in the elderly with the chronic use of nonsteroidal analgesics.[49,50] The relative roles of nonsteroidal analgesic use and *Helicobacter pylori* infection in peptic ulcer in the elderly remains a matter of controversy.

Peptic ulcers have long been associated with dietary factors, and these presumably impact on mucosal protection mechanisms. A low-fiber diet has been one of the factors associated with peptic ulcer disease. Two prospective studies of large cohorts, and a study of a smaller cohort, have addressed this issue. In one cohort of 34,198 Seventh-Day Adventists in the U.S., the strongest associations for peptic ulcer prevalence or incidence were found for nonsteroidal analgesic use.[51] However, ulcer prevalence also showed a statistically significant positive association with a low-fiber diet (Relative Risk (RR) >1.4).

In another prospective cohort of 47,806 adult men, higher consumption of fruits and vegetables was negatively associated with the risk of development of duodenal ulcer (RR = 0.67) after adjustment for age, body mass index, smoking, and use of aspirin or other nonsteroidal analgesic drugs.[52] Soluble dietary fiber showed a strong inverse association (RR = 0.40) with risk of duodenal ulcer, while vitamin A intake also showed a negative association with duodenal ulcer risk (RR = 0.46).

In a third cohort study, of 7624 Hawaiian men followed for an average of nearly 20 years, consumption of fruit had a mild, but nonsignificant negative association (RR = 0.8, $p = .19$) with development of duodenal or gastric ulcer.[53] Consumption of fresh vegetables was not assessed in this study.

In a cross-sectional community-based study of 46,693 subjects in Italy, consumption of vegetables showed a statistically significant inverse association with peptic ulcer prevalence (Odds Ratio = 0.74).[54] A case-control study comparing 78 duodenal ulcer patients with 160 healthy controls showed a positive association of duodenal ulcer with refined sugar intake.[55] This study also revealed that the relative risk of ulcer approximately halved in those with a higher intake of vegetable, but not cereal, fiber. It is possible that vegetable fiber in these studies was only a surrogate marker for other factors that may have provided the true protective effect against duodenal ulcer. Addition of fiber to the diet did not heal gastric ulcers faster.[56] However, a high-fiber diet was effective in preventing relapse in 73 patients with recently healed duodenal ulcers. Ulcer recurrence over 6 months was significantly lower in patients randomized to a high-fiber diet (45%) compared to those on a low-fiber diet (80%).[57] The same authors found that addition of wheat fiber to a traditional Norwegian diet did not significantly affect the relapse rate of duodenal ulcer,[58] suggesting either that fiber had only a threshold effect or that the type of fiber was important in determining the effect.

The components of a vegetable fiber diet that help prevent duodenal ulcers remain to be identified, but a variety of explanations are possible. Viscous soluble fiber has been reported to slow gastric emptying, an effect thought to be relevant to ulcer formation.[59] Ingestion of lentils reduced gastric emptying of a subsequent meal, and has been attributed to intestinal inhibition mediated through ileal receptors.[60,61] Vegetable oils containing linoleic acid may exert a cytoprotective effect on the gastric mucosa, and have been suggested as a possible cause for a decline in ulcer disease in recent years.[62,63] Vitamin A may also enhance mucosal cytoprotection.[64]

Studies in experimental ulcers in rats suggested that vegetables and pulses exerted a protective effect on ulcer formation.[65] Banana is a fruit that has been reported to decrease experimental ulcer formation in the stomach.[66] It was shown to increase mucosal prostanoids nonspecifically, and it was speculated that this was through increased mucosal availability of arachidonic acid.[67] Chilli, and its active ingredient capsaicin, were found to exert a cytoprotective effect on the stomach of both animals and humans.[68,69] A case-control study in peptic ulcer patients revealed that chilli intake prior to development of the ulcer was an apparent protective factor.[70] It was speculated that capsaicin present in chilli stimulated capsaicin receptors in the gastric mucosa and increased mucosal blood flow. Chilli also has been shown to delay gastric emptying.[71]

15.3.3.2 Gallstones

Prevalence of gallstone disease increases with age, although only a small proportion of patients may become symptomatic. The most important factor determining formation of cholesterol gallstones is the composition of bile with regard to cholesterol, bile salts, and lecithin. In a few predisposed populations, such as Pima Indians, inborn metabolic factors determine the composition of bile and lead to a very high prevalence of gallstones. In most other populations, dietary factors are thought to be the primary determinant of bile composition and gallstone disease.

A number of epidemiologic studies have examined the role of diet as a potential risk factor for gallstone formation. As with all studies that aim to determine the relationship between dietary factors and chronic gastrointestinal disease, there are potential pitfalls in these. Where only symptomatic gallstone disease was studied, it is difficult to ascertain whether changes in diet predated the development of gallstones or were secondary to symptoms of gallstone disease. Secondly, gallstone disease probably resulted from longstanding dietary habits that were prevalent at a younger age in the individual, and current dietary patterns that were identified may not have had any relationship to the previous diet. In a study from the U.K. of women 40–69 years of age, gallstones were found to be twice as prevalent in nonvegetarians (25%) as in vegetarians (12%).[72] The same investigators later confirmed a consistent negative association of vegetarianism with risk of gallstones.[73] Dietary fiber intake in the vegetarian group was much higher than in the nonvegetarian group. A negative association (with a Relative Risk of 0.4) was reported between the frequent intake of green beans (8 days per month) and gallstones.[74] This may have reflected the fiber content of green beans (from the pods). The investigators hypothesized that saponins from the seeds may have had effects on lipoprotein metabolism.

In a recent population-based case-control study, dietary intake of refined sugars and saturated fat were found to be associated with increased risk of gallstones, while consumption of monounsaturated fat and dietary fiber from cellulose were found to be protective.[75] In experimental animals, psyllium, a dietary fiber, was shown to increase fecal excretion of bile acids fourfold, and to decrease the lithogenic index of bile.[76] Gallstones and abnormal bile saturation indices have been related to low stool weight and slow intestinal transit, indicating a lack of dietary fiber.[77,78] The anti-lithogenic effect of fiber may primarily result from reduced deoxycholic acid absorption from the colon.[79]

It has been suggested that the risk of developing gallstones may be reduced by three factors — avoiding obesity that causes excessive cholesterol biosynthesis; a high-calcium, high-fiber diet to decrease deoxycholic acid input from the colon; and decreased intake of saturated fatty acids.[80] The net effect of these would be to avoid supersaturated bile, and reduce gallstone formation. These recommendations have only a speculative basis, and would need to be implemented from an early age to avoid the risk of gallstone disease.

15.3.3.3 Gastrointestinal Cancer

Cancer is primarily a disease of the elderly. Dietary factors are thought to play a considerable role in determining the risk of gastrointestinal cancer. Gastric cancer and colorectal cancer both involve a multistep origin, while the pathogenesis of other gastrointestinal cancers remains unclear. A strong and consistent inverse relationship has been found between the occurrence of gastrointestinal cancer and the ingestion of vegetables and fruits.[81-83] The sum of the evidence from a number of case control studies suggests that both fruits and vegetables are protective against a number of gastrointestinal cancers.

Some studies have shown a stronger protective effect for fruits against upper digestive tract cancers including oral cavity, pharynx, esophagus, and stomach, while vegetables had a greater protective effect against intestinal and colorectal cancer. Because of the tremendous variation in the types and amounts of fruit and vegetable consumed, and in the manner in which these have been quantitated, it is not easily possible to synthesize results from different studies to obtain a clear picture of the protective associations. Protective associations have been described for allium vegetables (onions, garlic, shallots, and chives), tomatoes, dark green vegetables, cruciferous vegetables (cabbage, cauliflower, broccoli, Brussels sprouts), citrus fruits, and yellow fruits against gastrointestinal cancers. Such associations do not necessarily hold across different population groups. The relationship between fruit and vegetable intake and cancer is dealt with in detail in other chapters in this book, and the following paragraphs will only briefly outline the association with cancer of the gastrointestinal tract.

Frequent consumption of vegetables, citrus fruit, fish, and vegetable oil appear to protect against cancers of the oral cavity and pharynx.[84] Several studies have reported protective effects of fruit and vegetable consumption against esophageal cancer.[85-88] Gastric cancer is the result of a complex multistep process, in which atrophic gastritis induced by *Helicobacter pylori* is thought to play an important part. In Western populations, carcinoma of the distal stomach (linked epidemiologically to *H. pylori*) has declined, and this is explained on the basis of domestic refrigeration and the increased availability of fresh fruit and vegetables.[89] Intake of fruit, particularly citrus fruit, was found to be protective against stomach cancer in a number of studies.[87,90-92] The effect of fruits and vegetables may reflect an antioxidant function, since depletion of mucosal antioxidants may be important in pathogenesis of gastric cancer.[93] Data from case control studies of intestinal cancer suggest that vegetable and fruit ingestion protect (the former twice as much as the latter) against the development of small intestinal adenocarcinoma.[94] Consumption of fruits and vegetables was also reported to have a protective effect against pancreatic cancer.[95,96]

Colon cancer is primarily a disease of the elderly, with a median age at diagnosis of about 70 years. Incidence of this cancer is particularly high (25 to 35 per 100,000) in the Western world. A number of studies have shown that intake of fruit and vegetables is protective against colon cancer, the relative risks varying between 0.07 to 0.6.[97-102] The association is stronger for vegetables than for fruits. A recent analysis showed that only current intake of vegetables was protective, and that intake of vegetables early in life seemed to offer no protection.[103] On the other hand, calorie restriction in early life provided protection against colorectal cancer. Fiber intake appears to best indicate that part of plant food consumption that is relevant to lowered risk.[102] However, one recent study suggested that fiber had no important protective association against colon cancer.[104]

Fiber has a multitude of effects, most prominent of which is fermentation in the colon to short-chain fatty acids. These have effects on colonic cell differentiation, and also reduce luminal pH, a factor associated with reduced risk for colon cancer. High fiber is associated with faster colonic transit, reducing exposure to potentially carcinogenic substances. Fiber facilitates a higher excretion of primary bile acids, with lower levels of tumor-promoting secondary bile acids. There is a decrease in production of mutagens in the stool. In addition to fiber, lignans (phytoestrogens) found in vegetables and fruits can potentially be converted to mammalian lignans by colonic bacteria. Urinary phytoestrogen excretion was highest in vegetarians, especially subjects consuming carotenoid and cruciferous vegetable diets.[105] The affinity of these molecules for estrogen receptors may partly underlie the protective effect of vegetable and fruit intake on colon cancer, in which estrogen receptors may be important.

15.3.3.4 Constipation

Constipation is common in the aging population, affecting approximately a quarter of free-living individuals over the age of sixty, and leading to considerable use of over-the-counter laxatives.[106] Constipation of short duration is usually due to pathology in the colon, including colon cancer. Chronic constipation occurs in hypothyroidism and with many drugs, including narcotic analgesics, and in those with neurological disease. Chronic idiopathic constipation, common in the elderly, is usually due to multiple factors, being related to low dietary fiber ingestion and debility. In such individuals, factors that have been found to correlate with constipation include inactivity, little leisure exercise, and poor food intake. Disease and confinement to bed worsens constipation in these individuals.[107,108]

Constipation is rare in populations consuming vegetarian diets high in dietary fiber. In a study from Singapore, for instance, constipation was reported by only 11% of elderly individuals, and was often associated with multiple illnesses and the use of medication for these.[109] Dietary factors that correlated with constipation included reduced intake of rice, fruit, and vegetables and increased intake of Chinese tea. Constipation in the elderly is associated particularly with distal colon dysfunction with or without associated anorectal dysfunction.[110] Transit within the colon accounts for the bulk of total intestinal transit time, which in turn correlates inversely with fecal weight. Bulk within the colon stimulates motor activity; in general, the greater the bulk the more rapid the transit.[34] In a meta-analysis of 11 studies, fecal weight was shown to correlate very well ($r = 0.84$) with the intake of dietary fiber (nonstarch polysaccharides).[111] On the basis of the regression line obtained, it was calculated that fecal weight would be in the range of 38 g/day on a diet free of nonstarch polysaccharides, while a fiber intake of 12.5 g/day would give fecal weight of 104 g/day.

Addition of plant fiber to the diet (in the region of 25 to 30 g/day) significantly relieves symptoms of constipation.[112-114] Adequate water intake is essential during dietary fiber supplementation.[114] In a study specifically of elderly constipated persons, oligosaccharides clinically improved the bowel habit, although fecal weight was not measured in these individuals.[115] Increased intake of fruit and vegetables, in addition to legumes and whole wheat bread, is commonly recommended in the constipated elderly individual. In healthy volunteers, administration of 20 g/day of fiber from different vegetable and fruit sources showed that fecal weight increased most with cabbage (69%), followed by carrot (59%), apple (40%), and guar gum (20%), while bran provided the least increase (12%).[116] A significant inter-individual variation was noted in the colonic response to various fiber sources. Addition of fiber shortened mean transit time through the gut.

Chronic anal fissures are associated with constipation, and may be common in the elderly. It has been shown that recurrent anal fissures can be partly avoided by increased consumption of dietary fiber and fluids.[117] A significant negative association was detected between consumption of raw fruits and vegetables and occurrence of anal fissure.[118]

15.3.3.5 Diverticular Disease

Diverticulosis of the colon is common in Western populations. While rare in the young, the prevalence increases with age to reach 50 to 75% in those over 80.[119,120] On the basis of geographic correlations and time trends, it was suggested that this condition may be caused by an inadequate intake of dietary fiber, leading to decreased fecal bulk and increased intraluminal pressure in the sigmoid colon.[121] A number of studies supported the association of low fiber intake with colonic diverticulosis. Crude fiber intake in the diet, and fecal excretion of beta-sitosterol (an unabsorbed plant sterol used as a marker of dietary fiber) were low in patients with diverticulosis.[119,122] Epidemiologic observations suggest that prevalence of diverticulosis increased in Japanese and African populations at the same time as their diet became more Westernized and deficient in fiber.[123,124] A study from Hong Kong showed a high prevalence of diverticular disease in individuals aged 50–79, while older adults had less diverticular disease.[125] Although hospital-based, the latter finding was cited as evidence for a recent increase in the prevalence of diverticular disease, possibly related to changes in dietary habits to a more Western-style diet.

Vegetarians in the U.K. with a higher dietary intake of fiber (41.5 g/day) than nonvegetarians (21.4 g/day) had less than half the expected prevalence of asymptomatic diverticulosis (12% compared to 33%).[120] A case control study in Greece demonstrated a very significant negative association between consumption of vegetables and the risk of diverticular disease, while meat consumption showed a very significant positive association.[126] In this study, the relative risk of developing diverticulosis was 50-fold less in those people frequently consuming vegetables but rarely consuming meat compared to people frequently consuming meat but rarely consuming vegetables. All the above observations refer only to the preventive effect of diet and fiber on the development of colonic diverticulosis. Fecal bulking is also used as therapy in symptomatic diverticular disease, but its effect remains controversial.[127-129]

Unraveling the nature of the protective effect of fiber on development of colonic diverticulae was facilitated by the development of an animal model. Rats that were fed less dietary fiber developed more diverticulae in the colon.[130] Recently, it was shown that rats fed a fiber-deficient diet had abnormalities in the colonic collagen, with increased cross-linking of collagen.[131] This correlated with the presence of diverticulae in fiber-deficient rats. Since the only dietary manipulation involved the amount of fiber contained in the feed, it may be presumed that some attribute of fiber (nonstarch polysaccharide) was important in determining development of colonic diverticulae. Fiber administration increased fecal weights and fecal short-chain fatty acids, and native collagen was preserved. These investigators also showed that fiber deficiency in the mother accentuated the collagen abnormality and the development of diverticulae in offspring when they were fed fiber-deficient diets.[132] These studies provide experimental evidence for the use of dietary fiber in prevention of colonic diverticulosis.

15.3.3.6 Inflammatory Bowel Disease

The incidence of inflammatory bowel disease in the elderly has increased over the last three decades.[133] The majority of epidemiological studies show a bimodal peak of distribution of both Crohn's disease and ulcerative colitis, with the second mode usually near age 70.[133] The etiology of inflammatory bowel disease remains unknown, but clearly there are predisposing genetic factors. In addition, dietary or infective agents are thought to provide an antigenic stimulus for the development of Crohn's disease in susceptible individuals. Increased intestinal and colonic permeability is noted in Crohn's disease, both in diseased individuals and in their asymptomatic relatives.[134] Luminal nutritive factors (glutamine in the small intestine and short-chain fatty acids in the large intestine) decrease mucosal permeability, and may be of relevance to protection from development of clinical disease. In the case of ulcerative colitis, metabolic abnormalities in colonic epithelial cells, as well as increased mucosal permeability, may perpetuate mucosal inflammation.[135] Both these attributes are beneficially affected by luminal short-chain fatty acids in the colon. Since the colonic epithelium obtains over 70% of its energy requirement from short-chain fatty acids, it has been suggested that the defect in epithelial metabolism may be overcome by providing luminal nutrition. This has been successfully accomplished by the use of short chain fatty acids as enemas in the treatment of distal ulcerative colitis.[136] An alternative way of increasing colonic short-chain fatty acids would be to provide more fiber that could be fermented in the colon. Another consideration in inflammatory bowel disease is that oxidative damage mediates inflammation. In ulcerative colitis, vitamin A and cysteine levels decreased during active inflammation, returning to normal when inflammation was controlled.[137] It is not known whether augmentation of vitamin A and cysteine will prevent or alter the course of an acute attack of ulcerative colitis. It is tempting to speculate that the increased incidence of inflammatory bowel disease in the elderly is related to changes in nutrition (specifically intestinal mucosal nutrition, which is dependent on luminal nutrients) and immunity in these individuals. One study detected significantly less fruit and vegetable intake among patients with ulcerative colitis, but it is not clear that this was not an effect of the disease.[138]

15.3.3.7 Diarrheal Disease

Diarrheal illness is common in the elderly and carries a high risk of morbidity and mortality.[139] Outbreaks of viral diarrhea are especially common in geriatric care facilities. It is important to maintain hydration during diarrhea, to prevent complications related to ischemia of the brain or heart. In addition to oral hydration, the provision of fermentable substrate in the colon helps the colon to conserve water during diarrhea, reducing fecal fluid loss and shortening illness. Short-chain fatty acids produced by bacterial fermentation of carbohydrate increase absorption of sodium and water from the colon, both in the basal state and even during secretion induced by diarrheal disease.[140] Thus, provision of fermentable fiber from fruit and vegetables may help in recovery from a diarrheal illness. Easily fermentable carbohydrates are now used as prebiotics, to favorably alter the colonic bacterial flora,[38] one application being to prevent attacks of diarrhea. In the elderly there is reduction of fecal bifidobacteria, and it has been suggested that this may account for the increased fatality rate in the elderly during epidemics of diarrhea.[38] Restoration of fecal bifidobacteria and normalization of the colonic flora by providing carbohydrate may be expected to have a preventive effect, although this remains to be tested.

15.4 CONCLUSIONS

This chapter reviews the relationship between the intake of vegetables and fruits and the health and nutrition of the gastrointestinal tract in the elderly. Constituents of fruits and vegetables have significant beneficial effects on the nutrition and health of the gastrointestinal tract and, beyond this, exert preventive effects against gastrointestinal disease in the elderly. Potential mechanisms of action of these dietary constituents and the associations with specific gastrointestinal problems have been reviewed. It is likely that protective associations detected in various kinds of epidemiological studies are the result of synchronous action of a number of the constituents of fruit and vegetables. In most instances, a common single factor or mechanism does not appear to completely explain the observed protective effect. In fact, use of a single agent in prevention may have unexpected effects, as was shown by the finding that supplementation with beta-carotene for lung cancer prevention had a deleterious effect on smokers in three out of four supplementation studies.[141] It is expected that following the current recommendations to include adequate quantities of a variety of vegetables and fruits in the diet[142] will preserve many aspects of gastrointestinal function and provide an optimal level of protection against a number of gastrointestinal diseases in the elderly.

REFERENCES

1. Chandra, R.K., Nutritional regulation of immunity and risk of infection in old age. *Immunology,* 67: 141, 1989.
2. Samal, S.C. and Ramakrishna, B.S., Gastrointestinal problems in the elderly. *Indian J. Med. Res.,* 106: 295, 1997.
3. Saltzman, J.R. and Russell, R.M., The aging gut: Nutritional issues. *Gastroenterol. Clin. North Am.,* 27: 309, 1998.
4. Hurwitz, A., Brady, D.A., Schaal, S.E., Samloff, I.M., Dedon, J., and Ruhl, C.E., Gastric acidity in older adults. *J. Am. Med. Assoc.,* 278: 659, 1997.
5. Carrere, J., Serre, G., Vincent, C., Croute, F., Soleilhavoup, J.P., Thouvenot, J.P., and Figarella, C., Human serum pancreatic lipase and trypsin I in ageing: Enzymatic and immunoenzymatic assays. *J. Gerontol.,* 42: 315, 1987.
6. Einarsson, K., Nilsell, K., Leijd, B., and Angelin, B., Influence of age on secretion of cholesterol and synthesis of bile acids by the liver. *N. Engl. J. Med.,* 313: 277, 1982.
7. Goidl, E.A., *Ageing and Immune Responses: Cellular and Humoral Aspects.* New York: Marcel Dekker, 1987.

8. Arranz, E., O'Mahony, S., Barton, J.R., and Ferguson, A., Immunosenescence and mucosal immunity: Significance of effects of old age on secretory IgA concentrations and intraepithelial lymphocyte counts. *Gut,* 33: 882, 1992.
9. Haboubi, N.Y. and Montgomery, R.D., Small bowel bacterial overgrowth in elderly people: Clinical significance and response to treatment. *Age Ageing,* 21: 13, 1992.
10. Chandra, R.K., Imbach, A., Moore, C., Skelton, D., and Woolcott, D., Nutrition of the elderly. *Can. Med. Assoc. J.,* 145: 1475, 1991.
11. Ahmed, F.E., Effect of nutrition on the health of the elderly. *J. Am. Diet. Assoc.,* 92: 1102, 1992.
12. Buttriss, J., Nutrition in older people — the findings of a national survey. *J. Hum. Nutr. Dietet.,* 12: 461, 1999.
13. Scythes, C.A., Zimmerman, S.A., Pennell, M.D., and Yeung, D.L., Nutrient intakes of a group of independently living elderly individuals in Toronto. *J. Nutr. Elderly,* 8: 47, 1989.
14. Robeothan, B. and Chandra, R.K., Nutritional status of an elderly population. *Age,* 14: 39, 1991.
15. Bates, C.J., Prentice, A., Cole, T.J., van der Pols, J.C., Doyle, W., Finch, S., Smithers, G., and Clarke, P.C., Micronutrients: highlights and research challenges from the 1994-5 National Diet and Nutrition Survey of people aged 65 years and over. *Br. J. Nutr.,* 82: 7, 1999.
16. Cid-Rufaza, J., Caulfield, L.E., Barron, Y., and West, S.K., Nutrient intakes and adequacy among an older population on the eastern shore of Maryland: the Salisbury eye evaluation. *J. Am. Diet. Assoc.,* 99: 564, 1999.
17. Nieman, D.C., Underwood, B.C., Sherman, K.M., Arabatzis, K., Barbosa, J.C., Johnson, M., and Shultz, D., Dietary status of Seventh Day Adventist vegetarian and nonvegetarian elderly women. *J. Am. Diet. Assoc.,* 89: 1763, 1989.
18. Sandstead, H.H., Henriksen, L.K., Greger, J.L., Prasad, A.S., and Good, R.A., Zinc nutriture in the elderly in relation to taste acuity, immune response and wound healing. *Am. J. Clin. Nutr.,* 36: 10, 1982.
19. Watson, R.R., Prabhala, R.H., and Plezia, P.M., Beta-carotene on lymphocyte subpopulations in elderly humans: evidence for a dose-response relationship. *Am. J. Clin. Nutr.,* 53: 90, 1991.
20. Olson, J.A., Vitamin A, in *Handbook of Vitamins: Nutritional, Biochemical and Clinical Aspects*, L.J. Machlin, Ed., New York: Marcel Dekker, 1985, pp. 1-43.
21. Iber, F.L., Blass, J.P., Brin, M., and Leevy, C.M., Thiamin in the elderly: relation to alcoholism and to neurological degenerative disease. *Am. J. Clin. Nutr.,* 6: 1067, 1982.
22. Roe, D.A., Geriatric Nutrition, 3rd ed., Englewood Cliffs, NJ, Prentice-Hall. 1992.
23. Burkitt, D.P., Epidemiology of cancer of the colon and rectum. *Cancer,* 28: 3, 1971.
24. Burkitt, D.P., Walker, A.R.P., Painter, N.S., Effect of dietary fibre on stools and transit times, and its role in the causation of disease. *Lancet,* 2: 1402, 1972.
25. Cummings, J.H. and Englyst, H.N., Gastrointestinal effects of food carbohydrates. *Am. J. Clin. Nutr.,* 61: 938S, 1995.
26. Joint FAO/WHO Expert Consultation: Carbohydrates in human nutrition. Food and Agriculture Organization, FAO Food and Nutrition Paper 66, World Health Organization, Geneva, 1998.
27. Ramakrishna, B.S. and Roediger, W.E.W., Bacterial short-chain fatty acids: their role in gastrointestinal disease. *Dig. Dis.,* 8: 337, 1990.
28. Slavin, J.L., Dietary fiber classification, chemical analyses, and food sources. *J. Am. Diet. Assoc.,* 87: 1164, 1987.

29. Stephen, A.M. and Cummings, J.H., The microbial contribution to human faecal mass. *J. Med. Microbiol.,* 13: 45, 1980.
30. Chen, H.L., Haack, V.S., Janecky, C.W., Vollendorf, N.W., and Marlett, J.A., Mechanisms by which wheat bran and oat bran increase stool weight in humans. *Am. J. Clin. Nutr.,* 68: 711, 1998.
31. Brown I., Complex carbohydrates and resistant starch. *Nutr. Rev.,* 54: S115, 1996.
32. Gibson, G.R., Dietary modulation of the human gut microflora using the prebiotics oligofructose and inulin. *J. Nutr.,* 129: 1438S, 1999.
33. Moshfegh, A.J., Friday, J.E., Goldman, J.P., and Ahuja, J.K.C., Presence of inulin and oligofructose in the diets of Americans. *J. Nutr.,* 129: 1407S, 1999.
34. Salminen, S., Bouley, C., Boutron-Ruault, M.C., Cummings, J.H., Franck, A., Gibson, G.R., Isolauri, E., Moreau, M.C., Roberfroid, M., and Rowland, I., Functional food science and gastrointestinal physiology and function. *Br. J. Nutr.,* 80: S147, 1998.
35. Rothstein, R.D. and Rombeau, J.L., Nutrient pharmacotherapy for gut mucosal diseases. *Gastroenterol. Clin. North Am.,* 27: 387, 1998.
36. McCord, J.M., Radical explanations for old observations. *Gastroenterology,* 92: 2026, 1987.
37. Bulger, E.M. and Helton, W.S., Nutrient antioxidants in gastrointestinal diseases. *Gastroenterol. Clin. North Am.,* 27: 403, 1998.
38. Diplock, A.T., Charleux, J.L., Crozier-Willi, G., Kok, F.J., Rice-Evans, C., Roberfroid, M., Stahl, W., and Vina-Ribes, J., Functional food science and defence against reactive oxidative species. *Br. J. Nutr.,* 80: S77, 1998.
39. Allard, J.P., Royall, D., Kurian, R., Muggli, R., and Jeejeebhoy, K.N., Effects of B-carotene supplementation on lipid peroxidation in humans. *Am. J. Clin. Nutr.,* 59: 884, 1994.
40. Vasankari, T.J., Kujala, U.M., Vasankari, T.M., Vuorimaa, T., and Ahotupa, M., Increased serum and low-density lipoprotein antioxidant potential after antioxidant supplementation in endurance athletes. *Am. J. Clin. Nutr.,* 65: 1052, 1997.
41. Lampe, J.W., Health effects of vegetables and fruit: assessing mechanisms of action in human experimental studies. *Am. J. Clin. Nutr.,* 70: 475S, 1999.
42. Young, J.F., Nielsen, S.E., Haraldsdottir, J., Daneshvar, B., Lauridsen, S.T., Knuthsen, P., Crozier, A., Sandstrom, B., and Dragsted, L.O., Effect of fruit juice intake on urinary quercetin excretion and biomarkers of antioxidative status. *Am. J. Clin. Nutr.,* 69: 87, 1999.
43. Hertog, M.G.L., Hollman, P.C.H., and van de Putte, B., Content of potentially anticarcinogenic flavonoids in tea infusions, wines and fruit juices. *J. Agric. Food Chem.,* 41: 1242, 1993.
44. Krishnaswamy, K. and Raghuramulu, N., Bioactive phytochemicals with emphasis on dietary practices. *Indian J. Med. Res.,* 108: 167, 1998.
45. Weisburger, J.H., Evaluation of the evidence on the role of tomato product in disease prevention. *Proc. Soc. Exp. Biol. Med.,* 218: 140, 1998.
46. Wargovich, M.J., Uda, N., Woods, C., Velasco, M., and McKee, K., Allium vegetables: their role in the prevention of cancer. *Biochem. Soc. Trans.,* 24: 811, 1996.
47. Tham, D.M., Gardner, G.D., and Haskell, W.L., Potential health benefits of dietary phytoestrogens: a review of the clinical, epidemiological and mechanistic evidence. *J. Clin. Endocrinol. Metab.,* 83: 2223, 1998.
48. Bernersen, B., Johnsen, R., and Straume, B., Non-ulcer dyspepsia and peptic ulcer: the distribution in a population and their relation to risk factors. *Gut,* 38: 822, 1996.
49. Somerville, K., Faulkner, G., and Langman, M., Non-steroidal anti-inflammatory drugs and bleeding peptic ulcer. *Lancet,* 1: 462, 1986.

50. Langman, M.J.S., Epidemiologic evidence on the association between peptic ulceration and antiinflammatory drug use. *Gastroenterology,* 96: 640, 1989.
51. Kurata, J.H., Nogawa, A.N., Abbey, D.E., and Petersen, F., A prospective study of risk for peptic ulcer disease in Seventh-Day Adventists. *Gastroenterology,* 102: 902, 1992.
52. Aldoori, W.H., Giovannucci, E.L., Stampfer, M.J., Rimm, E.B., Wing, A.L., and Willett, W.C., Prospective study of diet and the risk of duodenal ulcer in men. *Am. J. Epidemiol.,* 145: 42, 1997.
53. Kato, I., Nomura, A.M.Y., Stemmermann, G.N., and Chyou, P.H., A prospective study of gastric and duodenal ulcer and its relation to smoking, alcohol and diet. *Am. J. Epidemiol.,* 135: 521, 1992.
54. La Vecchia, C., Decarli, A., and Pagano, R., Vegetable consumption and risk of chronic disease. *Epidemiology,* 9: 208, 1998.
55. Katschinski, B.D., Logan, R.F., Edmond, M., and Langman, M.J., Duodenal ulcer and refined carbohydrate intake: a case-control study assessing dietary fibre and refined sugar intake. *Gut,* 31: 993, 1990.
56. Rydning, A., Weberg, R., Lange, O., and Berstad, A., Healing of benign gastric ulcer with low-dose antacids and fiber diet. *Gastroenterology,* 91: 56, 1986.
57. Rydning, A., Berstad, A., Aadland, E., and Odegaard, B., Prophylactic effect of dietary fibre in duodenal ulcer disease. *Lancet,* 2: 736, 1982.
58. Rydning, A., Børkje, B., Lange, O., Aadland, E., Bell, H., Odegaard, B., Myklestad, B., and Hansen, T., Effect of wheat fibre supplements on duodenal ulcer recurrence. *Scand. J. Gastroenterol.,* 28: 1051, 1993.
59. Schwartz, S.E., Levine, R.A., Singh, A., Scheidecker, J.R., and Track, N.S., Sustained pectin ingestion delays gastric emptying. *Gastroenterology,* 83: 812, 1982.
60. Lin, H.C., Moller, N.A., Wolinsky, M.M., Kim, B.H., Doty, J.E., and Meyer, J.H., Sustained slowing effect of lentils on gastric emptying of solids in humans and dogs. *Gastroenterology,* 102: 787, 1992.
61. Lin, H.C., Zhao, X.T., Chu, A.W., Lin, Y.P., and Wang, L., Fiber-supplemented enteral formula slows intestinal transit by intensifying inhibitory feedback from the distal gut. *Am, J. Clin. Nutr.,* 65: 1840, 1997.
62. Hollander, D. and Tarnawski, A., Dietary fatty acids and the decline in peptic ulcer disease — a hypothesis. *Gut,* 27: 239, 1986.
63. Kearney, J., Kennedy, N.P., Keeling, P.W., Keating, J.J., Grubb, L., Kennedy M., Gibney, M.J., Dietary intakes and adipose tissue levels of linoleic acid in peptic ulcer disease. *Br. J. Nutr.,* 62: 699, 1989.
64. Mahmood, T., Tenenbaum, S., Niu, X.T., Levenson, S.M., Seifter, E., and Demetriou, A.A., Prevention of duodenal ulcer formation in the rat by dietary vitamin A supplementation. *J. Parenteral Enteral Nutr.,* 10: 74, 1986.
65. Jayaraj, A.P., Tovey, F.I., and Clark, C.G., The possibility of dietary protective factors in duodenal ulcer. II. An investigation into the effect of pre-feeding with different diets and of instillation of foodstuffs into the stomach on the incidence of ulcers in pylorus-ligated rats. *Postgrad. Med. J.,* 52: 640, 1976.
66. Goel, R.K., Gupta, S., Shankar, R., and Sanyal, A.K., Anti-ulcerogenic effect of banana powder (Musa sapientum var. paradisiaca) and its effect on mucosal resistance. *J. Ethnopharmacol.,* 18: 33, 1986.
67. Goel, R.K., Tavares, I.A., and Bennett, A., Stimulation of gastric and colonic mucosal eicosanoid synthesis by plantain banana. *J. Pharm. Pharmacol.,* 41: 747, 1989.
68. Kang, J.Y., Teng, C.H., Wee, A., and Chen, F.C., Effect of capsaicin and chilli on ethanol induced gastric mucosal injury in the rat. *Gut,* 36: 664, 1995.

69. Yeoh, K.G., Kang, J.Y., Yap, I., Guan, R., Tan, C.C., Wee, A., and Teng, C.H., Chili protects against aspirin-induced gastroduodenal mucosal injury in humans. *Dig. Dis. Sci.,* 40: 580, 1995.
70. Kang, J.Y., Yeoh, K.G., Chia, H.P., Lee, H.P., Chia, Y.W., Guan, R., and Yap, I., Chili — protective factor against peptic ulcer? *Dig. Dis. Sci.,* 40: 576, 1995.
71. Horowitz, M., Wishart, J., Maddox, A., and Russo, A., The effect of chilli on gastrointestinal transit. *J. Gastroenterol Hepatol.,* 7: 52, 1992.
72. Pixley, F., Wilson, D., McPherson, K., and Mann J., Effect of vegetarianism on development of gallstones in women. *Br. Med. J.,* 2: 11, 1985.
73. Pixley, F. and Mann, J., Dietary factors in the aetiology of gallstones: a case-control study. *Gut,* 29: 1511, 1988.
74. Thijs, C. and Knipschild, P., Legume intake and gallstone risk: results from a case-control study. *Int. J. Epidemiol.,* 19: 660, 1990.
75. Misciagna, G., Centonze, S., Leoci, C., Guerra, V., Cisternino, A.M., Ceo, R., and Trevisan, M., Diet, physical activity, and gallstones — a population-based, case-control study in southern Italy. *Am. J. Clin. Nutr.,* 69: 120, 1999.
76. Trautwein, E.A., Siddiqui, A., and Hayes, K.C., Modeling plasma lipoprotein-bile lipid relationships: differential impact of psyllium and cholestyramine in hamsters fed a lithogenic diet. *Metabolism*, 42: 1531, 1993.
77. Marcus, S.N. and Heaton, K.W., Intestinal transit, deoxycholic acid and the cholesterol saturation of bile — three inter-related factors. *Gut,* 27: 550, 1986.
78. Brydon, W.G., Eastwood, M.A., and Elton, R.A., The relationship between stool weight and the lithocholate/deoxycholate ratio in faeces. *Br. J. Cancer,* 57: 635, 1988.
79. Marcus, S.N. and Heaton, K.W., Deoxycholic acid and the pathogenesis of gallstones. *Gut,* 29: 522, 1988.
80. Hofmann, A.F., Primary and secondary prevention of gallstone disease: implications for patient management and research priorities. *Am. J. Surg.,* 165: 541, 1993.
81. Steinmetz, K.A. and Potter, J.D., Vegetables, fruit, and cancer prevention: a review. *J. Am. Diet. Assoc.,* 96: 1027, 1996.
82. La Vecchia, C. and Tavani, A., Fruits and vegetables and human cancer. *Eur. J. Cancer Prev.,* 7: 3, 1998.
83. Hensrud, D.D. and Heimburger, D.C., Diet, nutrients and gastrointestinal cancer. *Gastroenterol. Clin. North Am.,* 27: 325, 1998.
84. Franceschi, S., Favero, A., Conti, E., Talamini, R., Volpe, R., Negri, E., Barzan, L., and La Vecchia, C., Food groups, oil, butter, and cancer of the oral cavity and pharynx. *Br. J. Cancer,* 80: 614, 1999.
85. Brown, L.M., Swanson, C.A., Gridley, G., Swanson, G.M., Silverman, D.T., Greenberg, R.S., Hayes, R.B., Schoenberg, J.B., Pottern, L.M., Schwartz, A.G., Liff, J.M., Hoover, R., and Fraumeni, J.F., Dietary factors and the risk of squamous cell esophageal cancer among black and white men in the United States. *Cancer Causes Control,* 9: 467, 1998.
86. Yokokawa, Y., Ohta, S., Hou, J., Zhang, X.L., Li, S.S., Ping, Y.M., and Nakajima, T., Ecological study on the risks of esophageal cancer in Ci-Xian, China: The importance of nutritional status and the use of well water. *Int. J. Cancer,* 83: 620, 1999.
87. Gao, C.M., Takezaki, T., Ding, J.H., Li, M.S., and Tajima, K., Protective effect of allium vegetables against both esophageal and stomach cancer: a simultaneous case-referent study of a high-epidemic area in Jiangsu Province, China. *Jpn. J. Cancer Res.,* 90: 614, 1999.
88. De Stefani, E., Deneo-Pellegrini, H., Mendilaharsu, M., and Ronco, A., Diet and risk of cancer of the upper aerodigestive tract — I. Foods. *Oral Oncol.,* 35: 17, 1999.

89. Palli, D., Gastric cancer and Helicobacter pylori: a critical evaluation of the epidemiological evidence. *Helicobacter,* 2(Suppl. 1) S50, 1997.
90. Terry, P., Nyren, O., and Yuen, J., Protective effect of fruits and vegetables on stomach cancer in a cohort of Swedish twins. *Int. J. Cancer,* 76: 35, 1998.
91. Jansen, M.C., Bueno-de-Mesquita, H.B., Rasanen, L., Fidanza, F., Menotti, A., Nissinen, A., Feskens, E.J., Kok, F.J., and Kromhout, D., Consumption of plant foods and stomach cancer mortality in the seven countries study. Is grain consumption a risk factor? Seven Countries Study Research Group. *Nutr. Cancer,* 34: 49, 1999.
92. Ward, M.H. and Lopez-Carrillo, L., Dietary factors and the risk of gastric cancer in Mexico City. *Am. J. Epidemiol.,* 149: 925, 1999.
93. Eapen, C.E., Madesh, M., Balasubramanian, K.A., Pulimood, A., Mathan, M., and Ramakrishna, B.S., Mucosal mitochondrial function and antioxidant defences in patients with gastric carcinoma. *Scand. J. Gastroenterol.,* 33: 975, 1998.
94. Negri, E., Bosetti, C., La Vecchia, C., Fioretti, F., Conti, E., and Franceschi, S., Risk factors for adenocarcinoma of the small intestine. *Int. J. Cancer,* 82: 171, 1999.
95. Gold, E.B. and Goldin, S.B., Epidemiology of and risk factors for pancreatic cancer. *Surg. Oncol. Clin. North Am.,* 7: 67, 1998.
96. Mori, M., Hariharan, M., Anandakumar, M., Tsutsumi, M., Ishikawa, O., Konishi, Y., Chellam, V.G., John, M., Praseeda, I., Priya, R., and Narendranathan, M., A case-control study on risk factors for pancreatic diseases in Kerala, India. *Hepatogastroenterology,* 46: 25, 1999.
97. Trock, B., Lanza, E., and Greenwald, P., Dietary fiber, vegetables, and colon cancer: critical review and meta-analyses of the epidemiologic evidence. *J. Natl. Cancer Inst.,* 82: 650, 1990.
98. Steinmetz, K.A. and Potter, J.D., Food-group consumption and colon cancer in the Adelaide Case-Control Study. I.Vegetables and fruit. *Int. J. Cancer,* 53: 711, 1993.
99. Slattery, M.L., Potter, J.D., Coates, A., Ma, K.N., Berry, T.D., Duncan, D.M., and Caan, B.J., Plant foods and colon cancer: an assessment of specific foods and their related nutrients (United States). *Cancer Causes Control,* 8: 575, 1997.
100. Slattery, M.L., Berry, T.D., Potter, J., and Caan, B., Diet diversity, diet composition, and risk of colon cancer (United States). *Cancer Causes Control,* 8: 872, 1997.
101. Franceschi, S., Parpinel, M., La Vecchia, C., Favero, A., Talamini, R., and Negri, E., Role of different types of vegetables and fruit in the prevention of cancer of the colon, rectum, and breast. *Epidemiology,* 9: 338, 1998.
102. Jansen, M.C., Bueno-de-Mesquita, H.B., Buzina, R., Fidanza, F., Menotti, A., Blackburn, H., Nissinen, A.M., Kok, F.J., and Kromhout, D., Dietary fiber and plant foods in relation to colorectal cancer mortality: the Seven Countries Study. *Int. J. Cancer,* 81: 174, 1999.
103. Caygill, C.P., Charlett, A., and Hill, M.J., Relationship between the intake of high-fibre foods and energy and the risk of cancer of the large bowel and breast. *Eur. J. Cancer Prev.,* 7 (Suppl. 2): S11, 1998.
104. Fuchs, C.S., Giovannucci, E.L., Colditz, G.A., Hunter, D.J., Stampfer, M.J., Rosner, B., Speizer, F.E., and Willett, W.C., Dietary fiber and the risk of colorectal cancer and adenoma in women. *N. Engl. J. Med.,* 340: 169, 1999.
105. Adlercreutz, H., Fotsis, T., Heikkinen, R., Dwyer, J.T., Woods, M., Goldin, B.R., and Gorbach, S.L., Excretion of the lignans enterolactone and enterodiol and of equol in omnivorous and vegetarian postmenopausal women and in women with breast cancer. *Lancet,* 2: 1295, 1982.
106. Sandler, R.S., Jordan, M.C., and Shelton, B.J., Demographic and dietary determinants of constipation in the US population. *Am. J. Public Health,* 80: 185, 1990.

107. Kinnunen, O., Study of constipation in a geriatric hospital, day hospital, old people's home and at home. *Aging (Milano)* 3: 161, 1991.
108. Towers, A.L., Burgio, K.L., Locher, J.L., Merkel, I.S., Safaeian, M., and Wald, A., Constipation in the elderly: influence of dietary, psychological, and physiological factors. *J. Am. Geriatr. Soc.,* 42: 701, 1994.
109. Wong, M.L., Wee, S., Pin, C.H., Gan, G.L., and Ye, H.C., Sociodemographic and lifestyle factors associated with constipation in an elderly Asian community. *Am. J. Gastroenterol.,* 94: 1283, 1999.
110. Whitehead, W.E., Drinkwater, D., Cheskin, L.J., Heller, B.R., and Schuster, M.M., Constipation in the elderly living at home: Definition, prevalence and relationship to lifestyle and health status. *J. Am. Geriatr. Soc.,* 37: 423, 1989.
111. Cummings, J.H., Bingham, S.A., Heaton, K.W., and Eastwood, M.A., Fecal weight, colon cancer risk, and dietary intake of nonstarch polysaccharides (dietary fiber). *Gastroenterology,* 103: 1783, 1992.
112. Astrup, A., Vrist, E., and Quaade, F., Dietary fibre added to very low calorie diet reduces hunger and alleviates constipation. *Int. J. Obes.,* 14: 105, 1990.
113. Lambert, J.P., Brunt, P.W., Mowat, N.A., Khin, C.C., Lai, C.K., Morrison, V., Dickerson, J.W., and Eastwood, M.A., The value of prescribed 'high-fibre' diets for the treatment of the irritable bowel syndrome. *Eur. J. Clin. Nutr.,* 45: 601, 1991.
114. Anti, M., Pignataro, G., Armuzzi, A., Valenti, A., Iascone, E., Marmo, R., Lamazza, A., Pretaroli, A.R., Pace, V., Leo, P., Castelli, A., and Gasbarrini, G., Water supplementation enhances the effect of high-fiber diet on stool frequency and laxative consumption in adult patients with functional constipation. *Hepatogastroenterology,* 45: 727, 1998.
115. Kleessen, B., Sykura, B., Zunft, H.J., and Blaut, M., Effects of inulin and lactose on fecal microflora, microbial activity, and bowel habit in elderly constipated persons. *Am. J. Clin. Nutr.,* 65: 1397, 1997.
116. Cummings, J.H., Branch, W., Jenkins, D.J., Southgate, D.A., Houston, H., and James, W.P., Colonic response to dietary fibre from carrot, cabbage, apple, bran. *Lancet,* 1: 5, 1978.
117. Jensen, S.L., Maintenance therapy with unprocessed bran in the prevention of acute anal fissure recurrence. *J. R. Soc. Med.,* 80: 296, 1987.
118. Jensen, S.L., Diet and other risk factors for fissure-in-ano: prospective case control study. *Dis. Colon Rectum,* 31: 770, 1988.
119. Brodribb, A.J.M. and Humphreys, D.M., Diverticular disease: three studies. *Br. Med. J.,* 1: 424, 1976.
120. Gear, J.S., Ware, A., Fursdon, P., Mann, J., Nolan, D.J., Brodribb, A.J., and Vessey, M.P., Symptomless diverticular disease and intake of dietary fibre. *Lancet,* 1: 511, 1979.
121. Painter, N.S. and Burkitt, D.P., Diverticular disease of the colon: a deficiency disease of Western civilisation. *Br. Med. J.,* 2: 450, 1971.
122. Miettinen, T.A. and Tarpila, S., Fecal B-sitosterol in patients with diverticular disease of the colon and in vegetarians. *Scand. J. Gastroenterol.,* 13: 573, 1978.
123. Ohi, G., Minowa, K., Oyama, T., Naahashi, M., Yamazaki, N., Yamamoto, S., Nagasake, K., Hayakawa, K., Kimura, K., and Mori, B., Changes in dietary fiber intake among Japanese in the 20th century: a relationship to the prevalence of diverticular disease. *Am. J. Clin. Nutr.,* 38: 115, 1983.
124. Madiba, T.E. and Mokoena, T., Pattern of diverticular disease among Africans. *East Afr. Med. J.,* 71: 644, 1994.

125. Chan, C.C., Lo, K.K., Chung, E.C., Lo, S.S., and Hon, T.Y., Colonic diverticulosis in Hong Kong: distribution pattern and clinical significance. *Clin. Radiol.,* 53: 842, 1998.
126. Manousos, O., Day, N.E., Tzonou, A., Papadimitriou, C., Kapetanakis, A., Polychronopoulou-Trichopoulou, A., Trichopoulous, D., Diet and other factors in the aetiology of diverticulosis: an epidemiological study in Greece. *Gut,* 26: 544, 1985.
127. Brodribb, A.J.M., Treatment of symptomatic diverticular disease with a high fibre diet. *Lancet,* 1: 664, 1977.
128. Eastwood, M.A., Smith, A.N., Brydon, W.G., and Pritchard, J., Comparison of bran, ispaghula, and lactulose on colon function in diverticular disease. *Gut,* 19: 1144, 1978.
129. Ornstein, M.H., Littlewood, E.R., Baird, I.M., Fowler, J., North, W.R.S., and Cox, A.G., Are fibre supplements really necessary in diverticular disease of the colon? A controlled clinical trial. *Br. Med. J.,* 282: 1353, 1981.
130. Berry, C.S., Fearn, T., Fisher, N., Gregory, J.A., and Hardy, J., Dietary fibre and prevention of diverticular disease of colon: evidence from rats. *Lancet,* 2: 294, 1984.
131. Wess, L., Eastwood, M.A., Edwards, C.A., Busuttil, A., and Miller, A., Collagen alteration in an animal model of colonic diverticulosis. *Gut,* 38: 701, 1996.
132. Wess, L., Eastwood, M.A., Busuttil, A., Edwards, C.A., and Miller, A., An association between maternal diet and colonic diverticulosis in an animal model. *Gut,* 39: 423, 1996.
133. Grimm, I.S. and Friedman, L.S., Inflammatory bowel disease in the elderly. *Gastroenterol. Clin. North Am.,* 19: 361, 1990.
134. Unno, N. and Fink, M.P., Intestinal epithelial hyperpermeability: Mechanisms and relevance to disease. *Gastroenterol. Clin. North Am.,* 27: 289, 1998.
135. Gibson, P.R., Ulcerative colitis: An epithelial disease? *Bailliere's Clin. Gastroenterol.,* 11: 17, 1997.
136. Scheppach, W., Sommer, H., Kirchner, T., Paganelli, G.M., Bartram, P., Christl, S., Richter, F., Dusel, G., and Kasper, H., Effect of butyrate enemas on the colonic mucosa in distal ulcerative colitis. *Gastroenterology,* 103: 51, 1992.
137. Ramakrishna, B.S., Varghese, R., Jayakumar, S., Mathan, M., and Balasubramanian, K.A., Circulating antioxidants in ulcerative colitis and their relationship to disease severity and activity. *J. Gastroenterol. Hepatol.,* 12: 490, 1997.
138. Matthew, J.A., Fellows, I.W., Prior, A., Kennedy H.J., Bobbin, R., and Johnson, I.T., Habitual intake of fruits and vegetables amongst patients at increased risk of colorectal neoplasia. *Cancer Lett.,* 114: 255, 1997.
139. Ratnaike, R.N., Diarrhoea in the elderly: epidemiological and etiological factors. *J. Gastroenterol. Hepatol.,* 5: 449, 1990.
140. Krishnan, S., Ramakrishna, B.S., and Binder, H.J., Stimulation of sodium chloride absorption from secreting rat colon by short chain fatty acids. *Dig. Dis. Sci.,* 44: 1924, 1999.
141. Paiva, S.A. and Russell, R.M., Beta-carotene and other carotenoids as antioxidants. *J. Am. Coll. Nutr.,* 18: 426, 1999.
142. Russell, R.M., Rasmussen, H., and Lichtenstein, A.H., Modified food guide pyramid for people over seventy years of age. *J. Nutr.,* 129: 751, 1999.

16 The Health Benefits of Cranberries and Related Fruits

Martin Starr and Marge Leahy

CONTENTS

16.1 INTRODUCTION

Cranberries, a fruit native to New England, belong to the Vaccinium family, which also includes *V. oxycoccus* (European cranberry or mooseberry, English mossberry, bogberry) and *V. vitis-idaea* (preseiberry, whortleberry, lingonberry). These latter varieties are generally not accepted as being identical to the North American cranberry because of size and compositional differences. Other related fruits in the Vaccinium family include *V. myrtillus* (bilberry), *V. augustifolium* (lowbush blueberry), *and V. corymbosum* (highbush blueberry).

Cranberries and cranberry products have long been associated with a variety of health benefits.[1-3] It is one of the very few native American fruits; there are reports of its use by American Indians to dress wounds and prevent inflammation. Cranber-

0-8493-0038-X/97/$0.00+$.50

ries were later used aboard ship to help prevent scurvy, although their level of vitamin C is well below that of most citrus fruits. In the early 20th century, cranberries were thought to help relieve the symptoms of urinary tract infections, or perhaps even prevent their occurrence. Much anecdotal information was generated on this issue, and was responsible for the "medical mystique" that surrounded the fruit and its products through much of the century. It was only in the late 1980s that science began to uncover what much of the population had long suspected — consumption of cranberry juice could help maintain a healthy urinary tract.

As the century closed, more information was published in this connection, patents regarding its use were filed and issued, and cranberry dietary supplements were manufactured and purchased for this benefit. In addition, scientists began looking more closely at other phytochemicals within the fruit and their possible benefits in human nutrition, totally apart from the urinary tract health (UTH) effect. As with virtually all fruits and vegetables, cranberries appear to have a relatively unique menu of components that will prove to have interesting value in human nutrition, particularly regarding maintaining health and wellness.

Cranberries, and particularly cranberry juice products, are best known for their effect on helping maintain UTH. Because they contain approximately 2% acid, this effect was thought due to these compounds, and possibly the acidification of the urine or urinary tract in some manner. However, as described below, there are excellent data which document that the level of organic acids present is at most a minor factor, and that the primary mechanism is one of inhibiting the adhesion of disease–causing bacteria (primarily *E. coli*) to urinary tract cells by interfering with the bacterial adhesins used by the organisms. By inhibiting or even reversing the adhesion of these bacteria, infection and the accompanying symptoms are reduced. This mechanism of the inhibition of bacterial adhesion is particularly interesting as it (1) may have applications elsewhere in the body, and (2) may have implications as a drug adjunct, thereby reducing drug duration and use, with a possible long-term reduction in the development of antibiotic-resistant bacteria, a growing problem of global proportions. Since the natural cranberry components appear to cripple rather than kill the bacteria, the selective pressure to mutate is likely less powerful.

Cranberries also are being shown to contain other classes of compounds and associated phytochemicals that may offer still other beneficial effects on human health and wellness.

16.2 BACTERIAL ANTI-ADHESION

16.2.1 Urinary Tract Infections

Estimates vary, but urinary tract infections (UTIs) affect at least 10% of the female population in the U.S. in any given year. This, combined with a 25% rate of recurrence[4] account for over 8,000,000 visits to doctors' offices annually in the U.S. alone.[5] Although women are roughly seven times more likely than men to develop UTI, older men have a far higher infection rate than younger men. Sexual activity, safe or otherwise, has been shown to be a major risk factor for women. Symptoms of the disease include frequent and painful urination, burning, lower back pain, and extreme discomfort.[6]

It is likely that a primary source of the causative *E. coli* bacteria is the patient themselves, as this organism is normally associated with the GI tract, and urine is normally sterile. This may account for the high association of UTI with sexual activity, and the attendant increased likelihood of the bacteria gaining entrance to the female urinary tract. The extraordinarily high incidence of UTIs in catheterized patients[7] may also be due to contamination from GI bacteria. While antibiotics are normally quite effective in combating UTIs, they are not universally effective and may deliver unwelcome side effects. They are ineffective for some groups (e.g., catheterized patients due to the growth of antibiotic-resistant bacteria), and are undesirable in other groups (e.g., pregnant women concerned about antibiotic resistance in themselves and their fetuses).

16.2.1.1 Intervention Trials

Several intervention trials regarding cranberry juice and urinary tract health have been reported in the literature. Many of these suffer from major experimental design limitations, including lack of untreated controls, unblinded, no use of placebo, and a low number of subjects. Key studies are reviewed here. Most focused on cranberry juice or cranberry cocktail and one focused on solid dietary supplements.

The most robustly designed study (randomized, double-blinded placebo-controlled, using a population of 153 elderly women in a 6-month trial) was conducted by Avorn et al.[8] Their findings suggested that daily consumption of 300 ml of a low-calorie cranberry juice cocktail can reduce bacteriuria and pyuria by nearly 50% in this population, and that it is more effective in moving subjects out of an infected state.

Walker et al. conducted an intervention trial using solid cranberry dietary supplements.[9] The study was a randomized double-blinded placebo-controlled crossover study using a population of 19 sexually active women (mean age of 37). A statistically significant reduction in risk for urinary tract infections when taking the cranberry supplement was found with the 10 subjects who completed the study.

Four other studies on cranberry juice suffered from design limitations, yielding anecdotal findings supporting a beneficial effect of cranberry juice on UTH. In these cases, cranberry juice was found to be beneficial for UTH in a mixed-gender study with 60 adults,[10] a mixed gender nursing home study with 538 patients,[11] a case study of an elderly woman,[12] and a study of 16 children with neurogenic bladders.[13]

Two pilot trials found a lack of effect of cranberry juice or concentrate on the incidence of bacteriuria in children with neurogenic bladders.[14,15] The authors of one study speculated on the reasons for this lack of an effect. They noted that the voiding dysfunction inherent to the neurogenic bladder may have overridden any clinical effect in this population highly prone to UTIs, or that the volume of cranberry concentrate ingested may have been too low.

16.2.1.2 Epidemiological Studies

One relevant epidemiological study has been conducted that reported on the relationship between sexual and health behaviors of women and first-time urinary tract infections.[16] The study used a population of women enrolled in a university health service, with 86 subjects experiencing first-time UTIs and 288 control subjects. After adjusting for frequency of vaginal intercourse, regular drinking of cranberry juice was found to be protective against UTI.

16.2.1.3 Mechanistic Studies

The considerable body of mechanistic research is highly compelling in substantiating cranberry juice's beneficial effect on urinary tract health. Early research focused on the cranberry's effect on acidification of the urine as the possible mechanism for cranberry's antibacterial effect in the urinary tract,[17-21] but this theory was not substantiated by other research.[8,14,22,23] Bacterial adherence to mucosal surfaces is generally considered to be an important prerequisite for colonization and infection.[24] Avorn et al.[8] found no evidence to support urinary acidification to be responsible for the bacteriostatic effect of cranberry juice: the median pH of urine samples from the cranberry subjects (pH 6.0) was actually higher from that of the placebo group (pH 5.5). Current theory supports the hypothesis that cranberry juice acts to promote UTH by inhibiting bacterial adherence to mucosal surfaces.[8,25-33]

Results from mechanistic studies measuring inhibition of bacterial adherence conducted by several researchers have provided great insight into cranberry's anti-adhesion effect. The mode of action of cranberry juice cocktail is associated with an interference of adherence, particularly by a surface component of *E. coli* and other Gram-negative bacteria to at least a few types of epithelial cells, including uroepithelial cells.[25,26] *In vitro* studies found that the strongest anti-adherence activity occurred when the bacteria were preincubated with cranberry juice. *In vivo* studies found that urine collected from both mice and humans after drinking cranberry juice cocktail significantly inhibited adherence when compared to control urine.[25,26]

It appears that cranberry juice cocktail contains at least two different inhibitors. One is fructose, common to many fruit juices. The second factor appears to inhibit certain adhesins (P-fimbriae) of some pathogenic strains of *E. coli*. Activity is a function of the concentration and the time of preincubation of the bacteria with cranberry juice cocktail. The P-fimbriae inhibitory activity of cranberry juice is dependent on the concentration and the time of preincubation of the bacteria with the cocktail. Evidence that the inhibitor is adsorbed by the bacteria was supported by the finding that inhibition occurred even when bacteria which had been preincubated in cranberry juice cocktail were extensively washed with phosphate buffer.[27]

While orange juice, pineapple juice, and cranberry juice cocktail exhibited antiadhesin activity against type 1 fimbriated *E. coli*, containing a mannose-sensitive (MS) adhesin, only those juices from the Vaccinium genus tested (cranberry and blueberry) contained the mannose-resistant (MR) adhesin inhibitor.[28,29]

Most recently, Howell et al. were the first to identify specific components responsible for cranberry juice's anti-adhesion activity against P-fimbriated *E. coli*.

Using bioassay directed fractionation techniques, these researchers were able to isolate and identify proanthocyanidins from cranberries as the compounds responsible for inhibiting adhesion to P-fimbriated *E. coli* in *in vitro* studies.[30,31] This supports the theory of Schmidt and Sobota,[26] who believed that the anti-adherence factor is of low molecular weight (<1000) and could conceivably move from the blood into the urine with little difficulty. There may be an additional P-fimbriated adhesin inhibitor in cranberry. Ofek et al.[28,29] believe this inhibitor to be a nondialyzable high molecular weight compound (>15,000) that is heat stable and resistant to trypsin.

Recent *in vitro* work by Ahuja et al.[32] using transmission electron microscopy confirmed growth in the control populations of *E. coli* and the presence of P-fimbriae, while growth of bacteria on a media containing cranberry juice was inhibited. Those grown on the cranberry-containing media also demonstrated a 95% reduction in their expression of fimbriae and exhibited extreme cellular elongation.

A recent study was conducted *ex vivo* to determine if vitamin C and cranberry supplements could help fight UTIs in catheterized patients.[33] Urine from healthy subjects was collected after ingestion of vitamin C, a cranberry dietary supplement, or water. The urine was then tested for its ability to act as a substrate for bacteria from silicone rubber, a common component of urinary medical devices. Intake of cranberry tablets (three times daily at 400 mg) reduced the risk of *E. coli* colonization. Though lack of an effect was found in the pilot trials involving children with neurogenic bladders, this work suggests potential benefits in catheterized patients. Future work addressing dose/response and temporal effects is in order.

Blueberries have also been found to contain anti-adhesion activity for P-fimbriated E. coli in animal studies. Howell et al.[30,31] found that, like cranberries, blueberries contain proanthocyanidins with anti-adhesion activity against P-fimbriated *E. coli*. However, no clinical trials have been conducted with blueberries to support this effect in humans.

16.2.2 Oral Cavity Health

The research team of Ofek et al. who had earlier[27-29,34,35] helped develop the theory of anti-bacterial adhesion as the mechanism of action of cranberry in the urinary tract, later turned their efforts to document the applicability of this theory elsewhere in the body. They quickly focused on the oral cavity, where dental plaque, which is composed in part of early and late bacterial colonizers adhering to cell surfaces, including teeth, harbors a variety of organisms important to human mouth health. Various bacteria appear to be major causative factors in the etiology of both dental caries and periodontal gum disease.

Weiss et al.[36] investigated the inhibition of interspecies coaggregation of plaque bacteria with a cranberry constituent. They describe in some detail the formation of dental plaque on tooth surfaces, and states that the adhesion of, in particular, streptococci and actinomyces to salivary glycoproteins appears to be an initial step.[37,38] This early colonization is subsequently followed by the colonization of primarily Gram-negative bacteria, and it is this group,[39] particularly *Porphyromonas gingivalis, P. intermedius, Actinobacillus actinomycetem-comitans*, and *Fusobacte-*

rium nucleatum, which appears to play the central role in both the initiation and subsequent progression of periodontal gum disease. The stability of this plaque appears largely to be a function of the strength of adhesion to the pellicle on tooth surfaces, and bacteria to each other.[40] A basic assumption of this model is that agents that disturb or disrupt or inhibit this bacterial coaggregation may improve oral hygiene.[41]

Of the hundreds of bacteria and bacterial pairs that could comprise the dental plaque, Weiss et al.[36] isolated a wide variety of bacteria from the human gingival crevice, and used a coaggregation assay[42] to measure both aggregation and the reversal of aggregation in the presence and absence of a selected cranberry fraction *in vitro*. Using this assay with over 80 pairs of the recovered bacteria, they reported that the isolated cranberry fraction was able to inhibit the coaggregation of 70% of the bacterial pairs tested when at least one was Gram negative. Also highly noteworthy was their finding that the fraction was able to actually reverse the coaggregation of 50% of those pairs. As an example, they showed that the cranberry fraction, but not apple juice, caused complete reversal of aggregation of *S. oralis* HI and *F. nucleatum* PK1594. The authors conclude that the cranberry fraction would be an excellent candidate for further animal and clinical studies to assess its ability to influence plaque development and the resultant effects on periodontal gum disease.

Although the researchers did not fully characterize the cranberry fraction, they found that it did not act preferentially on reactions that were lactose sensitive, so it appears the active material is not structurally similar to lactose.[42] They do, however, point out that polyphenols are being associated as a group of natural compounds which may have an ability to reduce dental plaque,[43,44] and as reported by Howell,[30,31] the condensed tannins identified in their work on bacterial anti-adhesion in the UT are in fact polyphenolic in character. Consequently it appears likely that the cranberry components responsible for bacterial adhesion at these two widely different sites are structurally quite similar, if not identical.

16.2.3 Other Applications

The mechanism of bacterial anti-adhesion could have a wide range of beneficial applications beyond the UT and the oral cavity. Patents and other intellectual property continues to be developed regarding both the identification of components with these properties, and for their specific and targeted application, both in human and animal nutrition, as well as on nonbiological surfaces. With continuing concern over the rapid proliferation of antibiotic-resistant bacterial strains, interest in alternative mechanisms to inhibit, prevent, or reduce bacterial invasions and infections will continue to rise.

16.3 CRANBERRY PHYTOCHEMICALS: ANTIOXIDANT AND OTHER BENEFITS

Epidemiological evidence supports the benefits of fruit consumption in maintaining health in a variety of ways. Diets rich in fruits and vegetables are protective against heart disease, stroke, and cancer.[45-47] All fruits, including cranberries, are composed of a mixture of phytochemicals that are believed to contribute to chronic disease prevention. While the bulk of evidence is currently epidemiological in nature, substantial work is focusing on understanding the biological mechanisms of chronic diseases, and the role that phytochemicals may play in preventing disease.

Cranberry and other related fruits contain many compounds that have been found to have antioxidant activity through *in vitro* and *in vivo* research. Antioxidants are essential for eliminating free radicals in the body. Free-radical reactions are believed to contribute to a number of chronic diseases including cancer, heart disease, stroke, cataracts, Parkinson's disease, arthritis, and some signs of aging. Free radicals result through normal metabolism. They have the ability to damage cell walls, some enzymes, and DNA. A balance between forming and eliminating free radicals must exist to suppress harmful effects to cells. Cranberries contain a number of phytochemicals that neutralize free radicals. It is believed that reduction of oxidative damage to lipids, proteins, and nucleic acids may reduce the risk of cardiovascular disease and cancer. Increases in human plasma antioxidant capacity have been found in diets high in fruits and vegetables.

The antioxidant activity of berries is the subject of some *in vitro* studies. Heinonen et al. examined 44 berry and fruit wines and liquors, including cranberry-based products. They measured antioxidant capacity as a function of the ability to inhibit methyl lineolate oxidation.[48] Cranberries and related fruits were found to exhibit varying degrees of activity.

Cranberries and related fruits contain many phenolics with antioxidant or other physiologically beneficial activities. These include flavonoids and phenolic acids. Classes of cranberry flavonoids include anthocyanins, flavonols, flavan-3-ols, and proanthocyanidins. Each of these classes of compounds has interesting physiological activities.

Anthocyanins are the pigments that give cranberries their rich, red color. Eight anthocyanins have been identified in cranberries, all glycosides of cyanidin, peonidin and malvidin. Those identified include cyanidin-3-arabinoside, cyanidin-3-galactoside, cyanidin-3-glucoside, peonidin-3-arabinoside, peonidin-3-galactoside, peonidin-3-glucoside, malvidin-3-arabinoside, and malvidin-3-glucoside. Preliminary evidence suggests that anthocyanins have great antioxidant capacity in *ex vivo* studies. Wang et al. found cyanidin-3-galactoside, an anthocyanin found in cranberries, had twice the oxygen radical-absorbing activity of trolox, a water-soluble vitamin E analog.[49] The human biological significance of much of the research on food phytochemical antioxidants is questionable, since this work has primarily been conducted *in vitro* or *ex vivo*. In a recent pilot human feeding study, Cao and Prior demonstrated absorption of anthocyanins from elderberry into the blood, signifying availability for biological activity.[50]

Cranberry flavonols include glycosides of quercetin, kaempferol, myricitin, and isorhamnetin. Flavonols are currently the subject of a high degree of interest with regard to their health effects. Cranberry flavan-3-ols include catechin, catechin gallate, epicatechin, epicatechin gallate, epigallocatechin gallate, and gallocatechin gallate. *In vitro* and *in vivo* animal studies have found anti-inflammatory, anticarcinogenic, antiplatelet aggregation, vasodilatory, and other effects of several of these compounds.

The health benefits of proanthocyanidins (condensed tannins) are of great current interest to researchers. Advances in analytical techniques, including NMR, are now allowing better structural elucidations of the many oligomers and polymers of this complex class of compounds. Cranberry proanthocyanidins are primarily oligomers and polymers of epicatechin. *In vitro* research has established cranberry proanthocyanidins as responsible for their anti-adhesion UTH benefits. Condensed tannins may be found in a number of plant materials, including grapeseed, cocoa beans, and maritime pine bark. Flavan-3-ol backbones and linkage types (A- and B-) of oligomers from these plants differ from those in cranberry. Preliminary research of various proanthocyanidins suggest that they may act as antioxidants, and have cardioprotective and anticarcinogenic activities.[51-55]

Phenolic acids have oxygen scavenging abilities, among other activities. Those identified in cranberries include benzoic acid, para-coumaric acid, caffeic acid, chlorogenic acid, ferulic acid, protocatechuic acid, cinnamic acid, benzoic acid, gallic acid, and para-hydroxybenzoic acid. *In vitro* testing and animal studies suggest that these phenolic acids may contain antibacterial, antifungal, anticancer effects and activity.

Cranberries contain ellagic acid, also found in strawberries and raspberries. Ellagic acid has been shown to have a broad range of anticarcinogenic activity. Both *in vitro* and *in vivo* studies have shown inhibition against a broad range of carcinogens in several different tissues.[56]

The significance of these phytochemicals in cranberries and related fruits to human health largely remains to be determined. Epidemiological evidence supports foods containing these components to reducing risk of many diseases. Considerable work is needed to understand factors affecting bioavailability of the various phytochemicals and interactions with other dietary components.

16.4 OTHER HEALTH BENEFITS OF CRANBERRIES AND RELATED FRUITS

16.4.1 ANTICARCINOGENESIS

Research suggests that cranberries and related fruits contain certain components that may reduce cancer risk. Further studies are needed to better understand the implications of the data available to date.

Bomser et al. attempted to determine the components of cranberry, bilberry, lowbush blueberry, and lingonberry that may possess anticarcinogenic activity *in vitro*.[57] Four fractions of each fruit were prepared: crude extract, extractable ethyl acetate fraction, purified total anthocyanins, and proanthocyanidins. Two assays were used in this study. One measured the induction of quinine reductase (QR). QR inactivates electrophilic forms of carcinogens. Induction of QR activity indicates that a compound may prevent the initial stages of carcinogenesis. The second assay measured induction of ornithine decarboxylase (ODC). ODC catalyzes the rate-limiting step in the synthesis of polyamines. Enhanced formation is associated with rapidly proliferating cancer cells. Therefore, inhibition of this enzyme may indicate prevention of the promotional stage of carcinogenesis. Only the ethyl acetate fraction had any activity on QR. Bilberry, lingonberry, cranberry, and blueberry each exhibited activity. With regard to ODC activity, the crude fractions of lowbush blueberry, cranberry, and lingonberry had greater activity than bilberry. Greatest activity was seen with the proanthocyanidin fractions from lowbush blueberry, cranberry, and lingonberry.

In another *in vitro* study, cranberry extract had moderate anticancer activity.[58] Natural fruit and vegetable colorant extracts were tested for antitumor-promoting effects on Epstein-Barr virus early antigen (EPV-EA) which was induced by 12-*O*-tetradecanoylphorbol-13-acetate (TPA), a tumor promoter. The most active extract was beet root (betanin), followed by short red bell peppers (carotenoids), red onion skin (anthocyanins), paprika (capsanthin), and cranberry (anthocyanins); the least active was long red bell peppers (carotenoids).

16.4.2 Cardiovascular and Stroke Benefits

Epidemiological studies strongly support a diet high in fruits and vegetables as reducing risk of cardiovascular diseases and stroke. Based on their phytochemical composition, cranberries and related fruits would be expected to have some inhibitory effects on LDL oxidation and platelet aggregation. Wilson et al.[59] investigated the effects of unsweetened cranberry juice on copper-induced oxidation of human LDL *ex vivo*. They found cranberry to protect against LDL oxidation in this model. They also found the cranberry juice helps dilate the blood vessels of rats. The flavonoid composition of cranberry likely contributes to this effect.

The inhibition of platelet aggregation may be beneficial to those with atherosclerosis. An anthocyanin complex from bilberry (*Vaccinium myrtillus*) was found to inhibit platelet aggregation both *in vitro* and *in vivo*.[60] *In vitro*, the anthocyanins cyanidin-3-glucoside, delphinidin-3-glucoside, and malvidin-3-glucoside inhibited platelet aggregation.

16.4.3 Bioavailability of Vitamin B12

In one pilot study, ingestion of cranberry juice was found to increase protein-bound vitamin B12 absorption in people undergoing omeprazole treatment and in people with low gastric hydrochloric acid.[61] Omeprazole is used in the treatment of gastroesophageal reflux disease and peptic ulcers. Omeprazole induces a low stomach acid condition. Both low stomach acid and bacterial overgrowth can lead to decreased absorption of vitamin B12. This can have implications for putting individuals at risk of a vitamin B12 deficiency. Further research in understanding cranberry's benefits in this area is warranted.

16.4.4 Aging

Researchers at the USDA Human Nutrition Center on Aging at Tufts University are investigating the antioxidant activity of fruits and vegetables and their potential effects on the aging process. A diet rich in blueberry extract reversed some loss of balance and coordination, and improved short-term memory in aging rats.[62] In another study, rats fed daily doses of blueberry extract for 5 weeks before being subjected to pure oxygen suffered much less damage to capillaries in and around their lungs.[63]

16.5 HEALTH CLAIM REGULATIONS

Cranberry products are widely available in a variety of food and beverage forms. Over the past 10 years, cranberry dietary supplements have become increasingly available as well. The passage of DSHEA in 1994 had a profound impact on the supplement industry, particularly regarding label statements acceptable to the FDA regarding the ability of these products to help maintain the structure of function of the body. While statements regarding specific diseases continued to be reserved for drugs (with the exception of formally approved "Health Claim Statements" for specific foods), such "structure/function" claims, as they have come to be known, were allowed by the government, although statements disclaiming FDA evaluation were required. Aggressive commercial activity on the part of supplement manufacturers was thought to put the food industry at a competitive disadvantage, since DSHEA, with its sole focus on dietary supplements, appeared to give supplements labeling permission specifically excluded from conventional foods.

However, this situation changed dramatically when the FDA, in the September 23, 1997 Federal Register, definitively stated that under specified conditions conventional foods could also make such structure/function claims, and further, were not required to include the disclaimer on the label. Of particular interest is that the FDA chose to use cranberry as the example of a conventional food that could make such a claim, i.e. "…cranberry products help maintain urinary tract health…," if it is truthful, not misleading, and derives from the nutritional value of the food.

Cranberry products have thus been generally included in the category of foods called Functional Foods, or Nutraceuticals, etc. due to their generally accepted beneficial effect on UT health. However, at this point this terminology exists only in the vernacular and has no regulatory status, although such status is under active consideration. At this time, however, there are no regulatory definitions for such products, nor are there specific requirements.

REFERENCES

1. Stang, E.J., The North American cranberry industry. *Acta Hortic.*, 346, 284, 1993.
2. Eck, P., History. In *The American Cranberry,* Rutgers University Press, New Brunswick, NJ, 1, 1990.
3. Crosby, C., A History of Cranberry Growing in Massachusetts. In *Cranberry Harvest* Thomas, J.D., Ed., Spinner, 18, 1990.
4. Hooton, T.M. and Stamm, W.E., Management of acute uncomplicated urinary tract infections in adults. *Med. Clin. N. Am.*, 75(2), 339, 1991.
5. Ambulatory care visits to physician offices, hospital outpatient departments, and emergency departments. NCHS, CDC, HHS. United States, 1996; (February 1998).
6. Pollack, H.M., *Clinical Urography*, W. B. Saunders, Philadelphia, PA, 788, 1990.

7. Reid, G., Denstedt, J.D., Kang, Y.S., Lam, D., and Nause, C.J., Microbial adhesion and biofilm formation on urethral stents *in vitro* and *in vivo*. *Urology,* 148, 1592, 1992.
8. Avorn, J., Monane, M., Gurwitz, J.H., Glynn, R.J., Choodnovskiy, I., and Lipsitz, L. Reduction of bacteriuria and pyruria after ingestion of cranberry juice. *J. Am. Med. Assoc.,* 271, 751, 1994.
9. Walker, E.B., Barney, D.P., Mickelsen, J.N., Walton, R.J., and Mickelsen, R.A., Jr., Cranberry concentrate: UTI prophylaxis. *J. Fam. Pract.,* 45(2), 167, 1997.
10. Papas, P.N., Brusch, C.A., and Ceresia, G.C., Cranberry juice in the treatment of urinary tract infections. *Southwest Med.,* 47, 17, 1966.
11. Dignam, R., Ahmed, M., Denman, S., Zayon, M., Wills, T., Shipman, C., Wolfert, R., and Kleban, M., The effect of cranberry juice on UTI rates in a long term care facility. *J. Am. Geriatr. Soc.,* 45(9), S53, 1997.
12. Moen, D.V., Observations on the effectiveness of cranberry juice in urinary infections. *Wisc. Med. J.,* 61, 282, 1962.
13. Rogers, J., Pass the cranberry juice. *Nursing Times,* 87(48), 36, 1991.
14. Schlager, T.A., Anderson, S., Trudell, J., and Hendley, J.O., *J. Pedriatr.,* 135(6), 698, 1999.
15. Foda, M.R., Middlebrook, P.F., Gatfield, C.T., Potvin, G., Wells, G., and Schillinger, J.F., Efficacy of cranberry in prevention of urinary tract infection in a susceptible pediatric population. *Can. J. Urol.,* 2(1), 98, 1995.
16. Foxman, B., Geiger, A.M., Palin, K., Gillespie, B., and Koopman, J.S., First-time urinary tract infection and sexual behavior. *Epidemiology,* 6(2), 162, 1995.
17. Blatherwick, N., The specific role of foods in relation to the composition of urine. *Arch. Intern. Med.,* 14, 409, 1914.
18. Blatherwick, N.R. and Long, M.L., Studies on urinary acidity. The increased acidity produced by eating prunes and cranberries. *J. Biol. Chem.,* 57, 815, 1923.
19. Fellers, C.R., Redmon, B.C., and Parrott, E.M., Effect of cranberries on urinary acidity and blood alkali reserve. *J. Nutr.,* 6, 455, 1933.
20. Nickey, K., Urine pH: effect of prescribed regimens of cranberry juice and ascorbic acid. *Arch. Phys. Med. Rehab.,* 56, 556, 1975.
21. Kinney, A. and Blount, M., Effect of cranberry juice on urinary pH. *Nursing Res.,* 28, 287, 1979.
22. Bodel, P.T., Cotran, R., and Kass, E.H., Cranberry juice and the antibacterial action of hippuric acid. *J. Lab. Clin. Med.,* 54, 881, 1959.
23. Kahn, H.D., Panariello, V.A., Saeli, J., Sampson, J.R., and Schwartz, E., Effect of cranberry juice on urine. *J. Am. Diet. Assoc.,* 51, 251, 1967.
24. Harber, M. and Asscher, A., Virulence of urinary pathogens. *Kidney Int.,* 28, 717, 1985.
25. Sobota, A.E., Inhibition of bacterial adherence by cranberry juice: potential use for the treatment of urinary tract infections. *J. Urol.,* 131(5), 1013, 1984.
26. Schmidt, D.R. and Sobota, A., An examination of the anti-adherence activity of cranberry juice on urinary and non-urinary bacterial isolates. *Microbios.,* 55, 173, 1988.
27. Zafriri, D., Ofek, I., Adar, R., Pocino, M., and Sharon, N., Inhibitory activity of cranberry juice on adherence of Type 1 and P fimbriated Escherichia coli to eukaryotic cells. *Antimicrob. Agents Chemother.,* 33, 92, 1989.
28. Ofek, I., Goldhar, J., Zafriri, D., Lis, H., Adar, R., and Sharon, N., Anti-Escherichia adhesin activity of cranberry and blueberry juices. *N. Engl. J. Med.,* 324, 1599, 1991.

29. Ofek, I., Zafiri, D., Goldhar, J., Heiber, R., Lis, H., and Sharon, N., Effect of various juices on activity of adhesins expressed by urinary and nonurinary isolates of Escheria coli. In *America's Foods: Health Messages and Claims*, Tillotson, J.E., Ed., CRC Press, Boca Raton, FL, 1993, pp. 193-201.
30. Howell, A.B., Vorsa, N., Der Marderosian, A., and Foo, L.Y., Inhibition of the adherence of P-fimbriated Escherichia coli to uroepithelial-cell surfaces by proanthocyanidin extracts from cranberries. *N. Engl. J. Med.,* 339(15), 1085, 1998.
31. Foo, Y.P., Lu, Y., Howell, A.B., and Vorsa, N., Characterization of cranberry proanthocyanidins that inhibit adherence of uropathogenic P-fimbriated Escherichia coli, *Phytochemistry,* in press.
32. Ahuja, S.K., Kaak, B., and Roberts, J.A., Loss of fimbrial adhesion with the addition of Vaccinium macrocarpon to the growth media of P-fimbriated E. coli. *J. Urol.,* 159, 559, 1998.
33. Habash, M.B., Van der Mei, H.C., Busscher, H.J., and Reid, G., The effect of water, ascorbic acid and cranberry dervied supplementation on human urine and uropathogen adhesion to silicone rubber. *Can. J. Microbiol.,* 45, 691, 1999.
34. Ofek, I. and Doyle, R.J., *Bacterial Adhesion to Cells and Tissues*, Chapman and Hall. New York, 523, 1994.
35. Ofek, I., Goldhar, J., and Sharon, N., Anti-E. coli adhesin activity of cranberry and blueberry juices. *Adv. Exp. Med. Biol.,* (408), 179, 1996.
36. Weiss, E.I., Lev-Dor, R., Kashman, Y., Goldhar, J., Sharon, N., and Ofek, I., Inhibiting interspecies coaggregation of plaque bacteria with a cranberry juice constituent. *J. Am. Dental Assoc.,* 129(12), 1719, 1997.
37. Gibbons, R.J. and Houte, J.V., Bacterial adherence in oral microbial ecology. *Ann. Rev. Microbiol.,* (29), 19, 1975.
38. Gibbons, R.J., Hay, D.I., and Schlesinger, D.H., Delineation of a segment of adsorbed salivary protein-rich proteins which promotes adhesion of Streptococcus gordonii to apatitic surfaces. *Infect. Innun.,* (59), 2948, 1991.
39. Moore, W.E. and Moore, L.V., The bacteria of periodontal disease. *Periodontol 2000,* (5), 66, 1994.
40. Kolenbrander, P.E. and London. J., Adhere today, here tomorrow: oral bacterial adherence. *J. Bacteriol.,* (175), 3247, 1993.
41. Kolenbrander, P.E., Ganeshkumar, N., Carrels, F.J., and Hughes, C.J., Coaggregation: specific adherence among human and plaque bacteria. *FASEB J.,* (7), 406, 1993.
42. Kolenbrander, P.E., Coaggregations among oral bacteria. *Methods Enzymol,* (253), 385, 1995.
43. Sakanaka, S., Aizawa, M., Kim, M., and Yamamoto, T., Inhibitory effects of green tea polyphenols on growth and cellular adherence of an oral bacterium Porphyromonas gingivalis. *Biosci. Biotech. Biochem.,* 60(5), 745, 1996.
44. Ooshima, T., Minami, T., Aona, W., Tamura, Y., and Hamada, S., Reduction of dental plaque deposition in humans by oolong tea extract. *Caries Res.,* (28), 146, 1994.
45. Block, G., Patterson, B., and Subhar, A., Fruit, vegetables and cancer prevention: A review of the epidemiological evidence. *Nutr. Cancer,* 18, 1, 1992.
46. Howard, B.V. and Kritchevsky, D., Phytochemicals and cardiovascular disease: A statement for healthcare professionals from the American Heart Association. *Circulation,* 95(11), 2591, 1997.
47. Joshipura, K.J., Ascherio, A., Manson, J.E., Stampfer, M.J., Rimm, E.B., Speizer, F.E., Hennekens, C,H., Spiegelman, D., and Willett, W.C., Fruit and vegetable intake in relation to risk of ischemic stroke. *J. Am. Med. Assoc.,* 282(13), 1233, 1999.
48. Heinonen, I.M., Lehtonen, P.J., and Hopia, A.I., *J. Agr. Food Chem.,* 46(1), 25, 1998.

49. Wang, H., et al., Oxygen radical absorbing capacity of anthocyanins. *J. Agric. Food Chem.,* 45, 304, 1997.
50. Cao, G. and Prior, R.L., Anthocyanins are detected in human plasma after oral administration of an elderberry extract. *Clin. Chem.,* 45(4), 574, 1999.
51. Ho, K.Y., Huang, J.S., Tsai, C.C., Lin, T.C., Hsu, Y.F., and Lin, C.C., Antioxidant activity of tannin components from Vaccinium vitis-idaea L. *J. Pharm. Pharmacol.,* 51(9), 1075, 1999.
52. Ye, X., Krohn, R.L., Liu, W., Joshi, S.S., Kuszynski, C.A., McGinn, T.R., Bagchi, M., Preuss, H.G., Stohs, S.J., and Bagchi, D., The cytotoxic effects of a novel IH636 grape seed proanthocyanidin extract on cultured human cancer cells. *Mol. Cell Biochem.,* 196(1-2), 99, 1999.
53. Fremont, L., Belguendouz, L., and Delpal, S., Antioxidant activity of resveratrol and alcohol-free wine polyphenols related to LDL oxidation and polyunsaturated fatty acids. *Life Sci.,* 64(26), 2511, 1999.
54. Sato, M., Maulik, G., Ray, P.S., Bagchi, D., and Das, D.K., Cardioprotective effects of grape seed proanthocyanidin against ischemic reperfusion injury. *J. Mol. Cell Cardiol.,* 31(6), 1289, 1999.
55. Bomser, J.A., Singletary, K.W., Wallig, M.A., and Smith, M.A., Inhibition of TPA-induced tumor promotion in CD-1 mouse epidermis by a polyphenolic fraction from grape seeds. *Cancer Lett.,* 135(2), 151, 1999.
56. Barch, D.H., Rundhaugen, L.M., Stoner, G.D., Pillay, N.S., and Rosche, W.A., Structure-function relationships of the dietary anticarcinogen ellagic acid. *Carcinogenesis,* 17(2), 265, 1996.
57. Bomser, J., Madhavi, D.L., Singletary, K., and Smith, M.A., *In vitro* anticancer activity of fruit extracts from Vaccinium species. *Planta Med.,* 62(3), 212, 1996.
58. Kapadia, G.J., Tokuda, H., Konoshima, T., and Nishino, H., Chemoprevention of lung and skin cancer by Beta vulgaris (beet) root extract. *Cancer Lett.,* 100(1-2), 211, 1996.
59. Wilson, T., Porcari, J.P., and Harbin, D., Cranberry extract inhibits low density lipoprotein oxidation. *Life Sci.,* 62(24), PL381-6, 1998.
60. Morazzoni, P. and Mgaistretti, M.J., Activity of Myrtocyan, an anthocyanoside complex from Vaccinium myrtillus (VMA), on platelet aggregation and adhesiveness. *Fitoterapia,* LXI(1), 13, 1990.
61. Saltzman, J.R., Kemp, J.A., Golner, B.B., Pedrosa, M.C., Dallal, G.E., and Russell, R.M., Effect of hypochlorhydria due to omeprazole treatment or atrophic gastritis on protein-bound vitamin B12 absorption. *J. Am. Coll. Nutr.,* 13(6), 584, 1994.
62. Joseph, J.A., Shukitt-Hale, B., Denisova, N.A., Bielinski, D., Martin, A., McEwen, J.J., and Bickford, P.C., Reversals of age-related declines in neuronal signal transduction, cognitive, and motor behavioral deficits with blueberry, spinach, or strawberry dietary supplementation. *J. Neurosci.,* 19(18), 8114, 1999.
63. Cao, G., Shukitt-Hale, B., Bickford, P.C., Joseph, J.A., McEwen, J., and Prior, R.L., Hyperoxia-induced changes in antioxidant capacity and the effect of dietary antioxidants. *J. Appl. Physiol.,* 86(6), 1817, 1999.

Section V

Overview and Approaches to the Use of Vegetables in Maintaining Optimum Health

17 Diet and Carcinogenesis

Cindy D. Davis

CONTENTS

17.1 INTRODUCTON

It has been estimated that up to 70% of all cancers are attributed to diet.[1] It is often believed that food and nutrition affect cancer risk only because diets may contain specific carcinogenic substances. Although various carcinogens have been identified in foods and beverages, these appear to contribute only slightly to the overall impact of diet on cancer risk. The most important effect of diet may be mediated by substances present in food that inhibit the cancer process. Nearly 200 studies in the epidemiologic literature have been reviewed and relate, with great consistency, the lack of adequate consumption of fruits and vegetables to the incidence of cancer.[2-4] The quarter of the population with the lowest dietary intake of fruits and vegetables compared to the quarter with the highest intake has roughly twice the cancer rate for most types of cancer (lung, larynx, oral cavity, esophagus, stomach, colon and rectum, bladder, pancreas, cervix and ovary).[5] Many components of fruits and vegetables may be responsible for the protective effect: bioactive compounds, micronutrients, fiber, and low caloric intake.

0-8493-0038-X/97/$0.00+$.50

Bioactive compounds and micronutrients can affect carcinogen metabolism. Virtually all dietary or environmental carcinogens to which humans are exposed require enzymatic transformation, known as metabolic activation, to exert their carcinogenic effects. The most common enzymatic process is the addition of oxygen catalyzed by cytochrome P450 enzymes. This type of transformation is referred to as Phase I metabolism and generally makes the molecule more polar and consequently more readily excreted. Some of the intermediates formed in this process may be electrophiles, which can react with nucleophilic sites in critical macromolecules such as DNA, RNA, and protein. Reaction with these macromolecules results in covalent binding products called adducts. DNA adducts that persist unrepaired can cause miscoding and thus produce mutations in critical genes such as oncogenes and tumor suppressor genes. Competing with metabolic activation is detoxification. Some of the Phase 1 metabolites are detoxified because the addition of oxygen renders them less reactive toward macromolecules than the parent carcinogen. Numerous constituents of plant foods, including flavonoids, isothiocyanates, and allyl sulfides, have been found to be potent modulators of the cytochrome P450 monooxygenases *in vitro* and in animal models. Dietary components can impede carcinogenesis by blocking metabolic activation, increasing detoxification, or by providing alternative targets for the electrophilic metabolites. A second group of enzymes known as Phase II enzymes adds polar moieties to the oxygenated carcinogen, generally producing highly polar molecules that are readily excreted. Examples include acetyltransferases, glutathione-*S*-transferases, UDP- glucoronyl transferases, and sulfotransferases. Various components of fruits and vegetables have been shown to affect Phase II enzyme activities.

17.2 DIETARY CARCINOGENS

Carcinogens present in food or as a result of cooking practices include aflatoxins, *N*-nitroso compounds, polycyclic aromatic hydrocarbons, and heterocyclic amines. Aflatoxin is a generic term for a group of fungal metabolites produced by *Aspergillus flavus* and *A. parasiticus*.[6] The most widely studied of the aflatoxin compounds is aflatoxin B_1, which can be found in moldy peanuts. Consumption of aflatoxin B_1 has been associated with an increased risk of liver cancer in humans.[7-9] Furthermore, the discovery of an aflatoxin-bound guanine adduct in human DNA and the high correlation between urinary excretion of this adduct and aflatoxin B_1 intake further support the relationship between aflatoxin intake and cancer susceptibility.[10,11]

Nitrites and nitrates are often used as preservatives in meats and other "cured" products. Nitrites and nitrates are not carcinogenic in experimental animals. However, nitrate can be reduced to nitrite, which can interact with dietary substances such as amines or amides to produde *N*-nitroso compounds. *N*-nitroso compounds are potent carcinogens in animals.[12] In a study in 24 countries, high urinary nitrate concentrations were associated with increased stomach cancer mortality.[13] Nitrate is also present in large quantities in vegetables. However, concomitant intake of various antioxidants in fresh vegetables prevents oxidation of nitrate to nitrite and counteracts any cancer risk.[9]

Two cooking-derived classes of carcinogens have been shown to induce cancer in animal models. The first class is the polycyclic aromatic hydrocarbons associated with barbecued meats. These compounds are formed from the pyrolysis of fats that occurs when fat drips from the meat onto the coals, forming smoke that is redeposited on the meat surface. A fairly consistent association between grilled fish and meat and stomach cancer suggests that dietary exposure to polycyclic aromatic hydrocarbons may be involved in human gastric carcinogenesis.[9]

Another class of compounds found in cooked meats are the heterocyclic amines. Amino acid and creatine precursors in meat react chemically to produce these carcinogens during high-temperature cooking by a variety of methods such as broiling, frying, barbecuing, and baking. The major carcinogenic heterocyclic amine found in the Western diet is 2-amino-1-methyl-6-phenylimidazo[4,5-*b*]pyridine (PhIP); it has been shown to induce cancer in the mammary gland, colon, and prostate gland of rat — three organ sites that show a relatively high incidence of cancer in the Western world.[14-17] Although the concentration of heterocyclic amines in the diet of individuals consuming cooked meat are in the part per billion range, significantly lower than the concentration shown to induce cancer in laboratory animals, heterocyclic amines are regarded as possible human carcinogens.[16,17]

17.3 ALLIUM COMPOUNDS

The allium vegetable family includes onions, garlic, scallions, chives, and leeks. These vegetables have high concentrations of compounds such as diallyl sulfide and allyl methyl trisulfide.[18] These compounds have been shown to inhibit cell proliferation and growth, enhance the immune system, alter carcinogen activation, stimulate detoxification enzymes, and reduce carcinogen-DNA binding.[19-22] The direct effect of diet on DNA adduct formation has been tested by using supplemental garlic. Hageman et al.[23] examined the effects of supplemental garlic consumption on *ex vivo* production of benzo[a]pyrene-DNA adducts in lymphocytes. In a nonrandomized pilot study of 9 men, isolated lymphocytes from the blood of participants eating garlic (3 g raw garlic per day for 8 days) developed fewer adducts when incubated with benzo[a]pyrene.[23] Various studies have shown that garlic can slow the development of bladder, skin, stomach, and colon cancers. A prospective study of 42,000 Iowa women aged 55 to 69 revealed that garlic consumption was inversely associated with cancer risk. Risk of cancer in the distal colon was 50% lower in women with the highest consumption of garlic than in women who did not consume garlic.[24]

Several lines of evidence support the ability of allium compounds present in garlic to inhibit the synthesis of *N*-nitroso compounds.[25,26] Habitual consumption of garlic has been reported to correlate with a reduction in gastric nitrite content and reduction in gastric cancer mortality.[27,28] Additional support for an effect of garlic on nitrosamine formation comes from a human study in which 5 g of fresh garlic consumption markedly surpressed urinary excretion of *N*-nitrosoproline in individuals given supplemental nitrate and proline.[25] Two ecological studies showed that, in areas where garlic or onion production is very high, mortality rates for stomach cancer is very low.[9]

17.4 ISOTHIOCYANATES AND INDOLES

Isothiocyanates and indoles are released upon chewing of certain cruciferous vegetables, in which they occur as thioglucoside conjugates called glucosinolates. Vegetables of the *Brassica* genus, including cabbage, kale, broccoli, cauliflower, Brussels sprouts, and root crops such as turnips and rutabagas contribute most to the intake of glucosinolates. Many experimental studies have shown that indoles and isothiocyanates given to animals after a carcinogen insult reduced tumor incidence and multiplicity at a number of sites including the liver, mammary gland, and colon.[29-31] For example, phenethyl isothiocyanate, benzyl isothiocyanate, and sulforaphane are effective inhibitors of cancer induction in rodents treated with carcinogens.[32] A possible inhibitory activity of isothiocyanates and indoles against tumorigenesis apparently stems from their ability to influence Phase I and Phase II biotransformation enzyme activites.[33-35] Sulforaphane, which is present in broccoli, is a potent inducer of the Phase II detoxification enzymes quinone reductase and glutathione transferase, and an inhibitor of the carcinogen-activating cytochrome P4502E1.[36,37] The effectiveness of sulforaphane in blocking the formation of mammary tumors in rats administered a chemical carcinogen has been demonstrated.[38]

Indole-3-carbinol can lead to marked increases in the activities of cytochrome P450-dependent monooxygenases as well as induction of glutathione transferase.[39,40] Recent studies have shown that estrogens are metabolized by specific isozymes of cytochrome P450. Indole-3-carbinol has been shown to have beneficial effects because of alterations in estrogen metabolism. Because the formation of different estrogen metabolites is linked to breast and uterine cancer, the use of indole-3-carbinol in women has produced a beneficial effect through a modification of estrogen metabolism. It appears that indole-3-carbinol may be a very useful preventive agent against hormone-related cancers. [41]

17.5 PHYTOESTROGENS

Phytoestrogens are naturally occurring plant compounds with estrogenic or anti-estrogenic activity. They are heterocyclic phenols with structural similarities to estrogenic steroids and are constituents of many foods including cabbage, spinach, soy beans, and other soy products, sprouts, grains, and hops.[42] There are three main groups of phytoestrogens, the isoflavones, coumestans, and lignans.[42] Isoflavones occur mainly in soybean and whole grain products, various seeds, and seed-containing berries. Some specific isoflavones include genistein, daidzen, and the precursors formononetin and biochanin A.[9] Phytoestrogens have been shown to bind to isolated estrogen receptors and cause proliferation and gene transactivation responses *in vitro*.[42] Some phytoestrogens are structurally similar to tamoxifen, a drug that is being used to successfully treat some types of breast cancer and is currently being tested for cancer prevention in high-risk women.[18] Genistein, which possesses weak estrogenic activity, has been shown to act in animal models as an anti-estrogen.[43] *In vitro*, genistein suppresses the growth of a wide range of cancer cells.[9] In humans, preliminary data indicate plasma concentrations of genistein can reach the low micormole per liter range, values similar to those required to inhibit *in vitro* cancer cell growth. [43]

Other biological activities of phytoestrogens have been described, in addition to their hormonal properties, which may be important in explaining their biological effects. For example, genistein and daidzein have antioxidant properties and are potent scavengers of hydrogen peroxide.[44] *In vitro*, genistein inhibits the action of several enzymes involved with tumor growth and development, including enzymes that phosphorylate tyrosine residues on key proteins involved in signal transduction events in normal and tumor cells; it also inhibits DNA topoisomerases and other critical enzymes involved in signal transduction.[45,46] Genistein and biochanin A have also been shown to induce apoptosis of tumor cells.[47]

17.6 FLAVONOIDS

Over 4000 flavonoids have been identified in plants. These universal plant pigments are responsible for the colors of flowers, fruits, and sometimes leaves.[48] Flavonoids are a group of polyphenolic antioxidant compounds with cancer-blocking properties. Flavonoids are present in a wide variety of fruits, vegetables, nuts, whole seeds, spices, tea, and wine. Flavonoids have a common skeleton of diphenyl pyrons, two benzene rings linked through a heterocyclic pyran or pyrone ring. The basic ring structure allows a multitude of substitution patterns giving rise to flavonoids, flavones, catechins, anthocyanadines, and isoflavonoids. Flavonoids have differing antioxidant properties depending upon the degree of hydoxylation of the benzene rings; this property may provide one anticarcinogenic mechanism.[9,49]

Quercetin is the major flavonoid in vegetables, fruits, and wine. Other common flavonoids include kaempferol, catechin, epicatechin gallate, chrysin, and cyanidin. Flavonoids may defend cells against carcinogens via their ability to increase the pump-mediated efflux of carcinogens from cells or via induction of detoxification enzymes.[49-51] Quercitin may also interact with specific carcinogens in the gastrointestinal tract, thereby reducing their bioavailability, and may reduce cell proliferation.[52]

17.7 LIMONENE

Monoterpenes are natural plant products found in the essential oils of many commonly consumed fruits and vegetables. They have been widely used for nearly 50 years as flavor and fragrance additives in food and beverages. A number of recent studies have shown that monoterpenes possess antitumorigenic activities and suggest that these compounds represent a new class of agents for cancer chemoprevention.[53,54] Limonene, the simplest monocyclic monoterpene, and perillyl alcohol, a hydroxylated limonene analog, have demonstrated chemopreventive and chemotherapeutic activity against mammary, skin, lung, pancreas, and colon tumors in rodent models.[54-57] They are capable of increasing tumor latency, decreasing tumor multiplicity, and causing regression of mammary carcinomas.[58,59] Because monoterpenes do not cause systemic toxicity at the doses required to induce regression of mammary tumors, they are currently being tested in Phase I clinical trials on advanced cancer patients in the U.S. and the U.K.[60,61]

17.8 HERBS

A variety of herbs and herbal extracts contain different phytochemicals that have been shown to be protective against cancer, including the flavonoids, lignans, sulfides, polyphenolics, carotenoids, coumains, saponins, cucumins, and phthalides.[62] The botanical term herb refers to seed-producing plants with nonwoody stems that die down at the end of the growing season.[62] As mentioned above, flavonoids are antioxidants and may induce carcinogen detoxification enzymes. Many commonly used herbs contain substantial amounts of flavonoid antioxidants. These include chamomile, dandelion, ginkgo, green tea, hawthorn, licorice, passionflower, milk thistle, rosemary, sage, thyme, and yarrow.[62] In addition to the flavonoids, a variety of phenolic compounds, are present in many herbs.[62] These phenolic compounds (such as caffeic, ellagic, and ferulic acids, sesamol, and vanillin) are also potent antioxidants and inhibit carcinogenic activity.[62]

Flaxseed contains a rich supply of lignans. These plant lignans are converted to mammalian lignans by bacterial fermentation in the colon and they can act as estrogens.[63] Mammalian lignans appear to be anticarcinogenic; lignan metabolites bear a structural similarity to estrogens and can bind to estrogen receptors and inhibit the growth of estrogen-stimulated breast cancer.[64-66] Urinary excretion of lignans is reduced in women with breast cancer, whereas the consumption of flaxseed powder increases urinary concentration of lignans severalfold.[67]

Eugenol is the principal constituent (70 to 90%) of the essential oil of clove and is also present in many essential oils of plants, especially basil, cinnamon, and nutmeg.[68] Eugenol has been shown to offer protection against liver cancer in rats and to inhibit lipid peroxidation.[68]

Turmeric is derived from the rhizome of a plant in the ginger family and is the major ingredient in curry powders.[9] Curcumin is the principal compound and the major yellow pigment in turmeric and curry. Curcumin is a phenolic compound that is a strong antioxidant, free-radical scavenger, and a potent inhibitor of nitrosation.[9] Tumeric/curcumin has been shown to suppress the development of stomach, breast, lung, and skin tumors.[69] Studies of humans at risk of palatal cancer because of reverse smoking showed that turmeric (1 g/day for 9 months) had a significant impact on the regression of precancerous lesions.[68]

Turmeric also contains a bioactive peptide, turmerin, which makes up 0.1% of its dry weight.[9] Turmerin has been shown, *in vitro*, to be a strong antioxidant, a DNA-protectant against oxidative injury, and an antimutagen. It has also been shown to decrease arachadonic release, which may be an important event in membrane-mediated chromosomal damage.[9]

17.9 CAROTENOIDS

Carotenoids constitute a class of over 600 natural compounds occurring predominantly in fruits and vegetables. Some carotenoids such as β-carotene are provitamin A compounds that can be converted into vitamin A *in vivo*. β-carotene is the most abundant carotenoid and is found notably in orange colored vegetables and fruits and in dark green leafy vegetables, including carrots, pumpkin, winter squash, sweet potatoes, cantaloupe, apricots, mangoes, kale, spinach, and collard greens.[18] Carotenoids are present in all foods that contain chlorophyll, and they appear to be the plants' main defense against singlet oxygen generated as a byproduct of the interaction of light and chlorophyll.[70] Many carotenoids are potent antioxidants enabling them to neutralize free radicals generated as byproducts of oxidative metabolism in the body or derived from exogenous sources such as cigarette smoking. Free radicals can attack and damage RNA and DNA in cells, as well as inactivate proteins and enzymes by reactions with amino acids. For example, Collins et al. observed an inverse correlation between the frequency of oxidized bases in lymphocyte DNA, an indicator of oxidative stress, and concentrations of carotenoids in blood.[71] Carotenoids have been shown to be anticarcinogens in rats and mice and may be anticarcinogens in humans.[72,73]

Although initially β-carotene was thought to exert antioxidant effects potentially suitable for chemoprevention, subsequent basic studies have shown that β-carotene can exert pro-oxidant effects under high oxygen pressures and oxidative stress, such as those occurring in the lung of smokers.[74,75] This latter finding may help explain the significantly increased risk of lung cancer that was associated with β-carotene in current smokers involved in recent epidemiologic studies.[76,77] For example, in a large trial carried out in Finland, a significant increase of 18% in lung cancer incidence was seen among those participants (all smokers) who received β-carotene over a period of 5 to 8 years, compared with those not receiving the carotenoids.[76] Soon after the publication of this report, another trial (the Beta-Carotene and Retinol Efficacy Trial [CARET], investigating a high-risk population of smokers and/or asbestos workers) was prematurely halted when a trend towards increased incidence of cancer with β-carotene supplementation became evident.[77]

Tomatoes, watermelon, pink grapefruit, and guava are particularly rich in a red pigment, lycopene, another antioxidant carotenoid.[78] Recent work demonstrates that lycopene is a more active inhibitor of human cancer cell proliferation than β-carotene.[73] *In vitro*, lycopene has been shown to be the most efficient quencher of singlet oxygen among the carotenoids. Investigators have also shown lycopene to inhibit the proliferation of breast, lung, and endometrial human cancer cells in culture.[73] Lycopene is a more potent inhibitor of human cancer cell proliferation than either α-carotene or β-carotene.[79]

Another potential mechanism whereby carotenoids may protect against cancer susceptibility involves the formation of retinol and its subsequent role in the regulation of epithelial cell differentiation.[18] Because lack of proper differentiation is a feature of cancer cells, adequate vitamin A (from either carotenoids or retinol) may allow normal cell differentiation and thus avoid the development of cancer.[9,18]

There are other biological functions of carotenoids that may be involved in cancer prevention. Many of the carotenoids (β-carotene, canthalxanthin, lutein, lycopene, and α-carotene) have been found to upregulate gap junctional intracellular communication via changes in gene expression.[80, 81] Enhanced cell-to-cell communication would restrict clonal expansion of initiated cells, decreasing the likelihood of cancer occurrence. Furthermore, β-carotene and α-carotene may inhibit cell proliferation and β-carotene may enhance immune function.[82-84]

17.10 VITAMIN C

Vitamin C is the most abundant water-soluble antioxidant in the body and is unique in that it can be regenerated when oxidized.[9] Specific food sources include citrus fruits, mangoes, papaya, banana, strawberries, melon, broccoli, cabbage, and other green leafy vegetables, peppers, tomatoes, pumpkin, and yams.[9] Epidemiologic studies have indicated relatively consistent inverse associations of vitamin C with stomach cancer, oral cancer, and cancer of the esophagus.[9,85] A cohort study of plasma antioxidant concentrations in Swiss men found that vitamin C concentrations were about 10% lower at baseline ($p < .01$) in men that subsequently died from any type of cancer than in those who did not.[86]

Via its antioxidant function, vitamin C is able to detoxify carcinogens and may protect cell membranes and DNA from oxidative damage.[9] In humans, supplementation with 100 mg/day has been shown to minimize oxidative damage in lymphocyte DNA.[87-89]

Vitamin C has also been shown to scavenge and reduce nitrite, thus reducing substrate availability for the formation of *N*-nitroso compounds. Ascorbic acid supplementation and addition of ascorbic acid-rich foods to a controlled experimental diet have been shown to inhibit endogenous formation of *N*-nitroso compounds in humans.[90] In a controlled dietary study conducted in China, supplements of 75 mg ascorbic acid for 2 days, reduced urinary excretion of *N*-nitrosoproline by 44%.[90]

17.11 VITAMIN E

Vitamin E, the most important antioxidant found within lipid membranes in the body, comes primarily from dietary vegetable oils (including safflower, corn, cottonseed, and soy bean oils) and nuts. Vitamin E occurs in food as compounds called tocopherols and tocotrienols. α-Tocopherol, the main form of Vitamin E in the U.S. diet, protects polyunsaturated fatty acids in cell membranes from oxidation by scavenging oxygen radicals and terminating free-radical chain reactions. Oxidation results in the production of malondialdehyde, which is possibly mutagenic, and free radicals, which can induce damage in DNA.[9] Vitamin E also functions to keep carotenoids in a reduced state, thereby enhancing their antioxidant capacity, and decreases the formation of nitrosamines in the stomach.[92,93] Finally, vitamin E also may prevent cancer progression by increasing production of humoral antibodies and enhancing cell-mediated immunity. Humans taking vitamin E supplements (200 U.I./day) for 10 years reduced their risk of colonic cancer by approximately half and evidence suggests a marked protective effect of a supplement (50 U/day) on prostate cancer.[94-96] Vitamin E also enhances the immune system in humans.[97]

17.12 FOLATE

Folate (folic acid) is so-called because it is abundant in foliage (green leafy vegetables). The importance of folate in cancer protection was first demonstrated in animal studies when folate deficiency was linked to enhanced chemically induced carcinogenesis and subsequently in humans in relation to cervical dysplasia and colon cancer.[98-100] More recently, the importance of folate for the maintenance of genetic stability and for control of gene expression has further highlighted the potential importance of folate in cancer protection.[98] Folate, which is central to methyl-group metabolism, may influence both methylation of DNA and the available nucleotide pool for DNA replication and repair. Inadequate intake of folic acid may lead to reduced methylation of cytosine in cytosine-guanine sequences of DNA which, if hypomethylated, may lead to enhanced expression of specific oncogenes.[99,100]

Folate deficiency, a common deficiency in people who eat few fruits and vegetables, causes chromosome breaks in human genes because of deficient methylation of uracil to thymine, and subsequent incorporation of uracil into human DNA.[101] Uracil in DNA is excised by a repair glycosylase with the formation of a transient single-strand break in the DNA; two opposing single-strand breaks cause a double-strand chromosome break, which is difficult to repair. Both high DNA uracil concentrations and chromosome breaks in humans are reversed by folate administration.[101] Folate supplementation above the Recommended Dietary Allowance value minimized chromosome breakage in human genes.[102] The potential role in human carcinogenesis of uracil misincorporation is supported by two recent studies that show a two- to fourfold lower risk of colon cancer in individuals who are homozygous for the mutant alleles of methylenetetrahydrate folate reductase.[103,104]

17.13 SELENIUM

Other potentially anticarcinogenic substances are not limited to one type of vegetable or fruit but are more widespread. Selenium is found in produce in amounts proportional to the selenium content of the soil in which it is grown. Plants are capable of converting inorganic selenium in soil to organic selenium compounds following the sulfur assimilatory scheme.[105] For example, seleniferous wheat is known to contain selenomethionine as a major source of selenium.[106] In some species of *Astragalus* that accumulate high concentrations of selenium, methylated derivatives such as Se-methylselenocysteine, have been isolated.[105] Selenium is an essential trace element for human health and has received considerable attention for its possible role as an effective, naturally occurring, anticarcinogenic agent. Epidemiologic studies reveal that selenium intake correlates inversely with the mortality from various types of cancer and suggest an increased risk of colon cancer in humans in geographic areas where selenium is low in the soil.[107-109] In a recent study by Clark et al.,[109] selenium supplementation reduced the incidence of, and mortality from, carcinomas at several sites in the body including the colon. Diets high in selenium have been shown to suppress carcinogenesis in many different animal tumor models.[110-115]

However, the chemopreventive effect of selenium depends on its chemical form. For example, we recently observed that 3,2'-dimethyl-4-aminobiphenyl (DMABP)-induced aberrant crypt formation (a preneoplastic lesion for colon cancer) decreased significantly in rats supplemented with 0.1 or 2.0 mg selenium per kilogram of diet as selenite or selenate, but not as selenomethionine, compared to animals fed a selenium-deficient diet (Figure 17.1).[114]

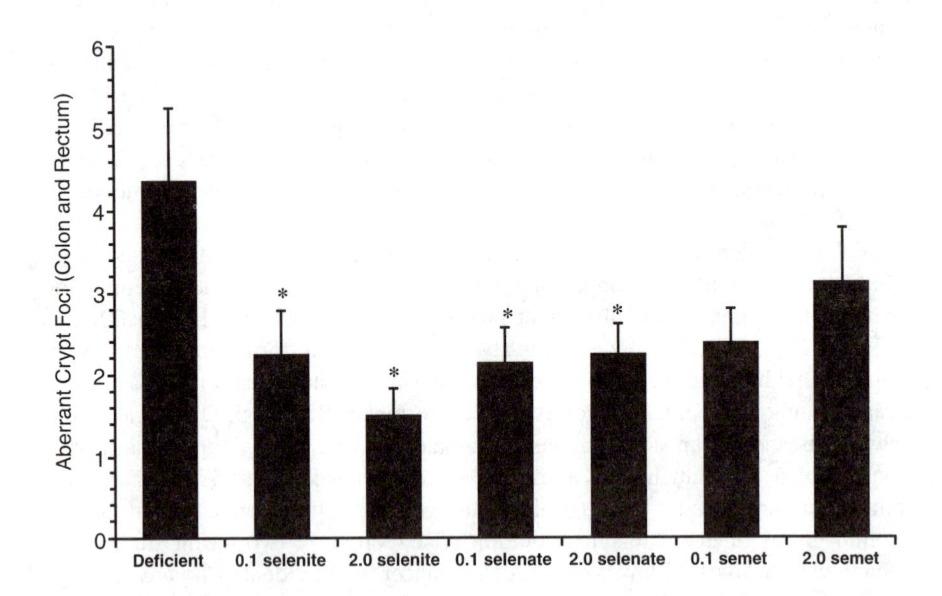

FIGURE 17.1 Total number of aberrant crypt foci in the colon and rectum of rats treated with 3,2'-dimethyl-4-aminobiphenyl and fed a selenium-deficient torula yeast-based diet supplemented with 0, 0.1, or 2 mg/kg Se diet as selenite, selenate, or selenomethionine. Values are mean ±SEM, n = 8. Asterisks indicate significantly ($p < .05$) different from 0 mg/kg selenium diet animals as determined by one-way analysis of variance followed by Dunnet's contrasts.

The biochemical basis for the protective effect of selenium in cancer is unknown. The selenium-containing antioxidant enzymes, glutathione peroxidase and thioredoxin reductase, may be involved.[116] Because of the role of glutathione peroxidase in reactive oxygen metabolism, it has been hypothesized by many that changes in glutathione peroxidase activity would provide the mechanism for the chemopreventive activity of selenium. However, it has been found that glutathione peroxidase activity was already at maximum concentrations in tissues of animals fed normal selenium and did not change appreciably as dietary selenium was increased to the ten-fold higher concentrations needed to observe chemopreventive effects in animal models.[117] In contrast, various studies have shown that selenite increases the activity of another antioxidant enzyme, thioredoxin reductase, in human cancer cells and in rats fed supranutritional concentrations of selenite.[117] In addition to its role in antioxidation, selenium has been shown to suppress cell proliferation and stimulate apoptosis.[118,119]

Various forms of selenium have also been shown to alter the metabolism of carcinogens and to inhibit the formation of carcinogen-DNA adducts.[120,121] We recently observed that supplementation with either a 0.1 or 2.0 mg selenium per kilogram diet as either selenite or selenate, but not as selenomethionine, resulted in significantly fewer (53 to 70%, $p < .05$) DMABP-DNA adducts in the colon, but not in the liver, than in rats fed a selenium-deficient diet.[121] This reduction in DMABP-DNA adduct formation in the colon correlates with a reduction in DMABP-induced aberrant crypt foci. The protective effect of selenite and selenate against DMABP-DNA adduct formation apparently is not a result of alterations in plasma or liver selenium concentrations or altered glutathione peroxidase or glutathione transferase activities, but may be related to differences in the metabolism of the different forms of selenium.[121]

Although most chemoprevention studies in animals have used inorganic selenite as the source of selenium, it should be noted that, in humans, the ingestion of selenium is mainly in the form of selenomethionine through the consumption of cereals, grains, fruits, and vegetables.

Plants are known to convert inorganic selenium in soil to organoselenium analogues of naturally occurring sulfur compounds.[105] Vegetables with a rich source of sulfur might, therefore, be expected to concentrate selenium if cultivated in a medium fertilized with selenium.[105] This idea was tested with garlic, which is abundant in a variety of sulfur compounds.[105] A major reason for choosing garlic as the experimental crop is because the allyl sulfides present in garlic are known to have anticarcinogenic activity, as discussed in Section 17.3 above. A number of studies have shown that selenium-enriched garlic is an effective anticarcinogen.[122-124] Furthermore, it has been reported that the chemopreventive activity of selenium-enriched garlic is likely to be accounted for by the effect of selenium rather than the effect of garlic per se.[125] Cai et al. have identified Se-methylselenocysteine as the predominant selenoamino acid in the selenium-enriched garlic.[126] A recent study has shown that the forms of selenium in garlic and broccoli are virtually identical and that broccoli can accumulate as much selenium as garlic.[125] We have recently observed that selenium-enriched broccoli is protective against chemically induced aberrant crypt formation (a preneoplastic lesion for colon cancer) in experimental animals;[127] this suggests that selenium-enriched broccoli is an effective anticarcinogen (Figure 17.2).

17.14 CONCLUSION

Epidemiologic studies consistently show an inverse relationship between fruit and vegetable intake and cancer susceptibility. Vegetables, fruits, and herbs are rich in many different substances that may decrease cancer risk. These include allium compounds, isothiocyanates, indoles, phytoestrogens, flavonoids, limonene, carotenoids, vitamin C, vitamin E, folate, and selenium. Different mechanisms whereby micronutrients and bioactive compounds exert their chemopreventive effects include: blocked metabolic activation of carcinogens, increased activity of enzymes that detoxify carcinogens, antioxidant effects, decreased cell proliferation, increased cell differentiation, increased apoptosis of cancer cells, blocked formation of *N*-nitrosamines, altered estrogen metabolism, and increased DNA methylation.

REFERENCES

1. Doll, R. and Peto, R. The causes of cancer. *J. Natl. Cancer Inst.*, 66, 1191, 1981.
2. Block, G., Patterson, B., and Subar, A. Fruit, vegetables and cancer prevention: A review of the epidemiologic evidence. *Nutr. Cancer,* 18, 1, 1992.

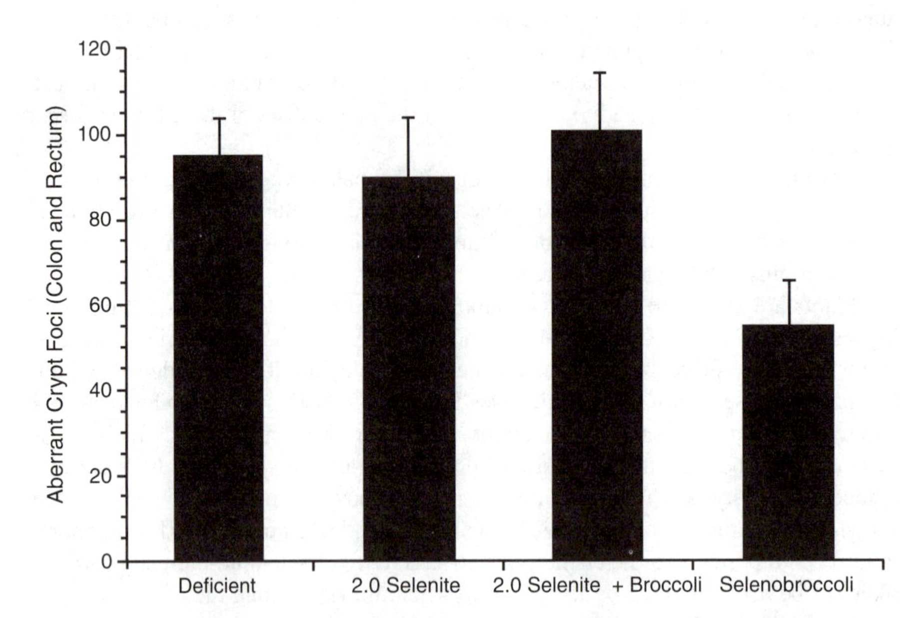

FIGURE 17.2 Total number of aberrant crypt foci in the colon and rectum of rats treated with dimethylhydrazine and fed either a selenium-deficient torula yeast-based diet, a diet supplemented with 2.0 mg/kg Se diet as selenite, a diet supplemented with 2.0 mg/kg Se diet as selenite and low-selenium broccoli, or a diet supplemented with 2.0 mg/kg Se diet as selenium-enriched broccoli. Values are mean ± SEM, n = 18.

3. Steinmetz, K.A. and Potter, J.D. Vegetables, fruit and cancer. I. Epidemiology. *Epidemiol. Cancer Causes Control,* 2, 325, 1991.
4. Hill, M.J., Giacosa, A., and Caygill, C.P.J., Eds. *Epidemiology of Diet and Cancer,* West & Sussex: Ellis Horwood, 1994.
5. Ames, B.N. and Gold, L.W. The causes and prevention of cancer: the role of the environment. *Biotherapy,* 11, 205, 1998.
6. Busby, W.F. and Wogan, G.N. Aflatoxins, in *Chemical Carcinogens,* Searle, C.E., Ed., American Cancer Society, Washington, D.C., 1984, 945.
7. Ross, R.K., Yuan, J.-M., Yu, M. C., Wogan, G.M., Qian, G.-S., Tu, J.-T., Groopman, J.D., Gao, Y.-T., and Henderson, B.E. Urinary aflatoxin biomarkers and risk of hepatocellular carcinoma. *Lancet,* 339, 943, 1992.
8. Qian, G.-S., Ross, R.K., Yu, M.C., Yuan, J.-M., Gao, Y.-T., Henderson, B.E., Wogan, G.N., and Groopman, J.D. A follow-up study of urinary markers of aflatoxin exposure and liver cancer risk in Shanghai, People's Republic of China. *Cancer Epidemiol. Biomed. Prev.,* 3, 3, 1994.
9. World Cancer Research Fund Food. Nutrition and the Prevention of Cancer: A Global Perspective. American Institute for Cancer Research, Washington, D.C., 1997.
10. Groopman, J.D., Zhu, J, Donahue, P.R., Pikul, A., Zhang, L., Chen, J., and Wogan, G.N. Molecular dosimetry of urinary aflatoxin-DNA adducts in people living in Guangxi Autonomous Region, People's Republic of China. *Cancer Res.,* 52, 42, 1992.
11. Sabbioni, G., Ambs, A., Wogan, G.N., and Groopman, J.D. The aflatoxin-lysine adduct quantified by high-performance chromatography from human serum albumin samples. *Carcinogenesis,* 11, 2063, 2066.

12. Mirvish, S.S. Effects of vitamins C and E on N- nitroso compound formation, carcinogenesis, and cancer. *Cancer,* 58, 1842, 1986.
13. Joosens, J.V., Hill, M.J., Elliott, P., Stamler, J., and Lesaffre, E. Stomach cancer, salt and nitrate in 24 countries. *Proc. 15th Int. Congr. Nutrition,* Sep. 27-Oct. 2; Adelaide, Australia, 381, 1993.
14. Ghoshal, A., Preisegger, K.-H., Takayama, S., Thorgeirsson, S.S., and Snyderwine, E.G., Induction of mammary tumors in female Sprague-Dawley rats by the food mutagen 2-amino-1-methyl-6-phenylimidazo[4,5-*b*]pyridine and the effect of dietary fat. *Carcinogenesis,* 15, 2429, 1994.
15. Layton, D.W., Bogen, K.T., Knize, M.G., Hatch, F.T., Johnson, V.M., and Felton, J.S. Cancer risk of heterocyclic amines in cooked foods: an analysis and implication for research. *Carcinogenesis,* 16, 39, 1995.
16. Sugimura, T. History, present and future, of heterocyclic amines, cooked food mutagens, in *Heterocyclic Amines in Cooked Foods: Possible Human Carcinogens,* Adamson, R.H., Gustafsson, J.A., Ito, N., Sugimura, T., Wakabayashi, K., and Yamazoe, Y., Eds., Princeton Scientific, Princeton, NJ, 1995, pp 214-231.
17. Snyderwine, E.G. Diet and mammary gland carcinogenesis. *Recent Results Cancer Res.,* 152, 3, 1998.
18. Steinmetz, K.A. and Potter, J.D. Vegetables, fruit and cancer prevention: a review. *J. Am. Diet. Assoc.,* 96, 1027, 1996.
19. Hatono, S., Jimenez, A., and Wargovich, M.J. Chemopreventive effect of *S*-allylcyseine and its relationship to the detoxification enzyme glutathione *S*-transferase. *Carcinogenesis,* 17, 1041, 1996.
20. Lin, X.Y., Liu, J.Z., and Milner, J.A. Dietary garlic suppresses DNA adducts caused by *N*-nitrosos compounds. *Carcinogenesis,* 15, 349, 1994.
21. Lee, E.S., Steiner, M., and Lin, R. Thioallyl compounds: potent inhibitors of cell proliferation. *Biochem. Biophys. Acta,* 1221, 73, 1994.
22. Amagase, J. and Milner, J.A. Impact of various sources of garlic and their constituents on 7,12-dimethylbenz[*a*]anthracene binding to mammary cell DNA. *Carcinogenesis,* 14, 1627, 1993.
23. Hageman, G., Krul, C., van Herwinjnen, M., Schilderman, P., and Kleinjans, J. Assessment of the anticarcinogenic potential of raw garlic in humans. *Cancer Lett.,* 114, 161, 1997.
24. Steinmetz, K.A., Kushi, L.H., Bostick, R.M., Folsom, A.R., and Potter, J.D. Vegetables, fruit and colon cancer in the Iowa women's health study. *Am. J. Epidemiol.,* 139, 1. 1994.
25. Mei, X., Lin, X., Liu, J.Z., Lin, X.Y., Song, P.J., Hu, J.F., and Liang, X.J. The blocking effect of garlic on the formation of *N*-nitrosoproline in humans. *Acta Nutrimenta Sinica*, 11, 141, 1989.
26. Liu, J.Z., Peng, S.S., Lin, X.Y., Song, P.J., and Hu, J.F. The blocking effect of garlic extract on the *in vitro* chemical formation of nitrosamines. *Acta Nutrimenta Sinica,* 8, 9, 1986.
27. Mei, X., Wang, M.L., Xu, H.X., Pan, X.Y., Gao, C.Y., Han, N., and Fu, M.Y. Garlic and gastric cancer. I. The influence of garlic on the level of nitrate and nitrite in gastric juice. *Acta Nutrimenta Sinica*, 4, 53, 1982.
28. You, W.C., Blot, W.J., Chang, Y.S., Ershow, A.G., Yang, Z.T., An, Q., Henderson, B., Xu, W.G., Fraumeni, J.F., and Wang, T.G. Allium vegetables and reduced risk of stomach cancer. *J. Natl. Cancer Inst.,* 81, 162, 1989.
29. Sugie, S., Okumura, A., Tanaka, T., and Mori, H. Inhibitory effects of benzylisothiocyanate and benzylthiocyanate on diethylnitrosamine-induced hepatocarcinogenesis in rats. *Jpn. J. Cancer Res.,* 84, 865, 1993.

30. Dashwood, R.H., Arbogast, D.N., Fong, A.T., Pereira, C., Hendricks, J.D., and Bailey, G.S. Quantitative inter-relationships between aflatoxin B1 carcinogen dose, indole-3-carbinol anti-carcinogen dose, target organ DNA adduction and final tumor response. *Carcinogenesis,* 10, 175, 1989.
31. Tanaka, T., Mori, Y., Morishita, Y., Hara, A., Ohno, T., Kojinna, T., and Mori, H. Inhibitory effect of sinigrin and indole-3-carbinol on diethylnitrosamine-induced-hepatocarcinogenesis in male ACN rats. *Carcinogenesis,* 11, 1403, 1990.
32. Hecht, S.S. Chemoprevention of cancer by isothiocyanates, modifiers of carcinogen metabolism. *J. Nutr.,* 129, 768s, 1999.
33. Zang, Y. and Talalay, P. Anticarcinogenic activities of organic isothiocyanates: chemistry and mechanisms. *Cancer Res.,* 50, 2, 1994.
34. Boone, C.W., Kelloff, G.J., and Malone, W.E. Identification of candidate cancer chemopreventive agents and their evaluation in animal models and human clinical trials: a review. *Cancer Res.,* 50, 2, 1990.
35. McDannell, R. and McLean, A.E.M. Chemical and biological properties of indole glucosinolates (glucobrassicins): a review. *Food Chem. Toxicol.,* 26, 59, 1988.
36. Zhang, Y., Talalay, P., Cho, C.-G., and Posner, G.H. A major inducer of anticarcinogenic protective enzymes from broccoli: isolation and elucidation of structure. *Proc. Natl. Acad. Sci. USA,* 89, 2399, 1992.
37. Barcelo, S., Gardiner, J.M., Gescher, A., and Chipman, J.K. CYP2E1-mediated mechanism of anti-genotoxicity of the broccoli constituent of sulforaphane. *Carcinogenesis,* 17, 277, 1996.
38. Zhang, Y., Kensler, T.W., Cho, C.-G., Posner, G.H., and Talalay, P. Anticarcinogenic activities of sulforaphane and structurally related synthetic norbornyl isothiocyanates. *Proc. Natl. Acad. Sci. USA,* 91, 3147, 1994.
39. Babish, J.G. and Stoewsand, G.S. Effect of dietary indole-3-carbinol on the induction of the mixed-function oxidases of rat tissue. *F. Cosmet. Toxicol.,* 16, 151, 1978.
40. Bradfield, C.A. and Bjeldanes, L.F. Effect of dietary indole 3-carbinol on intestinal and hepatic monooxygenase, glutathione *S*-transferase and epoxide hydrolase activities in the rat. *Food Chem. Toxicol.,* 22, 977, 1984.
41. Stoewsand, G.S., Bioactive organosulfur phytochemicals in *Brassica oleracea* vegetables — a review. *Food Chem. Toxicol.,* 33, 537, 1995.
42. Humfrey, C.D.N. Phytoestrogens and human health effects: weighing up the current evidence. *Nat. Toxins,* 6, 51, 1998.
43. Messina, M.J., Persky, V., Setchell, K.D.R., and Barnes, S. Soy intake and cancer risk: a review of the *in vitro* and *in vivo* data. *Nutr. Cancer,* 21, 113, 1994.
44. Wei, H., Bowen, R., Cai, Q., Barnes, S., and Wang, Y. Antioxidant and antipromotional effects of the soybean isoflavone genistein. *Proc. Soc. Exp. Biol. Med.,* 208, 124, 1995.
45. Knight, D.C. and Eden, J.A. A review of the clinical effects of phytoestrogens. *Obstet. Gynecol.,* 87, 897, 1996.
46. Kurzer, M.S. Dietary phytoestrogens. *Annu. Rev. Nutr.,* 17, 353, 1997.
47. Yanagihara, K., Ito, A., Toge, T., and Numoto, M. Antiproliferative effects of isoflavones on human cancer cell lines established from the gastrointestinal tract. *Cancer Res.,* 53, 5815, 1993.
48. Hollman, P.C.H. Bioavailability of flavonoids. *Eur. J. Clin. Nutr.,* 51, S66, 1997.
49. Phang, J.M., Poore, C.M., Lopaczynska, J., and Yeh, G.C. Flavonol-stimulated efflux of 7,12- dimethylbenz(a)anthracene in multidrug -resistant breast cancer cells. *Cancer Res.,* 53, 5977, 1993.

50. Descher, E.E., Ruperto, J., Wong, G., and Newmark, H.L. Quercetin and rutin as inhibitors of azoxymethanol-induced colonic neoplasia. *Carcinogenesis,* 12, 1193, 1991.
51. Dragsted, L.O., Strube, M., and Larsen, J.C. Cancer-protective factors in fruits and vegetables: biochemical and biological background. *Pharm. Toxicol.,* 72 (Suppl.), 116, 1993.
52. Stravic, B., Matula, T.I., and Klassen, R. Effect of flavonoids on mutagencity and bioavailability of xenobiotics in foods, in *Phenolic Compounds in Food and Their Effects on Health. II. Antioxidants and Cancer Prevention,* ACS Symp. Ser. 507, Huang, M.-T., Ho, C.-T., and Lee, C.Y., Eds., Washington, D.C., American Chemical Society, pp 239-249, 1992.
53. Kelloff, G.J., Boone, C.W., Crowell, J.A., Steele, V.E., Lubet, R.A, Doody, L.A., Maolone, W.F., Hawk, E.T., and Sigman, C.C. New Agents for cancer chemoprevention. *J. Cell Biochem.,* 26s, 1, 1996.
54. Crowell, P.L. and Gould, M.N., Chemoprevention and therapy of cancer by *d*-limonene. *Crit. Rev. Oncog.*, 5, 1, 1994.
55. Wattenberg, L.W. and Coccia, J.B. Inhibition of 4-(methylnitrosamino)-1-(3-pyridyl)-1-butanone carcinogenesis in mice by *d*-limonene and citrus fruit oils. *Carcinogenesis,* 12, 115, 1991.
56. Stark, M.J., Burke, Y.D., McKinzie, J.H., Ayoubi, A.S., and Crowell, P.L. Chemotherapy of pancreatic cancer with the monoterpene perillyl alcohol. *Cancer Lett.*, 96, 15, 1995.
57. Reddy, B.S., Wang, C.X., Samaha, H., Lubet, R., Steele, V.E., Kelloff, G.J., and Rao,, C.V. Chemoprevention of colon carcinogenesis by dietary perillyl alcohol. *Cancer Res.*, 57, 420, 1997.
58. Haag, J.D., Lindstrom, M.J., and Gould, M.N. Linonene-induced regression of mammary carcinomas. *Cancer Res.,* 52, 4021, 1992.
59. Haag, J.D. and Gould, M.N. Mammary carcinoma regression induced by perillyl alcohol, a hydroxylated analog of limonene. *Cancer Chemother. Pharmacol.*, 34, 477, 1994.
60. McNamee, D. Limonene trial in cancer. *Lancet*, 342, 801, 1993.
61. Gould, M.N. Cancer chemoprevention and therapy by monoterpenes. *Environ. Health Perspect. Suppl.,* 105, 977, 1997.
62. Craig, W.J. Health-promoting properties of common herbs. *Am. J. Clin. Nutr.*, 70, 491s, 1999.
63. Thompson, L.U., Robb, P., Serraino, M., and Cheung, F. Mammalian lignan production from various foods. *Nutr. Cancer,* 16, 43, 1991.
64. Serraino, M. and Thompson, L.U. The effect of flaxseed supplementation on the initiation and promotional stages of mammary tumorigenesis. *Nutr. Cancer,* 17, 153, 1992.
65. Hirano, T., Fukuoka, K., Oka, K., Naito, T., Hasaki, K., Mitshuhashi, H., and Matsumoto, Y. Antiproliferative activity of mammalian lignan derivatives against the human breast carcinoma cell line, ZR75-1. *Cancer Invest.,* 8, 595, 1990.
66. Serraina, M. and Thompson, L.U. The effect of flaxseed supplementation on early risk markers for mammary carcinogenesis. *Cancer Lett.*, 60, 135, 1991.
67. Lampe, J.W., Martini, M.C., Kurzer, M.S., Adlercreutz, H., and Slavin, J.L. Urinary, lignan and isoflavonoid excretion in premenopausal women consuming flaxseed powder. *Am. J. Clin. Nutr.,* 60, 122, 1994.

68. Krishnaswamy, K. and Raghuramulu, N. Bioactive phytochemicals with emphasis on dietary practices. *Indian J. Med. Res.*, 108, 167, 1998.
69. Nagabhushan, M. and Bhide, S.V. Curcumin as an inhibitor of cancer. *J. Am. Coll. Nutr.*, 11, 192, 1992.
70. Krinsky, N. Effects of carotenoids in cellular and animal models. *Am. J. Clin. Nutr.*, 53, 238s, 1991.
71. Collins, A.R., Olmedilla, B., Southon, S., Granado, F., and Duthie, S.J. Serum carotenoids and oxidative DNA damage in human lymphocytes. *Carcinogenesis,* 19, 2159, 1998.
72. Garland, M., Willett, W.C., Manson, J.E., and Hunter, D.J. Antioxidant, micronutrients and breast cancer. *J. Am. Coll. Nutr.,* 12, 400, 1993.
73. Singh, D.K. and Lippman, S.M. Cancer chemoprevention 1. Retinoids and carotenoids and other classic antioxidants. *Oncology,* 12, 1643, 1998.
74. Omenn, G.S. Chemoprevention of lung cancer: the rise and demise of beta-carotene. *Annu. Rev. Public Health,* 19, 73, 1998.
75. Burton, G.W. and Ingold, K.U. Beta-carotene: an unusual type of lipid antioxidant. *Science*, 224, 569, 1984.
76. The Alpha-Tocopherol, Beta-Carotene Cancer Prevention Study Group. The effect of vitamin E and beta-carotene on the incidence of lung cancer and other cancers in male smokers. *N. Engl. J. Med.,* 330, 1029, 1994.
77. Omenn, G.S., Goodman, G.E., Thronquist, M.D., Balmes, J., Cullen, M.R., Glass, A., Keogh, J.P., Meyskens, F.L., Valanis, B., Williams, J.H., Barnhart, S., and Hammar, S. Effects of a combination of beta carotene and vitamin A on lung cancer and cardiovascular disease. *N. Engl. J. Med.*, 334, 1150, 1996.
78. Mangels, A.R., Holden, J.M., Beecher, G.R., Forman, M.R., and Lanza, E. Carotenoid content of fruits and vegetables: an evaluation of the analytic data. *J. Am. Diet. Assoc.,* 93, 284, 1993.
79. Levy, J., Bosin, E., Feldman, B., Giat, Y., Miinster, A., Danilenki, M., and Sharoni, Y. Lycopene is a more potent inhibitor of human cancer cell proliferation than either α-carotene or β-carotene. *Nutr. Cancer,* 24, 257, 1995.
80. Zhang, L.-X., Cooney, R.V., and Bertram, J.S. Carotenoids enhance gap junctional communication and inhibit lipid peroxidation in C3H/T1/2 cells: relationship to their cancer chemopreventive action. *Carcinogenesis,* 12, 2109, 1991.
81. Zhang, L.-X., Cooney, R.V., and Bertram, J.S. Carotenoids up-regulate Connexin43 gene expression independent of their provitamin A or antioxidant properties. *Cancer Res.*, 52, 5707, 1992.
82. Murakoshi, M., Takayasu, J., Kimura, O., Kohmura, E., Nishino, H., Iwashima, A., Okuzumi, J., Sakai, T., Sugimoto, T., and Imanishi, J. Inhibitory effects of alpha-carotene on proliferation of the human neuroblastoma cell line. *J. Natl. Cancer Inst.*, 81, 1649, 1989.
83. Phillips, R.W., Kikendall, J.W., Luk, G.D, Willis, S.M., Murphy, J.R., Maydonovitch, C., Bowen, P.E. Stacewicz-Saputzakis, M., and Wong, R.K. β-Carotene inhibits rectal mucosal ornithine decarboxylase activity in colon cancer patients. *Cancer Res.*, 53, 3723, 1993.
84. Krinsky, N. Effects of carotenoids in cellular and animal models. *Am. J. Clin. Nutr.*, 53, 238, 1991.
85. Dorgan, J.F. and Schatzkin, A. Antioxidant micronutrients in cancer prevention. *Hematol. Oncol. Clin. North Am.*, 5, 43, 1991.

86. Stahelin, H.B., Gey, K.F., Eichholzer, M., Ludin, E., Bernasconi, F., Thurneysen, J., and Brucbacher, G. Plasma antioxidant vitamins and subsequent cancer mortality in the 12-year follow up of the prospective Basel study. *Am. J. Epidemiol.,* 133, 766, 1991.
87. Harats, D., Chevion, S., Nahir, M., Norman, Y., Sagee, O., and Berry, E.M. Citrus fruit supplementation reduces lipoprotein oxidation in young men ingesting a diet high in saturated fat: presumptive evidence for and interaction between vitamins C and E *in vivo. Am. J. Clin. Nutr.,* 67, 240, 1998.
88. Fraga, C.G., Motchnik, P.A., Shigenaga, M.K., Helbock, H.J., Jacob, R.A., and Ames, B.N. Ascorbic acid protects against endogenous oxidative damage in human sperm. *Proc. Natl. Acad. Sci. USA*, 88, 11003, 1991.
89. Duthie, S.J., Ma, A., Ross, M.A., and Collins, A.R. Antioxidant supplementation decreases oxidative DNA damage in human lymphocytes. *Cancer Res.,* 56, 1291, 1996.
90. Baratsch, H., Ohshima, H., and Pignatelli, B. Inhibitors of endogenous nitrosation mechanisms and implications in human cancer prevention. *Mutat. Res.*, 202, 307, 1988.
91. Xu, G.P., Song, P.J., and Reed, P.. Effects of fruit juices, processed vegetable juice, orange peel and green tea on endogenous formation of *N*-nitrosoproline in subjects from a high-risk area for gastric cancer in Moping County, China. *Eur. J. Cancer Prev.,* 2, 327, 1993.
92. Bertram, J.S., Kolonel, L.N., and Meyskens, F.L. Rationale and strategies for chemoprevention of cancer in humans. *Cancer Res.*, 47, 3012, 1987.
93. Fiala, E.S., Reddy, B.S., and Weisburger, J.H. Naturally occurring anticarcinogenic substances in foodstuffs. *Annu. Rev. Nutr.,* 5, 295, 1985.
94. White, E., Shannon, J.S., and Patterson, R.E. Relationship between vitamin and calcium supplement use and colon cancer. *Cancer Epidemiol. Biomarkers Prev.,* 6, 769, 1997.
95. Hartman, T.J., Albanes, D., Pietinen, P., Hartman, A.M., Rautalahti, A.M., Tangrea, J.A., and Taylor, P.R. The association between baseline vitamin E, selenium and prostate cancer in the alpha-tocopherol, beta-carotene cancer prevention study. *Cancer Epidemiol. Biomarkers Prev.,* 7, 335, 1998.
96. Heinonen, O.P., Albanes, D., Virtamo, J., Taylor, P.R., Hutenen, J.K., Hartman, A.M., Haapakoski, J., Malila, N., Rautalahti, M., Ripatti, S., Maenpaa, H., Teerenhovi, L., Koss, L., Viorlainen, M., and Edwards, B.K. Prostate cancer and supplementation with alpha-tocopherol and beta-carotene: incidence and mortality in a controlled trial. *J. Natl. Cancer Inst.*, 90, 440, 1998.
97. Meydani, S.N., Meydani, M., Blumberg, J.B., Leka, L.S., Siber, G., Loszewksi, R., Thompson, C., Pedroso, M.C., Diamond, R.P., and Stollar, B.P. Vitamin E supplementation and *in vivo* immune response in healthy elderly subjects: a randomized controlled trial. *J. Am. Med. Assoc.* 277, 1380, 1997.
98. Dreosti, I.E. Nutrition, cancer and aging. *Ann. N.Y. Acad. Sci.,* 854, 371, 1998.
99. Giovannucci, E., Stampfer, M.J., Colditz, G.A., Rimm, E.B., Trichopoulus, P., Rosner, B.A., Speizer, F.E., and Willett, W.C. Folate, methionine and alcohol intake and risk of colorectal adenoma. *J. Natl. Cancer Inst.,* 85, 875, 1993.
100. Mason, J.B. Folate and colonic carcinogenesis: searching for a mechanistic, understanding. *J. Nutr. Biochem.,* 5, 170, 1994.

101. Blount, B.C., Mack, M.M., Wehr, C.M., MacGregor, J.T., Hiatt, R.A., Wang, G., Wickromasinghe, S.N., Everson, R.B., and Ames, B.N. Folate deficiency causes uracil misincorporation into human DNA and chromosome breakage: implications for cancer and neuronal damage. *Proc. Natl. Acad. Sci USA,* 94, 3290, 1997.
102. Fenech, M., Aitken, C., and Rinaldi, J. Folate, vitamin B_{12}, homocysteine status and DNA damage in young Australian adults. *Carcinogenesis*, 19, 1163, 1998.
103. Chen, J., Giovannucci, E., Kelsey, K., Rimm, R.B., Stampfer, M.J., Colditz, G.A., Spiegelman, D., Willett, W.C., and Hunter, D.J. A methylenetetrahydrofolate reductase polymorphism and the risk of colorectal cancer. *Cancer Res.,* 56, 4862, 1996.
104. Tucker, K.L., Mahnken, B., Wilson, P.W., Jacques, P., and Selhum, J. Folic acid fortification of the food supply: Potential benefits and risks for the elderly population. *J. Am. Med. Assoc.,* 276, 1879, 1996.
105. Ip, C., Lisk, D.J., and Scimeca, J.A. Potential of food modification in cancer prevention. *Cancer Res.,* 54, 1957s, 1994.
106. Olson, O.E., Novacek, E.J., Whitehead, E.I., and Palmer, S. Investigations on selenium in wheat. *Phytochemistry,* 9, 1181, 1970.
107. Clark, L.C., Combs, G.F., Turnbull, B.W., Slate, E.H., Chalker, D.K., Chow, J., Davis, L.S., Glovar, R.A., Graham, G.F., Gross, E.G., Krongrad, A., Lesher, J.L., Park, K., Sanders, B.S., Smith, C.L., and Taylor, J.R. Effect of selenium supplementation for cancer prevention in patients with carcinoma of the skin. A randomized controlled trial. *J. Am. Med. Assoc.,* 276, 1957, 1996.
108. Kneckt, P., Aromaa, A., Maatela, J., Alfthan, G., Aaran, R.K., Hakama, M., Hakulinen, T., Peto, R., and Teppo, L. Serum selenium and subsequent risk of cancer among Finnish men and women. *J. Natl. Cancer Inst.*, 82, 864, 1990.
109. Clark, L.C., Cantor, K.P., and Allaway, W.H. Selenium in forage crops and cancer mortality in U.S. Counties. *Arch. Environ. Health,* 46, 37, 1991.
110. Chae, Y.-H., Upadhyaya, P., and El-Bayoumy, K. Structure-activity relationships among the ortho -, meta- and para-isomers of phenylenebis (methylene) selenocyanate (XSC) as inhibitors of 7,12-dimethylbenz(*a*)anthracene-DNA binding in mammary glands of female CD rats. *Oncol. Rep.,* 4, 1067, 1997.
111. El-Bayoumy, K., Chae, Y.-H., Upadhyaya, P., and Ip, C. Chemoprevention of mammary cancer by diallyl selenide, a novel organoselenium compound. *Anticancer Res.,* 16, 2911, 1996.
112. Ip, C. and Ganther, H.E. Activity of methylated forms of selenium in cancer prevention. *Cancer Res.,* 50, 1206, 1996.
113. Jao, S.-W., Shen, K.-L., Lee, W., and Ho, Y.-S. Effect of selenium on 1,2-dimethylhydrazine-induced intestinal cancer in rats. *Dis. Colon Rectum,* 39, 628, 1996.
114. Reddy, B.S., Wynn, T.T., El- Bayoumy, K., Upadhyaya, P., Fiala, E., and Rao, C.V. Evaluation of organoselenium compounds for potential chemopreventive properties in colon cancer. *Anticancer Res.,* 16, 1123, 1996.
115. Feng, Y., Finley, J.W., Davis, C.D., Becker, W.K., Fretland, A.J., and Hein, D.W. Dietary selenium reduces the formation of aberrant crypts in rats administered 3,2'-dimethyl-4-aminobiphenyl. *Toxicol. Appl. Pharmacol.*, 157, 36, 1999.
116. Gladyshev, V.N., Factor, V.M., Housseau, F., and Hatfield, D.L. Contrasting patterns of regulation of the antioxidant selenoproteins, thioredoxin reductase, and glutathione peroxidase in cancer cell. *Biochem. Biophys. Res. Commun.,* 251, 488, 1998.
117. Ganther, H.E. Selenium metabolism, selenoproteins and mechanisms of cancer prevention: complexities with thioredoxin reductase. *Carcinogenesis*, 20, 1657, 1999.

118. Lu, J., Jiang, C., Kaeck, M., Ganther, H., Vadhanavikit, S., Ip, C., and Thompson, H. Dissociation of the genotoxic and growth inhibitory effects of selenium. *Biochem. Pharmacol.,* 50, 213, 1995.
119. Stewart, M.J., Spallholz, J.E., Neldner, K.H., and Pence, B.C. Selenium compounds have disparate abilities to impose oxidative stress and induce apoptosis. *Free Rad. Biol. Med.*, 26, 42, 1999.
120. Shimada, T., El-Bayoumy, K., Upadhaya, P., Sutter, T.R., Guengrich, P., and Yamazaki, H. Inhibition of human cytochrome P450-catalyzed oxidations of xenobiotics and procarcinogens by synthetic organoselenium compounds. *Cancer Res.,* 4757, 1997.
121. Davis, C.D., Feng, Y., Hein, D.W., and Finley, J.W. The chemical form of selenium influences 3,2'-dimethyl-4-aminobiphenyl-DNA adduct formation in rat colon, *J. Nutr.,* 129, 63, 1999.
122. Ip, C., Lisk, D.J. and Stoewsand, G.S. Mammary cancer prevention by regular garlic and selenium enriched garlic. *Nutr. Cancer,* 17, 279, 1992.
123. Ip, C. and Lisk, D.J. Characterization of tissue selenium profiles and anticarcinogenic responses in rats fed natural sources of selenium-rich products. *Carcinogenesis*, 15, 573, 1994.
124. Ip, C. and Lisk, D.J. Enrichment of selenium in allium vegetables for cancer prevention. *Carcinogenesis,* 15, 1881, 1994.
125. Ip, C. and Lisk, D.J. Efficacy of cancer prevention by high selenium-garlic is primarily dependent on the action of selenium. *Carcinogenesis,* 16, 2649, 1995.
126. Cai, X.-J., Block, E., Uden, P.C., Zhang, X., Quimby, B.D., and Sullivan, J.J. Allium chemisty: identification of selenamino acids in ordinary and selenium-enriched garlic, onion and broccoli using gas chromatography with atomic emission detection. *J. Agric. Food Chem.*, 43, 1754, 1995.
127. Finley, J.W., Davis, C.D., and Feng, Y., Selenium from high-selenium broccoli is protective against colon cancer in rats, *J. Nutr.*, in press.

18 Raw Food Diets: Health Benefits and Risks

Ingrid Hoffmann and Claus Leitzmann

CONTENTS

18.1 HISTORICAL BACKGROUND

Humans have always pursued ways to improve health and prolong life. Besides other lifestyle factors, diet was always and is still a factor associated with desires and hopes in this connection. Pythagoras (570-500 B.C.) proclaimed vegetarianism to be an ideal way to fulfill this dream. During the nineteenth and twentieth century many movements for healthy and life prolonging lifestyles were initiated. Based on personal and clinical experiences a number of pioneers, most of whom were physicians, developed dietary therapy regimens which aimed to support healing and were not conceived as long-term diets. Most concepts were designed to bring people back to a natural way of life. One basic aspect of these diets was the recommendation for the consumption of exclusively or mostly natural food, meaning unheated and unprocessed food items.

One proponent of a natural diet was the Swiss physician Maximilian Bircher-Benner (1867-1939) who documented the healing effects of a diet consisting only of selected fresh and unprepared foods. He developed a holistic therapy going back to the principles of Hippocrates (460–370 B.C.). Bircher-Benner also tried to lead his patients to a natural lifestyle. The main focus of his therapy was a simple diet

0-8493-0038-X/97/$0.00+$.50

with foods that have a healing effect. He considered all natural raw and fresh food as wholesome and therefore adequate to support the self-healing ability of the body. It was his understanding that processing or heating food reduces its wholesomeness, since it leads to a loss of healing power. For severe illnesses Bircher-Benner recommended a strict vegan raw food diet. Two of the three meals per day, he advised, should comprise of only fruits and nuts; the other one of raw vegetables, fruits, and nuts (Leitzmann et al., 1999).

In the U.S. a group of physicians started a movement in 1822 that came to be known as Natural Hygiene. Herbert Shelton (1895–1985) made this movement very popular after World War II. His writings are still being read today (Shelton, 1964). His idea was that the deterioration of health occurs only when natural life laws are broken and that by means of a wholesome nutrition a self-cleaning process of the body is activated. Adherents of Natural Hygiene recommend a raw food diet consisting mainly of fruits. Apart from nutrition, other factors like physical activities, fresh air, and sunshine are claimed to be necessary to support health. There are many points of view within the Natural Hygiene movement. For example, one is that only the consumption of food items that have ripened in sunlight (fruits, vegetables, nuts, and seeds) is recommended.

Today the very popular Fit-for-Life program, developed by Marilyn and Harvey Diamond (Diamond and Diamond, 1985) is also based on Natural Hygiene. One basic element of this program is the concept of body cycles. According to that principle, the body prefers certain times of the day for the intake of food, for utilizing nutrients, and for excreting the metabolic products. The concept requires that before noon only fruits should be eaten. No other foods are allowed in the morning. Also, for the rest of the day foods with a high water content like raw fruits and vegetables are advised. In addition fruits should never be consumed simultaneously with other foods. The Diamonds recommend separate consumption of foods rich in protein and foods rich in carbohydrates. Processed and concentrated foods as well as meat, dairy products, cereals, and legumes are considered to be "dead" foods. The human being is seen as a frugivore. The Fit-for-Life program is predominantly a vegetarian raw food diet.

Today's raw food movement is very divergent. The diet can span from pure raw food to diets in which foods are not processed, chopped, or mixed with other food items. A study of the literature shows that raw food diets are subdivided into vegetarian and nonvegetarian type (Figure 18.1). Some regimens contain meat and meat products, others solely fruits. Staple foods like meat, dairy products, and cereals and cereal products are largely avoided. Therefore, fruits and vegetables make up a high percentage of the food consumed. The main reasons for practicing a raw food diet, as stated by its followers, are to attain health, to prevent illness, and to live in a natural and healthy way for a long time (Koebnick et al., 1995, 1997c).

Within the raw food movement, the theory of Guy-Claude Burger has a special position. According to his instincto-therapy, the body knows exactly what kind of food, and which and how much of a nutrient is needed in a certain situation. The smell and taste senses help the body to select the right food. Only if a food item smells and tastes good to a person may it be eaten at that time. The body indicates

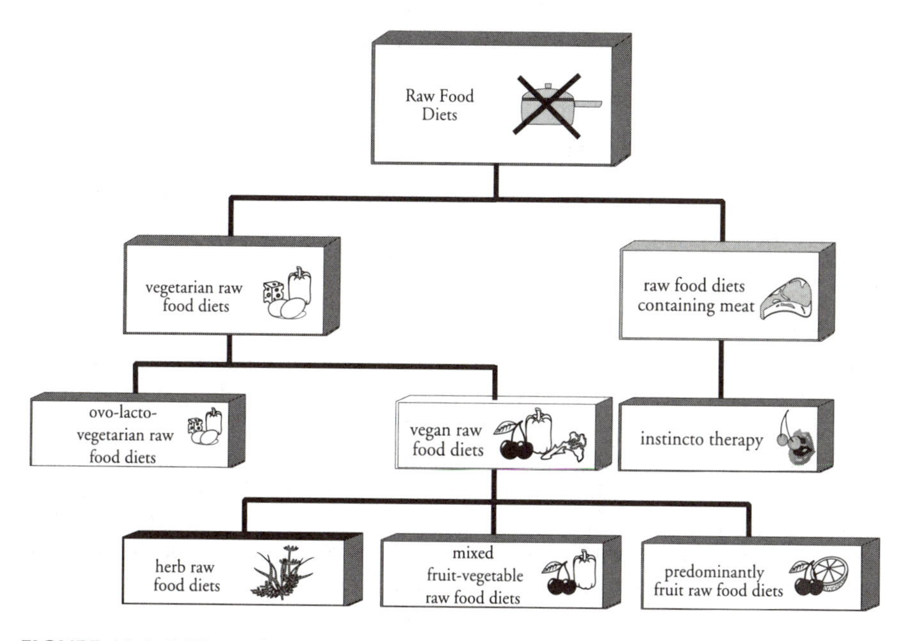

FIGURE 18.1 Different forms of raw food diets.

when enough of this food has been eaten since it then starts to tastes bitter. This instinct works only with natural, unprocessed foods. For all raw foods, even eggs, fresh meat, and fish, the body indicates whether it needs it or not. Burger's instincto-therapy is an omnivorous, strictly raw food diet (Burger, 1992).

The definition of raw food diets according to the Giessen Raw Food Working Group is an attempt to develop a basis for comparison of data reported in the literature (Table 18.1).

TABLE 18.1
Definition of Raw Food Diets

Raw food diets consist predominantly or exclusively of unheated foods, mainly of plant origin (partly of animal origin).

Some foods are included that require a certain degree of heating for their production (e.g., cold-pressed oils and honey) as well as foods that require a certain amount of heat during their processing (e.g., dried fruits, dried meat and fish, certain nuts).

Furthermore, cold-smoked produce (e.g., meat and fish) as well as pickled or fermented vegetables can be included in a raw food diet.

Source: Giessen Raw Food Working Group.

Even though raw food diets are claimed to improve health, the arguments for the different diets are not always in agreement with current scientific knowledge. However, persons following these diets report subjective improvements of their well-being. Since raw food diets — from a scientific point of view — can be very unbalanced, the question arises whether such a diet is suitable to guarantee or even improve the nutrition and health status when practiced on a long-term basis.

18.2 RESEARCH ON RAW FOOD DIETS

To evaluate the health benefits and risks of raw food diets it is necessary to examine the effects of such diets scientifically. Therefore, it is also essential to investigate persons following raw food diets on a long-term basis and also persons whose diets contain different amounts of raw food. So far, only a very few studies on raw food diets have been conducted. The few publications report only on selected aspects of the nutrition and health status of raw food dieters. Most of those studies are short-term interventions that include only small numbers of participants eating extreme forms of raw food diets.

Douglass et al. (1985) investigated 32 outpatients with essential hypertension of whom 28 were overweight. They were shifted to a diet with an average of 62% of their energy intake as uncooked food for a mean duration of 6.7 months. The results show a mean weight loss of 3.8 kg and a mean reduction of the diastolic blood pressure of 17.8 mmHg. Switching back to the cooked diets canceled the beneficial effects of the uncooked diet in some patients.

Ling and Hänninen (1992) examined the effect of eating an uncooked extreme vegan diet (living food diet) and then readapting to a Western-type diet on the enzyme activities of the fecal microflora and on toxic substances in the blood. Nine volunteers switched to an uncooked vegan diet for one month and switched back to their usual diet during the following month. During those two months, nine controls consumed the usual diet. The activity of bacterial enzymes, which were investigated in connection with colon cancer risk, decreased within the first week of dietary intervention: fecal urease by 66%, choloylglycine hydrolase by 55%, β-glucoronidase by 33%, and β-glucosidase by 40%. Those lower levels remained until the previous diet was reinstituted and then they returned to previous values within a fortnight. Phenol and *p*-cresol concentrations in serum and urine declined during the raw food period and increased to normal values within one month after returning to the usual diet. This study shows that an uncooked extreme vegan diet modifies the colonic environment, which may be related to a lower risk of colon cancer for raw food dieters.

The effect of a long-term adherence (5.2 ± 3.9 years) to an uncooked, strict vegan diet was investigated by Rauma et al. (1995a,b) in a cross-sectional study with 20 Finnish middle-aged women and 1 man and a longitudinal study with 9 women and 1 man. Compared to a matched group of omnivorous controls, the energy intake of the vegans did not differ. However, in vegans the proportion of energy derived from protein was lower and from carbohydrates was higher, whereas the fat intake did not differ.

Except for copper and zinc, the intake of the other nutrients (vitamin A, vitamin E, and selenium) met or exceeded the RDAs. While the intake of β-carotene, vitamin C, vitamin E, and copper was higher in the vegans, the controls had a higher selenium intake. Zinc and vitamin A intake did not differ between the study groups.

The blood concentrations of β-carotene, vitamin C, vitamin E, and the activity of erythrocyte superoxide dismutase were significantly higher in the vegans than in the omnivores. The better antioxidant status of persons adhering to a long-term and strict, uncooked vegan diet is due to a higher intake of the particular nutrients. The serum vitamin B_{12} levels in the living-food dieters were significantly lower than in the controls, reflecting a low vitamin B_{12} intake. During the longitudinal study six of the nine examined vegans showed a continuing deterioration of the serum vitamin B_{12} concentration. Vegans and omnivores did not differ in the activity of glutathione peroxidase even though the selenium intake of the vegans was lower. Parameters of iron status were also not different between the study groups.

To our knowledge, the only study investigating the effects of different forms of raw food diets — varying in the inclusion of animal products and the amount of raw food over a long-term and with a larger number of participants — is the Giessen Raw Food Study (Koebnick et al., 1994, 1997a,b,c, 1999; Strassner et al., 1997, 1998).

18.3 THE GIESSEN RAW FOOD STUDY

The objective of the Giessen Raw Food Study was the examination of the health behavior and nutrition status of raw food dieters. It was of special interest to investigate the effects of different consumption patterns. Therefore the participants were grouped either according to the inclusion of animal products (omnivores: include all food groups; ovo-lacto-vegetarians: exclude meat, fish, sea foods, and products thereof; vegans: omitting all animal foods from their diet) or according to the amount of raw food consumed (70 to 80%, 80 to 90%, or up to 100% of the total amount of food eaten) (Strassner et al., 1997).

Raw food dieters were recruited by call-ups for project participation in nine different nationwide magazines and by flyers at appropriate lectures, congresses, and self-help organizations. Over 2000 responders were screened by a short qualifying questionnaire. Criteria for further study participation were 25 to 64 years of age, raw food consumption for at least 14 months, proportion of raw food at least 70%, and nonsmokers. A group of 201 adults (94 men and 107 women) were selected for the study. Health habits were investigated by means of a detailed questionnaire. Primary areas of interest in addition to sociodemographic data were food preference and avoidance, health and diseases, as well as physical activity and recreational activities. The questionnaire included a food frequency table over a 1-month period for assessing food intake patterns. A 7-day estimated food record was especially developed and validated for this study (Strassner, 1998).

The participants had followed a raw food diet for at least 14 months, on average for 3.5 years, and with a maximum duration of 38 years. Thus their metabolism had most likely adapted to their new diet. The age of the participants ranged from 25 to 64 years with an average age of 46 years. The group was characterized by a high level of education and a high per capita income. The participants were physically very active — almost half participated regularly in sport activities. Further health-consciousness behavior was also distinctive: all participants were nonsmokers (study criteria), almost 60% did not drink alcohol and the remainder drank only up to 15 g alcohol per day, less than 30% took medication or supplements and only a few female participants took oral contraceptives. Many of the participants regularly made use of a relaxation technique: 26% meditated for a minimum of 1 hour a week, 21% used self hypnosis, and 21% practiced yoga. About 47% of the participants stated that they fasted regularly. Of these, 57% followed a total fast while 31% followed a juice fast (Strassner et al., 1997; 1998).

Of the group, 64% indicated health concerns as the major reason for changing to a raw food diet, followed by the desire for better performance (9%) and ecological reasons (3%). More than half of the participants (61%) gave a disease as the reason for changing to a raw food diet. Illnesses most often mentioned in this connection were allergies (n = 12), gastrointestinal diseases (n = 9) and rheumatism (n = 8). Most of the participants were highly content with their raw food diet and 98% intended to follow it as a long-term regimen.

18.3.1 Dietary Habits

The food consumption pattern of the investigated raw food dieters showed considerable differences to other dietary regimens. Although the participants drank, on average, less than 1 l/d, they had a liquid intake of about 2.5 l/d from foods with a high water content and met the RDAs. The participants consumed about 2 kg of food a day, most of this raw and of plant origin. The food eaten consisted, on average, of two-thirds fruits (67.8%), almost one-quarter vegetables and legumes (23.3%), and four additional food groups, each making up 1.0–1.5% (cereals and cereal products 1.4%, nuts 1.3%, milk and dairy products 1.3%, seeds 1.0%). Apples, oranges, and bananas were the fruits most often eaten, however, the findings may well be influenced by the season in which the study was carried out (February to April). The daily amount of these fruits consumed (average 100 to 300 g/d) was more than twice as high as that of other fruits (Strassner, 1998).

The participants of the Giessen Raw Food Study adhered to several different raw food diets. This divergence becomes obvious when dividing the participants into subgroups according to the consumption of animal products (Table 18.2). Potatoes, bread, and baked goods as well as cereal products played a marginal role compared to the average Western diet. The consumption of soy products was less than in other alternative dietary regimens. Where foods of animal origin were consumed, these were preferred raw. A number of differences in the consumption of food groups is statistically significant mainly between the vegan diet and the other two diet groups (Strassner et al., 1997).

Instead of the inclusion of foods of animal origin as a criteria for differentiation, the study groups can be divided according to the amount of raw food eaten (expressed as percentage of the total amount of food eaten, without beverages). On this basis three raw food groups (RFG) were formed: 70 to 80% raw food = 75 RFG; 80 to 90% raw food = 85 RFG; 90 to 100% raw food = 95 RFG.

The higher the amount of raw food consumed the more confined was the food selection. The 95 RFG consumed less food of animal origin, cereal products, bread, and baked products but ate more fruits, vegetables, and raw legumes than the 75 RFG; the 85 RFG being in-between. A higher amount of raw food also meant a

TABLE 18.2
Mean Food Consumption (g/d) of the Participants Following Omnivore, Ovo-Lacto-Vegetarian, or Vegan Raw Food Diets

Foodstuffs	Total Participants	Omnivore	Ovo-Lacto-Vegetarian	Vegan
Food, total[2]	2098	2293	1948	2144
Raw foods, total[2]	1976	2159	1787	2098
Foods of plant origin[2]	2050	2190	1908	2141
Foods of animal origin[1,2,3]	49	109	40	0
Fruit and fruit products[2]	1423	1559	1279	1522
Vegetables and legumes	489	481	477	519
Nuts[1]	28	32	25	29
Seeds	20	21	15	27
Bread and baked goods[1,3]	19	27	25	2.2
Cereal products[1,3]	29	23	39	18
Soy products[2]	3.5	0	3.1	7.7
Dairy products[1,2,3]	28	40	38	0
Eggs, total[1,3]	3.6	7.1	3.6	0
Meat and meat products[1,2]	11	38	0	0
Seafood[1,2]	10	36	0	0

Test of significance according to Mann-Whitney (U-test): significant differences between (1) omnivore and vegans, (2) omnivore and ovo-lacto-vegetarians, (3) ovo-lacto-vegetarian and vegans.

higher weight of the daily consumption. The 75 RFG did not consume raw potatoes, raw meat, raw eggs, and raw milk, while the stricter raw food dieters did.

18.3.2 Energy and Nutrient Intake

In the ovo-lacto-vegetarian and vegan groups the majority of the participants did not achieve the RDAs for nutrient energy intake when age and gender are considered. The energy intake of the male participants was significantly higher than that of the females. Most of the participants (57%) did not meet the recommended energy intake according to their age.

Apparently, only with a mixed raw food diet did it seem possible for the participants to reach the recommendations for energy, even when the high dietary fiber concentration of the diet is considered. The chief source of dietary energy for the participants is fruit, followed by vegetables, and legumes. The food groups sweets/desserts, sweeteners, drinks, and fats/oils play a relatively unimportant role as energy sources.

The macronutrients ratio of the raw food diets corresponds to the recommendations. Since sufficient energy intake as a whole is problematic, the macronutrients are most likely utilized to a large extent directly as energy sources (Strassner, 1998).

The participants showed on average an insufficient protein intake. Only the more liberal forms of the raw food diets (concerning the amount of plant and raw foods) achieved the recommendations. The average protein intake of the participants corresponded to the region of the recommendations minus added safety factors. The protein sources of Western diets play a lesser role in the mixed or vegetarian raw food diets. Almost 50% of the protein intake results from fruits and vegetables; for vegan participants this amounts to about 60%. Nuts and seeds each contribute about 10% to the protein intake (Strassner, 1998).

The nutrient intakes of omnivore, ovo-lacto-vegetarian, and vegan participants showed distinct differences (Table 18.3). For vitamin A, E, B_1, B_6, and C, as well as for magnesium and iron, the median intake of all groups was above the recommendations. For vitamins D and B_{12}, as well as zinc and calcium, none of the groups reached the recommended intakes, whereas the participants following an omnivorous raw food diet had the highest intake of the three subgroups. For vitamins A, B_6, D, and the minerals magnesium and iron, there were statistically significant differences between the omnivore and ovo-lacto-vegetarian intake: the ovo-lacto-vegetarians having the lowest median intake for all nutrients mentioned other than iron (Strassner et al., 1997; National Research Council,1989; Food and Nutrition Board, 1997, 1998).

With a higher amount of raw food the intake of β-carotene, vitamins D, E, K, B_6, C, and folic acid increased, while the intake of vitamin B_{12} was extremely low (0.2 μg/d). The 85 RFG showed the lowest intake of carbohydrates, fat, vitamin B_1 and vitamin B_2, magnesium, calcium, phosphorus, iron, and zinc.

TABLE 18.3
Median Daily Nutrient Intake of Omnivore, Ovo-Lacto-Vegetarian, and Vegan Raw Food Diets

Nutrients	Total Participants	Omnivore	Ovo-Lacto-Vegetarian	Vegan
Nutrient energy (kcal)[1,2]	1976	2117	1852	1899
Vitamin A (mg RE)[2]	2.4	2.8	2	2.4
Retinol (μg)[1,2,3]	41	121	65	0
β-carotene (mg)	14	15	11	15
Vitamin D (μg)[2]	3.2	4.4	2.9	3.2
Vitamin E (mg)	19	21	19	19
Vitamin B_2 (mg)[1,2]	1.5	1.8	1.4	1.4
Vitamin B_6 (mg)[2]	3	3.7	2.8	3
Vitamin B_{12} (μg)[1,2,3]	0.3	1.4	0.3	0
Vitamin C (mg)	442	496	439	424
Magnesium (mg)[2]	596	646	570	618
Calcium	738	831	732	714
Iron (mg)[2]	19	21	18	18
Zinc (mg)[1,2]	8.8	9.9	8.6	8.1

Test of significance according to Mann-Whitney (U-test): significant differences between (1) omnivore and vegans, (2) omnivore and ovo-lacto-vegetarian, (3) ovo-lacto-vegetarian and vegan.

18.3.3 Blood Parameters

The low intake of some essential nutrients affects the nutrient supply of the body as observed in their concentration in blood samples (Koebnick et al., 1997b).

The consumption of raw fruits and vegetables results in a low bioavailability of carotenoids. The high intake of β-carotene has a negative influence on the absorption rate. Because of the low intake of vitamin A a high conversion rate of β-carotene into retinol may be expected. This results in a plasma retinol level at the lower end of the standard range. About 70% of the raw food dieters showed β-carotene concentrations within the standard range. The status of vitamin A was good, the one of β-carotene just sufficient.

The high intake of vitamin E did not lead to corresponding high blood concentrations. This may be due to the inhibition of vitamin E absorption because of high concentrations of polyunsaturated fatty acids in the diets.

The nutrient status of vitamins B_1, B_2, and B_6 were within the normal range. The high intake of folic acid led to high concentrations in the blood. But high plasma folate levels may also be due to the low vitamin B_{12} intake (Dagnelie, 1989). For vitamin B_{12}, critical values were found for about 20% of the raw food dieters. A clear relationship between low vitamin B_{12} concentrations and increased homocysteine levels are observed (Figure 18.2).

The supply of magnesium was adequate for about half of the group. The serum iron and ferritin concentrations were rather low. With increasing duration of a raw food diet the iron concentrations decreased further and 43% of the men and 15% of the women were anemic.

18.3.4 Body Weight

Even though most of the raw food diets are considered as a long-term form of nutrition, the Diamonds suggest that their raw food diet may additionally be used to reduce body weight (Diamond and Diamond, 1992; Koebnick et al., 1997c). Furthermore, fasting periods and regular enemas are often recommended by proponents of raw food diets as a method of body cleansing. About half of the participating raw food dieters fasted at least once a year, some of them for several weeks. It is reported that very long fasting periods (>100 days) can result in morphological changes in cardiac muscle, with ECG changes caused by protein deficiency. Even though none of the study participants fasted for such a long period of time, fasting for them could have been a risk because of their low energy stores and low body weight, particularly in association with their low-energy diet.

The results of the Giessen Raw Food Study showed a substantial reduction in body weight for participants during long-term consumption of a raw food diet. The body weight first decreased and then usually increased to a level below the initial weight. Consequently, the strict raw food dieters showed a greater loss of body weight than the moderate raw food dieters. Changes in body weight usually indicate a change in energy balance and reflect changes in energy stores and in active body tissues (Shetty and James, 1994). Decreasing body weight and concomitant under-

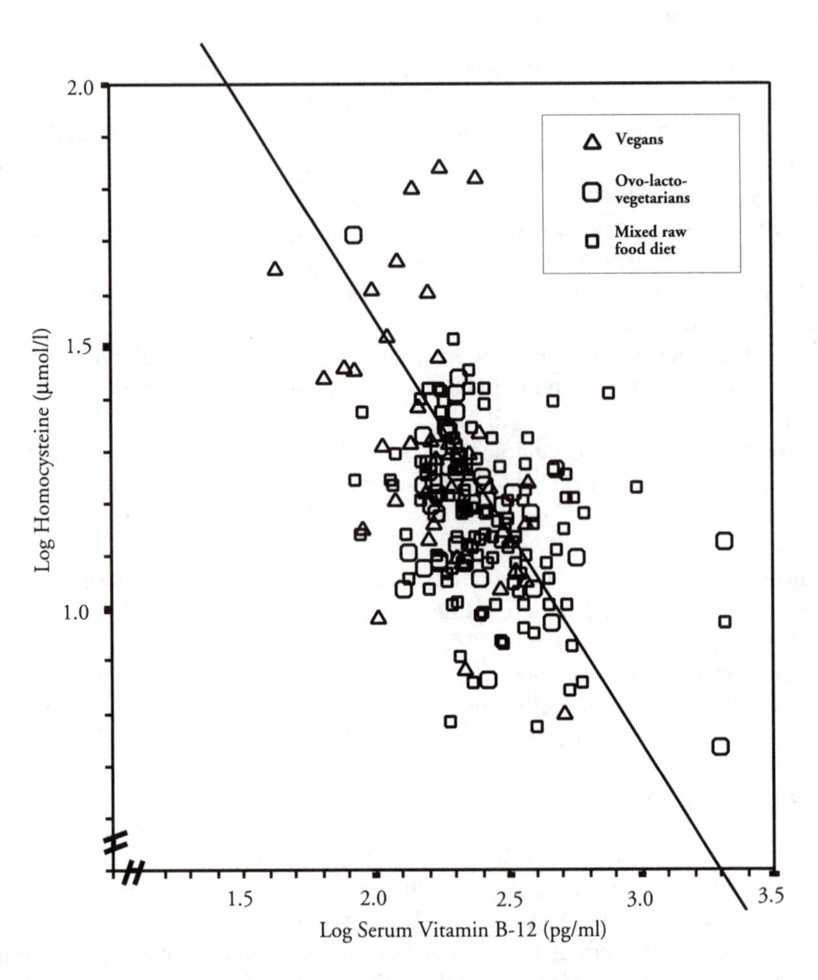

FIGURE 18.2 Relationship between serum vitamin B_{12} and homocyteine concentrations.

nutrition result in a greater visceral mass to muscle mass ratio (Soares and Shetty, 1991).

The body mass index (BMI) reflects body energy stores and is used as an indicator for chronic energy deficiency (Norgan and Ferro-Luzzi, 1982; Ferro-Luzzi et al., 1992; James, 1994) since it shows a strong correlation with body fat (Naidu and Rao, 1994; Shetty and James, 1994). Most participants of the Giessen Raw Food Study had BMI values within the normal range; however, 25% of the females and 14.7% of the males were below the normal range — in some cases the BMI reflecting a chronic energy deficiency. Undernutrition affects only a small group of the average German population — 5.6% of the females and 3.8% of the males, mostly under the age of 34 years, are underweight. The optimum range of BMI which is compatible with good health is 20.1 to 25.0 kg/m^2 for males and 18.7 to 23.8 kg/m^2 for females (WHO, 1985; Shetty and James, 1994). Low body weight is often reported for ovo-lacto-vegetarians and vegans (Hahn and Leitzmann, 1996), but a BMI reflecting chronic energy deficiency is rarely observed, in contrast to raw food dieters. The main reason for a low BMI for raw food dieters is the consumption of a strict raw food diet. Furthermore, BMI is correlated with the duration of the raw food diet and the vegan regimen (Koebnick et al., 1999).

Very strict raw food dieters have higher odds of becoming underweight than moderate raw food dieters. Therefore, a strict raw food diet has to be considered as a risk to health if practiced for a long time. The absence of obesity in raw food dieters should be seen positively, but their extreme low body weight may be a problem. While an energy restriction for many adults consuming an average Western diet is recommended, a strict raw food diet cannot guarantee an adequate energy supply (Strassner, 1998). A low BMI for raw food dieters indicates low body energy stores and chronic energy deficiency. In a mostly vegan diet like the raw food diets, with low protein and energy intake, protein metabolism can be affected to the point of protein energy malnutrition.

18.3.5 Menstruation

A high percentage of the women participating in the study (70%) had irregularities in their menstruation after changing to a raw food diet (Figure 18.3). A total absence of menstruation was observed in 23% of female raw food dieters of childbearing age. With increasing amounts of raw food the BMI decreased and the odds of amenorrhea increased. The participants judged this as a success of their diet, since proponents of raw food diets view menstruation as a process of cleansing. They claim that when eating enough raw food menstruation stops, so that the cleansing process is no longer required (Shelton, 1964; Burger, 1992). This attitude concerning amenorrhea has no scientific basis and ignores the possibility that amenorrhea may be an indicator of impaired health.

Nutritional deficiencies, low body fat stores, chronic energy deficiency, and low body weight which is related to changes in body composition are associated with amenorrhea (Shetty and James, 1994; Benson et al., 1996). Amenorrhea is also observed with eating disorders like bulimia and anorexia (Kopp et al., 1997; McIver et al., 1997).

A low BMI is indicative for chronic energy deficiency and is associated with amenorrhea. Amenorrhea can result in impaired fertility (Shetty and James, 1994; Fruth and Worrell, 1995; McIver et al., 1997). When estrogen levels are low, changes in mineral, glucose, and fat metabolism accompany amenorrhea. These metabolic changes affect bone and cardiovascular health, increasing the risk of osteoporosis and coronary heart disease in later life (Fruth and Worrell, 1995; McIver et al., 1997).

For the female raw food dieters of this study the odds of having amenorrhea increased with the strictness of the raw food diet. For women of childbearing age there may be further consequences for the unborn child in case of pregnancy.

The incidence of amenorrhea in female raw food dieters is also a sign for future functional problems in the long-term consumption of a raw food diet. As shown in this study, the main determinant for the BMI and the incidence of amenorrhea is the amount of raw food in the diet. On the basis of the obtained data and the reports

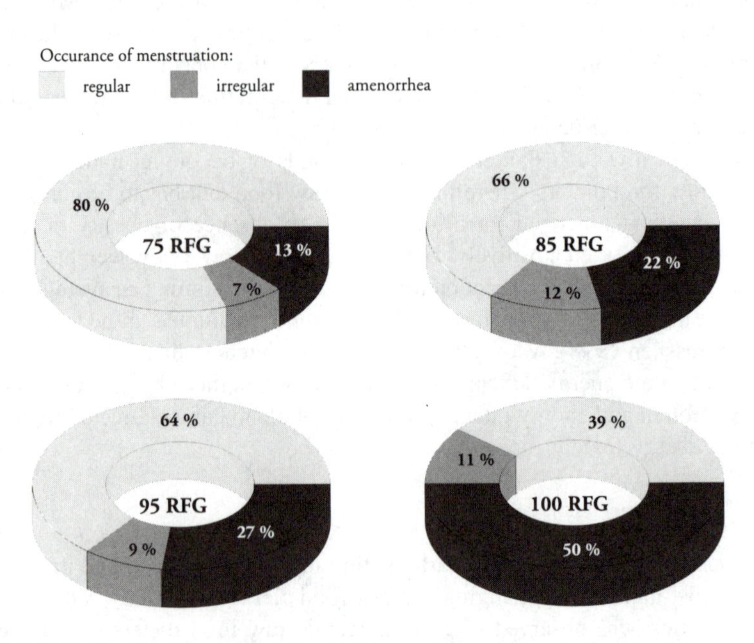

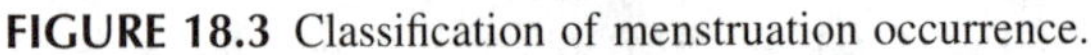
FIGURE 18.3 Classification of menstruation occurrence.

in the literature, a strict raw food diet with amounts of raw food over 90% cannot be recommended (Koebnick et al., 1999).

18.3.6 Dental health

Dental erosions are caused by chemical processes which may be due, among others, to dietary sources like acidic drinks or foods. Since raw food diets often contain large amounts of citrus fruits, they bear a certain risk of dental erosions. About half of the participants ate 9 to 23.5 kg fruit per week. Additionally, about half of the participants ate fruit from 5 up to 16 times a day. A high frequency of fruit intake is considered to be as a risk factor in erosion occurrence (Linkosalo and Markkanen, 1985; Järvinen et al., 1991; Lussi et al., 1991).

To determine the frequency and severity of erosions, a subgroup of 64 females and 66 males consuming more than 95% raw food was investigated using study models (Ganss et al., 1999). A control group of 76 sex- and age-matched outpatients were recruited from a dental clinic.

Compared to the control group subjects, those living on a raw food diet had significantly more dental erosions. Only 2.3% of the raw food group (13.2% of the controls) had no erosive defects, whereas 37.2% had at least one tooth with a moderate erosion (55.2% of the controls) and 60.5% had at least one tooth with a severe erosion (31.6% of the controls). Within the raw food group no significant correlation was found between nutrition or oral health data and the prevalence of erosions. Still, even at the lowest intake frequency, lowest amount of fruit eaten, or the shortest duration of the diet already means a risk factor for dental erosions. This corresponds with the finding that consuming citrus fruits more than twice a day may increase the risk of erosions 37-fold (Järvinen et al., 1991).

This study shows that following a raw food diet bears an increased risk of dental erosion. In the raw food group the median erosions index (percent of affected surfaces of surfaces at risk) was 24.2 compared to 7.4 in the control group (Ganss et al., 1999).

18.4 RAW FOOD DIET AND PREVENTIVE DIETARY RECOMMENDATIONS

Based on large epidemiological studies and other scientific knowledge, dietary recommendations for the prevention of nutrition-related diseases like cancer and coronary heart disease are promoted by experts and public health organizations such as the American Heart Association and the World Cancer Research Institute. The most important recommendations are eating a variety of foods, primarily based on foods of plant origin (vegetables, fruits, and whole grain products), maintaining or reducing body weight, and choosing a diet low in fat, saturated fatty acids, and cholesterol. Moreover, sugar and salt should be used in moderation, and alcohol, if used at all, should be consumed in moderate amounts (Nutrition Committee, American Heart Association, 1996; World Cancer Research Fund and American Institute of Cancer Research, 1997).

The data of the Giessen Raw Food Study show that the raw food dieters have a healthy life style — all participants were nonsmokers (selection criteria), almost 60% did not drink alcohol, less than 30% took medication or supplements, and only a few females who participated took oral contraceptives. Comparing their food consumption with national and international recommendations it becomes obvious that about half of their energy intake derives from fruits and vegetables — increasing with the strictness of the raw food diet. The official recommendation is that 7% or more of the energy intake should be provided by fruits and vegetables (World Cancer Research Fund and American Institute of Cancer Research, 1997). The absolute amount of fruits and vegetables consumed exceeds the recommendation of 400–800 g by at least three times. But the recommendation to eat 600–800 g of starchy or protein-rich foods of plant origin is not met. The study participants eat about half or one-third of it. Only few include meat in their diet.

A comparison with the Vegetarian Food Guide Pyramid is noteworthy. Unrefined and minimally processed foods as well as a variety and abundance of plant foods are emphasized (Haddad et al., 1999). Whole grains and legumes such as soybeans and soy-based products form the basis of the pyramid. On the next level (indicating smaller amounts) are fruits and vegetables, followed by nuts and seeds. This is in contrast to the consumption patterns of the raw food dieters in the study. On average, more than 90% of their diet derives from fruits and vegetables.

It becomes obvious that the food selection of the raw food dieters is too limited to meet the preventive recommendations to their full extent. The higher the amount of raw food the greater the risks. Even though the intake of protective nutrients is high, for some of the essential nutrients the intake is too low to cover the requirements and therefore several nutrient-based deficiencies are hard to avoid. The total nutrient supply is provided almost exclusively by fruits and vegetables. As a consequence, the intake of nutrients that are usually provided by cereal products and/or foods of animal origin, such as the vitamins D, B_2, B_{12}, and niacin, as well as the minerals zinc, calcium, and iodine, is insufficient (Strassner, 1998). This deficit may even be harmful. For example, the low intake of vitamin B_{12} may lead to an increase of homocysteine, which is an independent risk factor for coronary heart diseases.

In conclusion, for an evaluation of raw food diets it is necessary to compare them to other diets, including the amount of raw food eaten, the food selection, and the energy intake. On the basis of the data presented, a strict raw food diet is not recommended, especially not for groups at risk such as pregnant or lactating women, children, or the elderly.

Whereas a strict raw food diet cannot be recommended, with adequate nutritional knowledge a moderate raw food diet including foods like whole grain bread or other whole grain products as well as products of animal origin — especially dairy products — may guarantee good nutrition and health status in adults. However, the total amount of food eaten must be sufficient to supply enough energy and protein. The positive and preventive aspects of raw food diets are desirable, especially when practiced for a limited period (Koebnick et al., 1997b).

ACKNOWLEDGMENTS

Supported by a grant from the Stoll VITA Foundation, Waldshut, Germany.
We are indebted to Corinna Koebnick and Gunther Weiss for their expert help.

REFERENCES

Benson, J.E., Engelbert-Fenton, K.A., Eisenman, P.A., Nutritional aspects of amenorrhea in the female athlete triad, *Int. J. Sport Nutr.*, 6, 134, 1996.

Burger, G.C., *Die Rohkosttherapie*, Heyne, München, 1992.

Dagnelie, P.C., van Staveren, W.A., Vergote, F.J.V.R.A., Dingjan, P.G., van den Berg, H., Hautvast, J.G.A.J., Increased risk of vitamin B_{12} and iron deficiency in infants on macrobiotic diets. *Am. J. Clin. Nutr.*, 50, 818, 1989.

Diamond, H., Diamond, M., *Fit for Life*, Warner Books, New York, 1985.

Douglass, J.M., Rasgon, I.M., Fleiss, P.M., Schmidt, R.D., Peters, S.N., Abelmann, E.A., Effects of a raw food diet on hypertension and obesity, *Southern Med. J.*, 78 (7), 841, 1985.

Ferro-Luzzi, A., Sette, S., Franklin, M., James, W.P.T., A simplified approach of assessing adult chronic energy deficiency, *Eur. J. Clin. Nutr.*, 46, 173, 1992.

Food and Nutrition Board, Institute of Medicine, Dietary reference intakes for calcium, phosphorus, magnesium, vitamin D, and fluoride, National Academy Press, Washington, D.C., 1997.

Food and Nutrition Board, Institute of Medicine, Dietary reference intakes for thiamin, riboflavin, niacin, vitamin B_6, folate, vitamin B_{12}, pantothenic acid, biotin, and choline. Prepublications copy, National Academy Press, Washington, D.C., 1998.

Fruth, S.J., Worrell, T.W., Factors associated with menstrual irregularities and decreased bone mineral density in female athletes, *J. Orthop. Sports Phys. Ther.*, 22, 26, 1995.

Ganss, C., Schlechtriemen, M., Klimek, J., Dental erosions in subjects living on a raw food diet, *Caries Res.*, 33, 74, 1999.

Haddad, E.H., Sabaté, J., Whitten, C.G., Vegetarian food guide pyramid: a conceptual framework, *Am. J. Clin. Nutr.*, 70(Suppl.), 615S-9S, 1999.

Hahn, A., Leitzmann, C., *Vegetarische Ernährung.*, Ulmer, Stuttgart 1996.

James, W.P., Introduction: the challenge of adult chronic deficiency, *Eur. J. Clin. Nutr.*, 48 (Suppl. 3), 1, 1994.

Järvinen, V.K., Rytömaa, I., Heinonen, O.P., Risk factors in dental erosion *J. Dent. Res.*, 70, 927, 1991.

Koebnick, C., Doerries, S., Fuhrmann, P., Kwanbunjan, K., Strassner, C., Leitzmann, C., Die Giessener Rohkost-Studie — Ergebnisse zeigen Trend — Gesundheitliche Gründe stehen im Vordergrund, *Naturarzt,* 4, 44, 1994.

Koebnick, C., Strassner, C., Doerries, S., Kwanbunjan, K., Leitzmann, C., Ernährungs- und Gesundheitsverhalten von Personen mit überwiegender Rohkost-Ernährung, *Z. Ernährungswiss.,* 34, 53, 1995.

Koebnick, C., Strassner, C., Hoffmann, I., Leitzmann, C., Consequences of a long-term raw food diet on body weight and menstruation: results of a questionnaire survey, *Ann. Nutr. Metab.,* 43, 69, 1999.

Koebnick, C., Strassner, C., Leitzmann, C., Rohkost-Ernährung: Teil I — Überblick und Bewertung der theoretischen Grundlagen, *Verbraucherdienst,* 42(10), 244, 1997a.

Koebnick, C., Strassner, C., Leitzmann, C., Rohkost-Ernährung: Teil II — Die Giessener Rohkost-Studie, *Verbraucherdienst*, 42(11), 268, 1997b.

Koebnick, C., Strassner, C., Leitzmann, C., Bewertung der Rohkost-Ernährung in der Ernährungsberatung, Ernährungsumschau, 44(12), 444, 1997c.

Kopp, W., Blum, W.F., von Prittwitz, S., Ziegler, A., Luppert, H., Emons, G., Herzog, W., Herpertz, S., Deter, H.C., Remschmidt, H., Hedebrand, J., Low leptin levels predict amenorrhea in underweight and eating disorders of females, *Mol. Psychiatry,* 2, 335, 1997.

Leitzmann, C., Keller, M., Hahn, A., *Alternative Ernährungsformen*, Hippokrates, Stuttgart, 1999.

Ling, W.H., Hänninen, O., Shifting from a conventional diet to an uncooked vegan diet reversibly alters fecal hydrolytic activities in humans, *J. Nutr.,* 122, 924, 1992.

Linkosalo, E., Markkanen, H., Dental erosions in relation to lactovegetarian diet, *Scand. J. Dent. Res.,* 93, 436, 1985.

Lussi, A., Schaffner, M., Hotz, P., Suter, P., Dental erosions in a population of Swiss adults, *Community Dent. Oral Epidemiol.,* 19, 286, 1991.

McIver, B., Romanski, S.A., Nippoldt, T.B., Evaluation and management of amenorrhea, *Mayo Clin. Proc.,* 72, 1161, 1997.

Naidu, A.N., Rao, N.P., Body mass index: a measure of the nutritional status in Indian populations, *Eur. J. Clin. Nutr.,* 48(Suppl. 3), 131, 1994.

National Research Council, Recommended Dietary Allowances, National Academy Press, Washington, D.C., 1989.

Norgan, N.G., Ferro-Luzzi, A., Weight-height indices as estimators of fatness in men, *Hum. Nutr. Clin. Nutr.,* 36C, 363, 1982.

Nutrition Committee, American Heart Association, Dietary guidelines for healthy American adults, *Circulation*, 94, 1795, 1996.

Rauma, A.L., Törrönen, R., Hänninen, O., Mykkänen, H., Vitamin B-12 status in long-term adherents of a strict uncooked vegan diet ("Living Food Diet") is compromised, *J. Nutr.*, 125, 2511, 1995a.

Rauma, A.L., Törrönen, R., Hänninen, O., Verhagen, H., Mykkänen, H., Antioxidant status in long-term adherents to a strict uncooked vegan diet, *Am. J. Clin. Nutr.*, 62, 1221-7, 1995b.

Shelton, H.M., Principles of Natural Hygiene, Dr. Shelton's Health School, San Antonio, Texas, 1964.

Shetty, P.S., James, W.P.T., Body Mass Index. A Measure of Chronic Energy Deficiency in Adults, FAO Food and Nutrition Paper 56, Aberdeen, Rower Research Institute, 1994.

Strassner, C., Ernähren sich Rohköstler gesünder? Die Gieβener Rohkost-Studie, Verlag für Medizin und Gesundheit, Heidelberg, 1998.

Strassner, C., Doerries, S., Kwanbunjan, K., Leitzmann, C., Vegetarian raw food dietary regimens: health habits and nutrient intake, Poster, 3rd. Int. Congr. Vegetarian Nutrition, Loma Linda, CA, 1997.

WHO (World Health Organization), Energy and Protein Requirements; Report of a Joint FAO/WHO/UNU Expert Consultation Tech. Rep. Ser. No. 724. Geneva, WHO. 1985.

World Cancer Research Fund, American Institute of Cancer Research, Food, Nutrition and the Prevention of Cancer: A Global Perspective, American Institute for Cancer Research, Washington, D.C., 1997.

19 Effect of Nutrition on Stress Management

Ali Reza Waladkhani and Michael Roland Clemens

CONTENTS

ABSTRACT

Persistent mild to moderate hypothalamic-pituitary-adrenal axis activation associated with depressive illness is a well-documented phenomenon. Clinical studies have shown that during periods of depression this results in persistent hypercortisolism of varying degrees that is sufficiently chronic to induce adaptive changes in the hypothalamic-pituitary-adrenal axis function. Animal studies suggest that chronic stress causes high basal cortisol and low cortisol response to acute stressors and that such changes may contribute to disease states. Components of the diet such as protein and carbohydrate, even when the intakes of fat and energy remain unchanged, can produce consistent changes in concentrations of cortisol and its binding globulin, CBG. Further, the fat content of the diet plays a critical role in CBG and cortisol concentration. Also, addition of monounsaturated and polyunsaturated free fatty acids to purified human CBG enhances CBG binding activity in a concentration-dependent fashion. Other important factors are micronutrients, e.g., vitamins and phytochemicals. Studies indicate that persons who eat green or yellow vegetables every day show a lower incidence of stress

0-8493-0038-X/97/$0.00+$.50

syndrome (irritation, sleeplessness) than those who do not eat them regularly. Also, dietary modification may reduce stress susceptibility and improve the stress management.

19.1 INTRODUCTION

Persistent mild to moderate hypothalamic-pituitary-adrenal (HPA) axis activation associated with depressive illness is a well-documented phenomenon and can be demonstrated in approximately half of patients suffering from major depression.[1] Clinical studies have shown that during periods of depression this results in persistent hypercortisolism of varying degrees that is sufficiently chronic to induce adaptive changes in HPA axis function.[1] Many investigators have speculated that subtler, subclinical changes related to HPA axis activation may occur in depression.

Because cortisol is critically involved in the regulation of immune function, many investigations have focused on aspects of immune function in patients with depression.[2] Psychosocial stress may be associated with a process of premature aging in middle-aged males, corresponding to a hypogonadal state as well as to indirect signs of increased insulin resistance.[3] The steady-state blood glucose levels were significantly higher after stress, demonstrating impairment of the insulin sensitivity by mental stress.[4] It is documented from vitamin deprivation studies that alterations in behavior and mental performance arise in early stages of vitamin deficiency.[5]

The increase in the circulating glucocorticoid signal associated with acute stress endures well beyond the period of increased total corticosterone levels.[6] After an acute stressor termination, glucocorticoid-sensitive targets are exposed to high levels of free corticosterone for several days. The long-term increase in free corticosterone may play an important role in mediating some of the effects produced by acute stressor as well as those produced by other acute stressors.[7]

In most species, as much as 68% of plasma CBG remained free of cortisol under physiologic conditions.[8] Also, in addition to its role as a transport protein, CBG plays an active role in determining the disposition of cortisol in humans.[9] Acute exposure to a stressor is able to decrease CBG levels provided that duration of exposure to the stressor and its intensity are high and that the effect is tested at least 6 h after the onset of stress. The effect appears to be mediated by some adrenal factor(s) other than glucocorticoids.[10] Further, psychological stress seems to increase oxidative stress.[11] Early studies indicate that psychological stress decreases DNA repair[12] and inhibits radiation-induced apoptosis[13] in human blood cells. This may mean that oxidative damage may persist during psychological stress and may increase the likelihood of a pathological development.[11]

In contrast to the tendency of chronic stress to elevate baseline cortisol, it appears to decrease testosterone, both in animals and humans (Figure 19.1).[14,15]

19.2 MEAL FREQUENCY

Timing and the nutritional composition of the meal can influence the effects of meals on cognitive behavior. Using a cross-over design, Simeon and Grantham-McGregor[16] found that stunted and previously malnourished 9- and 10-year-old

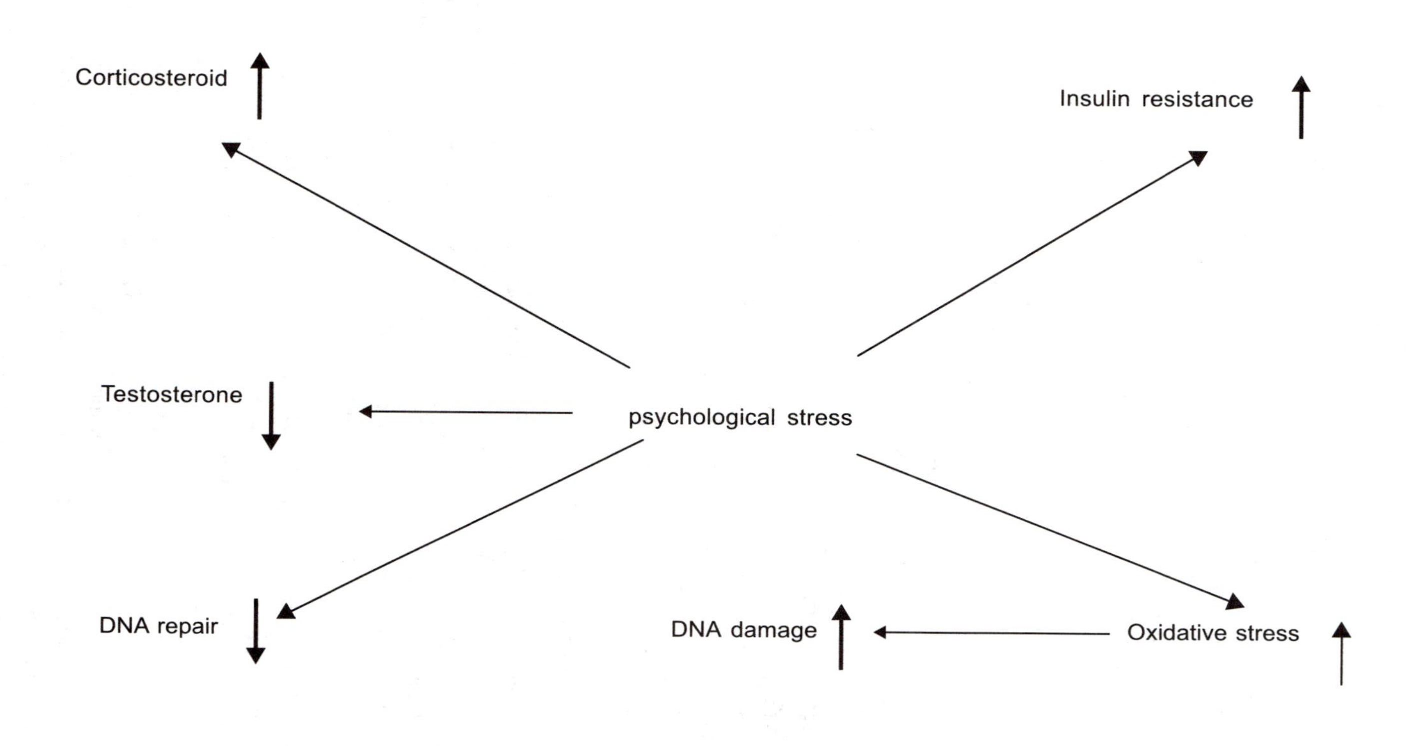
Corticosteroid
Insulin resistance
Testosterone
psychological stress
DNA repair
DNA damage
Oxidative stress

FIGURE 19.1

Jamaicans performed less well on tests of short-term memory and problem-solving ability when they had not eaten breakfast than when they had eaten a morning meal. Undernourished children's performance on a test of verbal fluency was significantly better when they had consumed a school breakfast than when they had not.[17] Experimental evidence suggests that omitting breakfast negatively affects cognitive functioning.[18]

The degree to which lunch moderates subsequent cognitive performance and mood may be mediated by a number of factors. One of the most obvious of these factors is meal size. In a study investigating the effect of meal size on attention and mood, Smith et al.[19] reported that subjects who ate a larger than usual lunch made more errors on attention and search tasks than those who ate a normal-sized lunch, or one smaller than usual. No differences in mood were noted as a function of meal size. Craig and Richardson[20] found that relative to their performance before lunch, young men made significantly more errors on a letter-cancellation project after eating a large lunch, but tended to make less errors after a small lunch. Changes in performance were greater when subjects ate a meal similar in size to their normal lunch. Performance improved to a greater degree after the small lunch in subjects who typically ate a heavy lunch than in those who ate a light lunch. Afternoon snacks may also have positive effects on cognitive performance.[21]

Smith et al.[22] addressed the effects of an evening meal on cognitive performance and mood. After 1-3 h, subjects who consumed the meal reported feeling stronger, more proficient, and more interested than subjects who did not consume the meal. Additionally, 90 min after the meal, the subjects who had eaten completed more sentences on a logical-reasoning task than those had not eaten.

19.3 CARBOHYDRATES

Components of the diet, such as protein and carbohydrate, even when the intakes of fat and energy remain unchanged, can produce consistent changes in concentrations of cortisol and its binding globulin. The isocaloric change from a high protein to a high carbohydrate intake was associated with decreases in plasma cortisol and corticosteroid binding globulin, with reciprocal changes in plasma testosterone and sex hormone binding globulin.[23] Also, a carbohydrate-rich, protein-poor diet may increase personal control in subjects with a high stress proneness.[24] An abnormal rhythm of glucocorticoids combined with elevated cortisol concentrations has also been reported in pathological situations involving an elevation of free fatty acid, such as in insulin-dependent diabetes mellitus or acquired immune deficiency syndrome.[25]

An improvement in memory in those who had eaten breakfast has been found to correlate with the levels of blood glucose.[26] The impression that memory, rather than other aspects of cognition, is more susceptible to changes in blood glucose levels is unavoidable. A glucose-containing drink has been found to improve memory in both young healthy adults[27] and the elderly.[28] The mechanism by which an enhanced provision of glucose might facilitate memory and the possibility that cholinergic activity is enhanced has attracted particular attention; an association between acetylcholine-mediated neurotransmission and memory is well documented.[29] Acetylcholine is formed by choline acetyltransferase from the precursors choline and acetyl-CoA; glucose is the main source of the acetyl groups used in the formation of acetyl-CoA.[30] One situation associated with a high demand for acetylcholine is learning. Durkin et al.[31] produced the first direct evidence that raised glucose levels facilitate acetylcholine synthesis, by measuring its release from the rat hippocampus under conditions of increased neuronal activity.

19.4 FAT

Fat content of the diet plays a critical role in CBG and cortisol concentration. Early studies in burn patients indicated patients fed the low-fat solutions (15% kcal as fat) had higher serum CBG than patients fed the standard solution (35% kcal as fat) and that higher levels of CBG resulted in a lower free serum cortisol.[32] Not only the fat amount but also the fat deposition is effective in corticosteroid bioavailability. Also, free fatty acids modulate the action of steroids mainly by inhibiting their binding to specific plasma and tissue proteins such as the human sex steroid binding protein.[33] *In vitro* studies have also shown that free fatty acids modulate the functionality of human CBG positively or negatively, depending on their molar ration to CBG.[34] *In vivo*, the release of free fatty acids consecutive to heparin-induced lipoprotein lipase activation mediates conformational changes, causing a reduction of CBG binding in suckling rats.[35] *In vitro* addition of physiological concentrations of exogenous free fatty acids confirms that the stimulation of CBG binding properties is mainly due to monounsaturated free fatty acid classes. Oleic acid alone mimicked the *in vivo* situation by increasing the affinity constant of CBG for cortisol (three-fold) and reducing the number of binding sites (two-fold), whereas saturated fats did not enhance the binding.[36] Addition of monounsaturated and polyunsaturated free fatty acids to purified human CBG enhanced CBG binding activity in a concentration-dependent fashion.[34] Garrel et al.[32] showed that CBG and cortisol levels did not indicate any changes by the consumption of n-3 and n-6 fatty acids (Figure 19.2).

19.5 VITAMINS

In the presence of a chronically insufficient vitamin supply verified by repeated measurements of the vitamin parameters, many unfavorable psychometric findings in the corresponding deficiency groups were obtained for vitamin C, thiamin, riboflavin, cobalamin, and folate, depending on the degree of insufficient vitamin supply.[5] Administration of folic acid, vitamin C, and to a lesser extent thiamin, as compared to placebos, in men with an initial suboptimal folate status, led to a decreased emotional lability, increased activeness and concentration, higher extroversion and lower introversion, greater self-confidence, and a markedly improved mood.[5] In volunteers with an initial mild-to-moderate vitamin C deficiency, supplementation led to decreased nervousness, less depression, and increased emotional lability.[5]

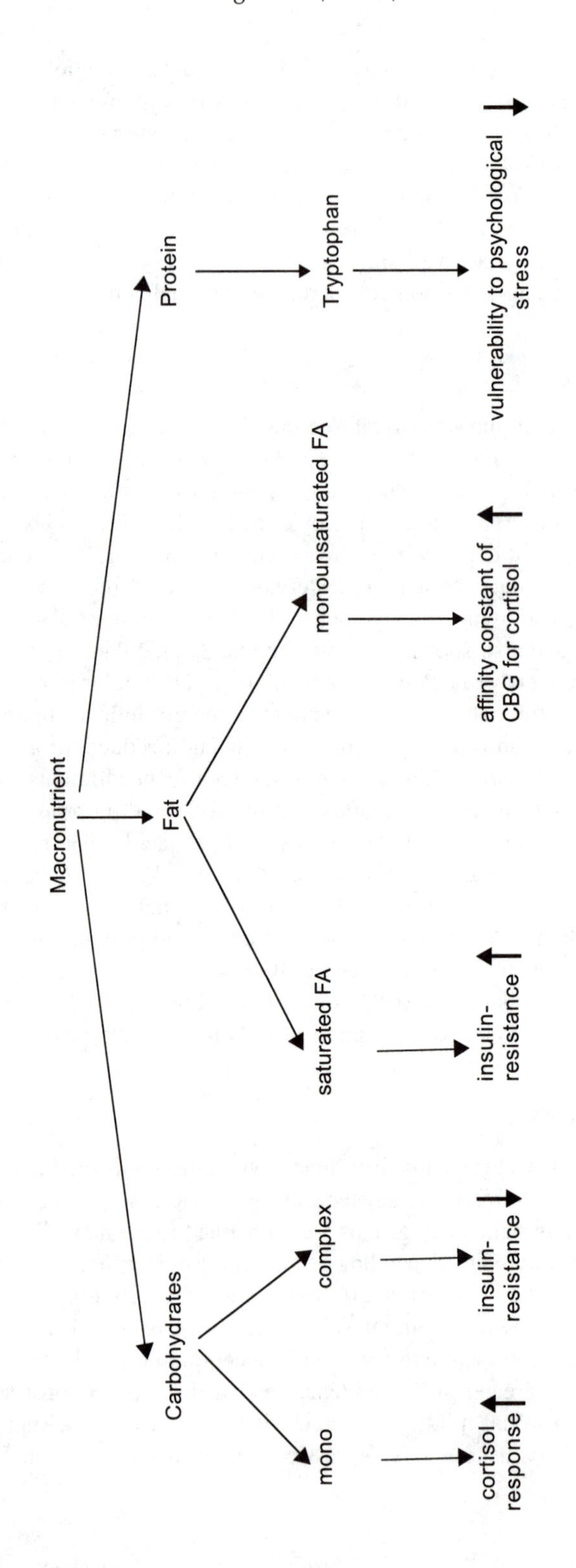
Macronutrient
Carbohydrates
Fat
Protein
mono
complex
saturated FA
monounsaturated FA
Tryptophan
cortisol response
insulin-resistance
insulin-resistance
affinity constant of CBG for cortisol
vulnerability to psychological stress

FIGURE 19.2

19.5.1 Vitamin C

It has long been known that endocrine organs are exceedingly high in the concentration of vitamin C per weight of tissue as compared with nonendocrine organs.[37] Ascorbic acid exceeds the functions of a vitamin, since it not only has its known cofactor roles for several enzymes, but also affects the regulation of the levels of the circulating thyroid and adrenal cortical hormones.[38] Differing plasma concentrations of ascorbic acid regulate *in vivo* steroidogenesis by altering the activity of the membrane-bound enzyme adenylate cyclase.[39] Ascorbic acid is essential for optimal steroid hormone functions and this suggests an involvement of ascorbic acid in steroid synthesis mechanisms.[40] Vitamin C depletion led to a significant increase in plasma cortisol without an increase in ACTH.[41] In animal studies, ascorbic acid deficiency caused an increase in plasma cortisol concentration.[42] In humans there was a distinct increase of plasma cortisol about 2 h after vitamin C application. This increase was concomitant with an increase in urinary 17-hydroxycorticosteroids.[43] In rats, vitamin C pretreatment enhanced the release of endogenous glucocorticoid such as to delay the turnover of the tracer cortisol in plasma.[44]

Vitamin C depletion led to a significant increase in plasma cortisol without an increase in ACTH.[41]

19.5.2 Vitamin B_6

There are *in vivo* effects of steroids that are altered depending on vitamin B_6 status. The *in vivo* action of pyridoxal phosphate does not appear to involve a change in receptor number or binding capacity of the hormone.[45] Evidence accumulated over the past decade suggests that vitamin B_6 may function as a physiological regulator of steroid hormone action.[46] Induction of vitamin B_6 deficiency in rats altered the function of the glucocorticoid receptor such that at low cellular concentrations of pyridoxal phosphate there was an increased translocation of the receptor complex to the nucleus, whereas at normal or high levels nuclear translocation of steroid receptor complex was diminished.[47]

High concentrations of pyridoxal phosphate suppress activation of transcription, while vitamin deficiency enhances responsiveness to steroid hormone.[48] Further, pyridoxine deficiency states are associated with decreased GABA and increased central nervous system irritability.[49] Also, pyridoxine is essential in the conversion of L-dihydroxyphenylalanine to dopamine. Side effects of excessive L-dihydroxyphenylalanine include dystonia and dyskinesia (Figure 19.3).[49]

19.5.3 Vitamin E

Vitamin E, as the major chain-breaking lipid-soluble antioxidant, would be expected to be important for functional integrity of all biological membranes. A deficiency of vitamin E results in an number of pathological changes in muscle, reproductive, cardiovascular, and nervous systems.[50] Animal studies indicated that chickens raised on a vitamin E-deficient diet developed cerebellar encephalomalacia.[51] Einarson and Telford[52] found that prolonged vitamin E-deficiency in the rat caused demyelination of axons and gliosis in the gracilis and cuneate nuclei.

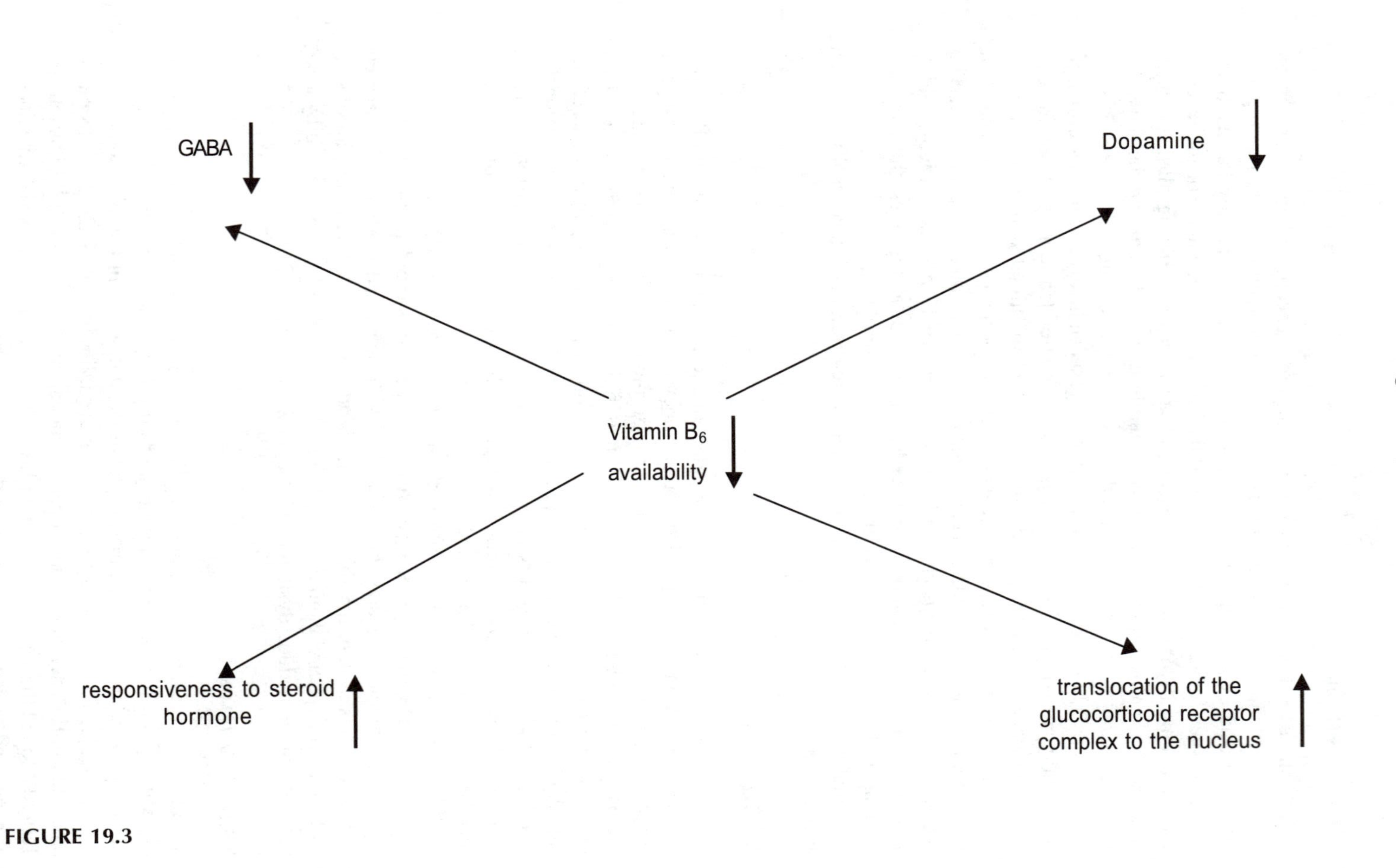
GABA
Dopamine
Vitamin B$_6$
availability
responsiveness to steroid
hormone
translocation of the
glucocorticoid receptor
complex to the nucleus

FIGURE 19.3

The importance of vitamin E for maintaining the structural and functional integrity of nervous system in humans has now been well established. Clinical data on the role of vitamin E in nervous system diseases indicate that even though a dietary vitamin E deficiency is very rare in humans, a symptomatic vitamin E deficiency exists in association with abetalipoproteinemia, chronic cholestatic hepatobilliary diseases, cystic fibrosis, short bowel syndrome, and isolated vitamin E deficiency syndrome.[53]

The neuropathologic changes of vitamin E deficiency in humans are very similar to those in rats and rhesus monkeys,[53] and the resulting neurological syndrome is characterized by areflexia, peripheral neuropathy, cerebellar involvement with gait and limbo ataxia, and decreased propioception and vibration sense.[54]

Nelson et al.[55] compared the neuropathologic changes in vitamin E-deficient rats and monkeys and described the process as a distal and dying-back type of axonopathy. Concentrations of α-tocopherol in the distal and proximal parts of the sciatic nerve are not different. This suggests that susceptibility of the distal portion of peripheral nerves to vitamin E deficiency must be due to reasons other than lower levels of tocopherol in distal regions.[56] A defect in the fast anterograde and retrograde axonal transport has been reported in vitamin E-deficient rats.[57]

Cerebellum seems to be active in the metabolic utilization of vitamin E. This could be the reason for cerebellar damage during experimental vitamin E deficiency and for the incidence of cerebellar symptoms in clinical vitamin E deficiency.[56]

19.6 PHYTOCHEMICALS

Persons who eat green or yellow vegetables every day show a lower incidence of stress syndrome (irritation, sleeplessness) than those who do not eat them daily.[58] Plant foods contain a wide variety of phytochemicals that have the potential to modulate stress, e.g., carotinoids, flavonoids, and sulfides.

Human studies indicated that β-carotene suppresses the secretion of CRH dose-dependently.[59] It is also suggested that the effective site of β-carotene is the hypothalamus, where β-carotene suppressed the secretion of CRH induced by exercise stress, and consequently the secretion of ACTH in the pituitary. As CRH stimulates the sympathetic neuron,[60] β-carotene also inhibited the stimulation of noradrenaline and adrenaline secretion through the suppression of CRH secretion.[59]

Rats fed diets containing extracts high in both flavonoid levels as well as total antioxidant activity for 6 weeks before being subjected to 48 h of exposure to 100% normobaric O_2 showed no loss in striatal muscarinic or cerebellar GABAergic receptor sensitivity.[61] These oxygen-induced decreases in neuronal function have been shown to be sensitive to aging and have been associated with behavioral deficits.[62]

Recent studies have indicated that garlic extract was effective in preventing brain atrophy[63] as well as learning and memory impairments[64] in the senescence-accelerated mouse.

19.7 VEGETARIAN DIETS

Nutritional studies suggest that the change from their customary vegetarian diet to a cafeteria-fed Western diet for 3 weeks in a group of 13 elderly black South African men was associated with a decrease in plasma testosterone.[65] Comparisons of hormone levels in vegetarians and omnivores[66] also indicate that steroid hormone metabolism can be influenced by diet. Not only diet but also stress influences testosterone level. Also, chronic stress appears to decrease testosterone both in animals and humans.[14,15] Furthermore, an increase of testosterone in response to acute stress is found in successful (low stress) male baboons, while subordinate (chronically stressed) males show a decrease.[67] Thus, changes in nutritional behavior could cause changes in endocrine balance and eventually in stress response.

19.8 ALCOHOL

Alcohol affects the endocrine system in healthy subjects. Earlier studies showed that a high dose of ethanol stimulates adrenal catecholamine secretion and urinary excretion[68] but inhibits luteinizing hormone (LH) secretion.[69] Also, alcohol affects cortisol[70] and dehydroepiandrosterone sulfate.[71] In the premenopausal women alcohol consumption did increase the concentrations of cortisol.[72] Detoxified alcoholics and controls had similar baseline cortisol levels; the alcoholics showed an attenuated cortisol response to the combined stressors. Therefore, higher stress cortisol values were seen in the patients with the most severe withdrawal symptoms.[73]

Animal models of alcohol dependence demonstrated decreased sensitivity to GABAergic agonists and enhanced sensitivity to GABA inverse agonists.[74]

19.9 CONCLUSION

Modification of the diet and changes in frequency of the diet intake may be helpful in stress management. It is of great importance to eat properly. A large part of the diet has to be of complex carbohydrates. In general, foods of plant origin have to be preferred. Reduction and modification of dietary fat may be helpful. In particular, a diet rich in monounsaturated and n-3 fatty acids is advisable. These modifications can produce consistent changes in concentrations of cortisol and its binding globulin. Further, plant foods are rich in phytochemicals, trace elements, and vitamins, which show a variety of positive effects on health. Also, consumption of green or yellow vegetables every day may lower the incidence of some stress syndromes (e.g., irritation and sleeplessness).

REFERENCES

1. Gold, P. W., Goodwin, F. K., and Chrousos, G. P., Clinical and biochemical manifestations of depression. Relation to the neurobiology of stress. *N. Engl. J. Med.*, 319, 348 and 413, 1988.

2. Michelson, D. and Gold, P. W., Pathophysiologic and somatic investigations of hypothalamic-pituitary-adrenal axis activation in patients with depression, in *Neuroimmuno-Modulation. Molecular Aspects, Integrative Systems, and Clinical Advances*, McCann, S. M., Sternberg, E. M., Lipton, J. M., Chrousos, G. P., Gold, P. W., and Smith, C. C., Eds., New York Academy of Sciences, New York, 1988, 722.
3. Nilsson, P. M., Moller, L., and Solstad, K., Adverse effects of psychosocial stress on gonadal function and insulin levels in middle-aged males. *J. Intern. Med.*, 237(5), 479, 1995.
4. Moberg, E., Kollind, M., Lins, P. E., and Adamson, U., Acute mental stress impairs insulin sensitivity in IDDM patients. *Diabetes,* 37(3), 247, 1994.
5. Heseker, H., Kübler, W., Pudel, V., and Westenhöffer, J., Psychological disorders as early symptoms of a mild-to-moderate vitamin deficiency, in *Beyond Deficiency. New Views on the Function and Health Effects of Vitamins*, Sauberlich, H. E. and Machlin, L. J., Eds., New York Academy of Sciences, New York, 1992, 352.
6. Tannenbaum, B., Rowe, W., Sharma, S., Diorio, J., Steverman, A., Walker, M., and Meaney, M. J., Dynamic variations in plasma corticosteroid-binding globulin and basal HPA activity following acute stress in adult rats. *J. Neuroendocrinol.,* 9(3), 163, 1997.
7. Fleshner, M., Deak, T., Spencer, R. L., Laudenslager, M. L., Watkins, L. R., and Maier, S. F., A long-term increase in basal levels of corticosterone and a decrease in corticosteroid-binding globulin after acute stressor exposure. *Endocrinology,* 136(12), 5336, 1995.
8. Gayrard, V., Alvinerie, M., and Toutain, P. L., Interspecies variations of corticosteroid-binding globulin parameters. *Domest. Anim. Endocrinol.,* 13(1), 35, 1996.
9. Bright, G. M., Corticosteroid-binding globulin influences kinetic parameters of plasma cortisol transport and clearance. *J. Clin. Endocrinol. Metab.* 80(3), 770, 1995.
10. Marti, O., Martin, M., Gavalda, A., Giralt, M., Hidalgo, J., Hsu, B. R., Kuhn, R. W., and Armario, A., Inhibition of corticosteroid-binding globulin caused by a severe stressor is apparently mediated by the adrenal but not by glucocorticoid receptors. *Endocrine,* 6(2), 159, 1997.
11. Moller, P., Wallin, H., and Knudsen, L. E., Oxidative stress associated with exercise, psychological stress and life-style factors. *Chem.-Biol. Interact.,* 102, 17, 1996.
12. Kiecolt-Glaser, J. K., Stephens, R. E., Lipetz, P. D., Speicher, C. E., and Glaser, R., Distress and DNA repair in human lymphocytes. *J. Behav. Med.,* 8, 311, 1985.
13. Tomei, L. D., Kiecolt-Glaser, J. K., Kennedy, S., and Glaser, R., Psychological stress and phorbol ester inhibition of radiation-induced apoptosis in human peripheral blood leukocytes. *Psychiat. Res.,* 33, 59, 1990.
14. Allen, P. I. M., Batty, K. A., Dodd, C. A. S., Herbert, J., Hugh, C. J., Moore, G. F., Seymour, M. J., Shiers, H. M., Stacey, P. M., and Young, S. K., Dissociation between emotional and endocrine responses preceding an academic examination in male medical students. *J. Endocrinol.,* 107, 163, 1985.
15. Leedy, M. G. and Wilson, M. S., Testosterone and cortisol levels in crewmen of U.S. Air Force fighter and cargo planes. *Psychosom. Med.,* 47(4), 333, 1985.
16. Simeon, D. T. and Grantham-McGregor, S., Effects of missing breakfast on the cognitive functions of school children of differing nutritional status. *Am. J. Clin. Nutr.,* 49, 646, 1989.
17. Chandler, A. M., Walker, S. P., Connolly, K., and Grantham-McGregor, S. M., School breakfast improves verbal fluency in undernourished Jamaican children. *J. Nutr.,* 125, 894, 1995.

18. Kanarek, R., Psychological effects of snacks and altered meal frequency. *Br. J. Nutr.,* 77(1), 105, 1997.
19. Smith, A., Ralph, A., and McNeill, G., Influences of meal size on post-lunch changes in performance efficiency, mood and cardiovascular function. *Appetite,* 16, 85, 1991.
20. Craig, A. and Richardson, E., Effects of experimental and habitual lunch-size on performance, arousal, hunger and mood. *Int. Arch. Occup. Environ. Health,* 61, 313, 1989.
21. Kanarek, R. B. and Swinney, D., Effects of food snacks on cognitive performance in male college students. *Appetite,* 14, 15, 1990.
22. Smith, A., Kendrick, A., Maben, A., and Salmon, J., Effects of breakfast and caffeine on cognitive performance, mood and cardiovascular functioning. *Appetite,* 22, 39, 1994.
23. Anderson, K. E., Rosner, W., and Khan, M. S., Diet-hormone interaction: Proteins/carbohydrate ratio alters reciprocally the plasma levels of testosterone and cortisol and their respective binding globulin in man. *Life Sci.,* 40, 1761, 1987.
24. Markus, C. R., Panhuysen, G., Tuiten, A., Koppeschaar, H., Fekkes, D., and Peters, M. L., Does carbohydrate-rich, protein-poor food prevent a deterioration of mood and cognitive performance of stress-prone subjects when subjected to a stressful task? *Appetite,* 31(1), 49, 1998.
25. Christeff, N., Michon, C., Goertz, G., Hassid, J., Martheron, S., Girard, P. M., Coulaud, J. P., and Nunez, E. A., Abnormal free fatty acids and cortisol concentrations in the serum of AIDS patients. *Eur. J. Cancer Res. Clin. Oncol.,* 24, 1179, 1988.
26. Benton, D. and Sargent, J., Breakfast, blood glucose and memory. *Biol. Psychiatry,* 33, 207, 1992.
27. Parker, P. Y. and Benton, D., Blood glucose levels selectively influence memory for word list dichotically presented to the right ear. *Neuropsychology,* 33, 843, 1995.
28. Craft, S., Dagogo-Jack, S. E., Wiethop, B. V., Murphy, C., Nevins, R. T., Fleischman, S., Rice, V., Newomer, J. W., and Cryer, P. E., Effects of hyperglycemia on memory and hormone levels in dementia of the Alzheimer type: a longitudinal study. *Behav. Neurosci.,* 107, 926 1993.
29. Kopelman, M. D., The cholinergic neurotransmitter system in human memory and dementia: a review. *Q. J. Exp. Psychol.,* 38A, 535, 1986.
30. Tucek, S., Acetylcoenzyme A and the synthesis of acetylcholine in neurones: a review of recent progress. *Gen. Phys. Biochem.,* 2, 313, 1983.
31. Durkin, T. P., Messier, C., de Boer, P., and Westernik, B. H. C., Raised glucose levels enhance scoplamine-induced acetylcholine overflow from the hippocampus: an in vivo microdialysis study in rat. *Behav. Brain Res.,* 49, 181, 1992.
32. Garrel, D. R., Razi, M., Larivire, F., Jobin, N., Bonneton, A., and Pugeat, M., Improved clinical status and length of care with low fat nutritional support in burn patients. *J. Parenteral Enteral Nutr.,* 19(6), 482, 1995.
33. Martin, M. E., Vranckx, R., Benassayag, C., and Nunez, E. A., Modifications of the properties of human sex steroid-binding protein by nonesterified fatty acids. *J. Biol. Chem.,* 261, 2954, 1986.
34. Martin, M. E., Benassayag, C., and Nunez, E. A., Selective changes in binding and immunological properties of human corticosteroid binding globulin by free fatty acids. *Endocrinology,* 123, 1178, 1988.
35. Haourigui, M., Vallette, G., Martin, M. E., Sumida, C., Benassayag, C., and Nunez, E. A., In vivo effect of free fatty acids on the specific binding of glucocorticoids to corticosteroid binding globulin and liver receptors in immature rats. *Steroids,* 59, 46, 1994.

36. Haourigui, M., Sakr, S., Martin, M. E., Thobie, N., Girard-Globa, A., Benassayag, C., and Nunez, E. A., Postprandial free fatty acids stimulate activity of human corticosteroid binding globulin. *Am. J. Physiol.,* 269(6, Pt. 1), E1067, 1995.
37. Giroud, A., Repartion de la vitamin C dans l'organisme. *Ergeb. Vitam. Hormonforsch.,* 1, 68, 1938.
38. Degkwitz, E., Neue Aspekte der Biochemie des Vitamins C. *Z. Ernahrungswiss,* 24(4), 219, 1985.
39. Doulas, N. L., Constantopoulos, A., and Litsios, B., Effect of ascorbic acid on guinea pig adrenal adenylate cyclase activity and plasma cortisol. *J. Nutr.,* 117(6), 1108, 1987.
40. Goralczyk, R., Moser, U. K., Matter, U., and Weiser, H., Regulation of steroid hormone metabolism requires L-ascorbic acid, in *Beyond Deficiency. New Views on the Function and Health Effects of Vitamins,* Sauberlich, H. E. and Machlin, L. J., Eds., New York Academy of Sciences, New York, 1992, 349.
41. Redmann, A., Mobius, K., Hiller, H. H., Oelkers, W., and Bahr, V., Ascorbate depletion prevents aldosterone stimulation by sodium deficiency in the guinea pig. *Eur. J. Endocrinol.,* 133(4), 499, 1995.
42. Enwonwu, C. O., Sawiris, P., and Chanaud, N., Effect of marginal ascorbic acid deficiency on saliva level of cortisol in the guinea pig. *Arch. Oral Biol.,* 40(8), 737, 1995.
43. Kodama, M., Kodama, T., Murakami, M., and Kodama, M., Autoimmune disease and allergy are controlled by vitamin C treatment. *In Vivo,* 8, 251, 1994.
44. Kodama, M., Inoue, F., Kodama, T., and Kodama, M., Intraperitoneal administration of ascorbic acid delays the turnover of 3H-labelled cortisol in the plasma of an ODS rat, but not in the Wistar rat. Evidence in support of the cardinal role of vitamin C in the progression of glucocorticoid synthesis. *In Vivo,* 10(1), 97, 1996.
45. Leklem, J. E. and Reynolds, R. D., *Clinical and Physiological Applications of Vitamin* B_6. Allan R. Liss, New York, 1988.
46. Compton, M. M. and Cidlowski, J. A., Vitamin B_6 and glucocorticoid action. *Endocrinol. Rev.,* 7, 140, 1986.
47. DiSorbo, D. M., Phelps, D. S., Ohl, V. S., and Litwack, G., Pyridoxine deficiency influences the behavior of the glucocorticoid receptor complex. *J. Biol. Chem.,* 255, 3866, 1980.
48. Allgood, V. E., Powell-Oliver, F. E., and Cidlowski, J. A., The influence of vitamin B_6 on the structure and function of the glucocorticoid receptor, in Vitamin B_6, Dakshinamurti, K., Ed., New York Academy of Sciences, New York, 1990, 452.
49. Bernstein, A. L., Viatmin B6 in clinical neurology, in *Vitamin* B_6, Dakshinamurti, K., Ed., New York Academy of Sciences, New York, 1990, 250.
50. Scot, M. L., Studies on vitamin E and related factors in nutrition and metabolism, in *Fat Soluble Vitamins*, Deluca, H. F. and Suttie, J. W., Eds., The University of Wisconsin Press, Madison, WI, 335, 1969.
51. Pappenheimer, A. M. and Goettsch, M., A cerebellar disorder in chicks, apparently of nutritional origin. *J. Exp. Med.,* 53, 11, 1931.
52. Einarson, L. and Teleford, I. R., Effect of vitamin E deficiency on the central nervous system in various laboratory animals. *Dan. Videnskabernes Selskab,* 11, 1, 1960.
53. Sokol, R. J., Vitamin E and neurologic function in man. *Free Rad. Biol. Med.*, 6, 189, 1989.
54. Muller, D. P. R., Lloyd, J. K., and Wolff, O. H., Vitamin E and neurological function. *Lancet,* 1(8318), 225, 1983.

55. Nelson, J. S., Fitch, C. D., Fischer, V. W., Broun, G. O., and Chou, A. C., Progressive neuropathological lesions in vitamin E-deficient rhesus monkeys. *J. Neuropathol. Exp. Neurol.,* 40, 166, 1981.
56. Vatassery, G. T., Vitamin E, neurochemistry and implications for neurodegeneration in Parkinson's disease, in *Beyond Deficiency. New Views on the Function and Health Effects of Vitamins,* Sauberlich, H. E. and Machlin, L., Eds., New York Academy of Sciences, New York, 1992, 97.
57. Southam, E., Thomas, P. K., King, R. H. M., Gross-Sampson, M. A., and Muller, D. P. R., Experimental vitamin E deficiency in rats. *Brain,* 114, 915, 1991.
58. Hirayama, T., Personal communication, 1992.
59. Hasegawa, T., Anti-stress effect of β-carotene, in *Carotenoids in Human Health,* Canfield, L. M., Krinsky, N. I., and Olson J. A., Eds., New York Academy of Sciences, New York, 1993, 281.
60. Kurosawa, M., Sato, A., Swenson, R. S., and Takahashi, Y., Sympatho-adrenal medullary functions in response to intracerebroventricularly injected corticotropin-releasing factor in anesthetized rats. *Brain Res.,* 367(1-2), 250, 1986.
61. Chadman, K., Joseph, J. A., Shukitt-Hale, B., Prior, R., Taglialatela, G., and Bickford, P. C., Diets high in antioxidant activity prevent deleterious effects of oxidative stress on signal transduction and nerve growth factor. *Soc. Neurosci. Abstr.,* 23, 348, 1997.
62. Joseph, J. A., Shukitt-Hale, B., Denisova, N. A., Prior, R. L., Cao, G., and Martin, A., Long-term dietary strawberry, spinach, or vitamin E supplementation retards the onset of age-related neuronal signal-transduction and cognitive behavioral deficits. *J. Neurosci.,* 18(19), 8047, 1998.
63. Moriguchi, T., Saito, H., and Nishiyama, N., Anti-aging effect of aged garlic extract in the inbred brain atrophy mouse model. *Clin. Exp. Pharmacol. Physiol.,* 24, 235, 1997.
64. Nishiyama, N., Moriguchi, T., and Saito, H., Beneficial effects of aged garlic extract on learning and memory impairment in the senescence-accelerated mouse. *Exp. Gerontol.,* 32, 149, 1997.
65. Hill, P., Wynder, E. L., Garbaczewski, L., and Walker, A. R. P., Effect of diet on plasma and urinary hormones in South African black men with prostatic cancer. *Cancer Res.,* 42, 3864, 1982.
66. Goldin, B. R., Adlercreutz, H., Gorbach, S. L., Warram, J. H., Dwyer, J. T., Swenson, L., and Woods, M. N., Estrogen excretion patterns and plasma levels in vegetarian and omnivorous women. *N. Engl. J. Med.,* 307, 1542, 1982.
67. Sapolsky, R. M., The endocrine stress-response and social status in the wild baboon. *Horm. Behav.,* 16, 279, 1982.
68. Adams, M. A. and Hirst, M., Ethanol-induced cardiac hypertrophy: correlation between development and the excretion of adrenal catecholamines. *Pharmacol. Biochem. Behav.,* 24, 33, 1986.
69. Pohl, C. R., Guilinger, R. A., and van Thiel, D. H., Inhibitory action of ethanol on luteinizing hormone secretion by rat anterior pituitary cells in culture. *Endocrinology,* 120, 849, 1987.
70. London, S., Willett, W., Longcope, C., and McKinlay, S., Alcohol and other dietary factors in realtion to serum hormone concentrations in women at climacteric. *Am. J. Clin. Nutr.,* 53, 166, 1991.
71. Longcope, C., Adrenal and gonadal androgen secretion in normal females. *Clin. Endocrinol. Metab.,* 15, 213, 1986.

72. Reichman, M. E., Judd, J. T., Longcope, C., Schatzkin, A., Clevidence, B. A., Nair, P. P., Campbell, W. S., and Taylor, P. R., Effect of alcohol consumption on plasma urinary hormone concentrations in premenopausal women. *J. Natl. Cancer Inst.,* 85, 722, 1993.
73. Bernardy, N. C., King, A. C., Parsons, O. A., and Lovallo, W. R., Altered cortisol response in sober alcoholics: an examination of contributing factors. *Alcohol,* 13(5), 493, 1996.
74. Buck, K. J. and Harris, R. A., Benzodiazepine agonist and inverse agonist actions on GABAa receptor-operated chloride channels II chronic effects of ethanol. *J. Pharmacol. Exp. Ther.,* 253, 713, 1990.

20 Legal Developments in Marketing Foods with Health Claims in the United States

Paul M. Hyman

CONTENTS

20.1 INTRODUCTION

The regulation of health claims in the U.S. for vegetables, fruits and herbs,* as with virtually all foods, is primarily the responsibility of the Food and Drug Administration (FDA), pursuant to the Food, Drug, and Cosmetic Act (FDC Act),[1] as amended by Nutrition Labeling and Education Act of 1990 (NLEA),[2] the Dietary Supplement Health and Education Act of 1994 (DSHEA),[3] and, to some extent, the Food and Drug Administration Modernization Act of 1997 (FDAMA).[4] The classification of a product under the law determines what claims can be made for the product. Such classification depends upon its intended use, which may be explained on its labels, labeling, promotional materials, or advertising. An ingested product intended to affect the health of consumers may be regulated as a conventional food,

* Meat, poultry, and eggs are regulated by the U.S. Department of Agriculture (Vol. 21, United States Code). Advertising of all foods is regulated by the Federal Trade Commission (Vol. 15, United States Code).

0-8493-0038-X/97/$0.00+$.50

a dietary supplement, a food for special dietary use, a medical food, or a prescription or over-the-counter drug. Each group is allowed varying permitted claims and must meet different regulatory burdens and risks.

Until 1990, the FDC Act did not explicitly provide for health claims for foods. It routinely treated health claims as drug claims.[5] Although FDA eventually allowed nutrition labeling in the 1970s and, reluctantly, a few health claims for foods in the late 1980s, these initiatives only became statutory law in 1990 when Congress enacted the NLEA, which amended the FDC Act expressly to "assist consumers in maintaining healthy dietary practices."[6] Four years later, in enacting the DSHEA, Congress found, among other things, that "the importance of nutrition and the benefits of dietary supplements to health promotion and disease prevention have been documented increasingly in scientific studies" and that "there is a growing need for emphasis on the dissemination of information linking nutrition and long-term good health."[7] As amended by these recent laws, the FDC Act now expressly mandates nutrition labeling for most foods subject to FDA's jurisdiction and authorizes nutrient content claims and health claims under specified conditions. Consumers are the beneficiaries of substantially more information concerning the nutritional values of the foods in their diets as well as the contributions some of these foods make to their health and well-being. From a legal viewpoint, the most important factor in providing health-related information for foods remains the need to avoid drug status, which triggers more onerous regulation.

20.2 PERTINENT DEFINITIONS

The FDC Act defines foods rather simply as (1) "articles used for food or drink for man or other animals, (2) chewing gum, and (3) [their] components . . . ."[8] Under the statute, a food also may be "intended to affect the structure or any function of the body of man or other animals."[9] In addition, the courts have noted that a food is consumed "primarily for taste, aroma, or nutritive value," but not always for those purposes, citing prune juice and coffee.[10]

A "dietary supplement" is defined in the FDC Act, as amended by DSHEA, to mean: a product (other than tobacco) intended to supplement the diet that bears or contains one or more of the following dietary ingredients:

(A) A vitamin
(B) A mineral
(C) An herb or other botanical
(D) An amino acid
(E) A dietary substance for use by man to supplement the diet by increasing the total dietary intake
(F) A concentrate, metabolite, constituent, extract, or combination of any ingredient described in clause (A), (B), (C), (D), or (E)[11]

Such products may be formulated as tablets, capsules, powders, softgels, gelcaps, liquid droplets, or as conventional foods, but may not be "represented for use as a conventional food or as a sole item of a meal or the diet."[12]

A "food for special dietary use" is represented to

(A) Supply a special dietary need that exists by reason of a physical, physiological, pathological, or other condition, including but not limited to the condition of disease, convalescence, pregnancy, lactation, infancy, allergic hypersensitivity to food, underweight, overweight, or the need to control the intake of sodium.
(B) Supply a vitamin, mineral, or other ingredient for use by man to supplement his diet by increasing the total dietary intake.
(C) Supply a special dietary need by reason of being a food for use as the sole item of the diet.[13]

The definition of dietary supplement in the DSHEA effectively superseded subsection (B) of the FDC act. The definition of "medical food" was included in the Orphan Drug Amendments of 1988. Medical foods are regulated by the FDA.

A "medical food" is defined as:

> a food which is formulated to be consumed or administered enterally under the supervision of a physician and which is intended for the specific dietary management of a disease or condition for which distinctive nutritional requirements, based on recognized scientific principles, are established by medical evaluation.[14]

Drugs are defined, in pertinent part, to include:

(A) Articles intended for use in the diagnosis, care, mitigation, treatment, or prevention of disease in man or other animals
(B) Articles (other than food) intended to affect the structure or any function of the body
(C) Components[15]

Drugs that are not generally recognized by qualified experts for their labeled uses are new drugs that may be marketed only after approval by FDA.[16] This more rigorous requirement does not apply to the marketing of most food products and makes it essential to avoid crossing the line between appropriate health claims for foods and therapeutic claims allowable only for drugs.

Vegetables, fruits, and herbs thus may be legally defined as foods or drugs (or both) depending upon the representations made in their labeling or advertising.

20.3 NUTRITION LABELING

In 1973, FDA responded to increased concern about issues of nutrition and health by Congress, the White House, consumer groups, the media, food scientists, and the general public by issuing voluntary nutrition labeling regulations for foods. The addition of nutrition information was required on food labels whenever a vitamin or mineral was added to the food or any nutrition claim or information was claimed in labeling or advertising. The nutrition information had to show caloric, protein, carbohydrate, fat, vitamin, and mineral content in a standard format.[17]

FDA issued the regulation without specific statutory authority, relying on its general authority to promulgate regulations for the efficient enforcement of the FDC Act and on the theory that failure to provide the information was a material omission of fact, rendering the food misbranded under the law.[18] The regulation was never directly challenged, however, and a substantial number of foods were marketed with this nutrition labeling over the next 20 years.

In 1990, Congress enacted the NLEA, which, among other things, specifically amended the FDC Act to require nutrition labeling in a standardized format to be established by FDA regulations for most foods subject to FDA's jurisdiction.[19] The law requires nutrition information to be based on serving size, which is an "amount customarily consumed and … expressed in a common household measure."[20] The nutrition information label must show the total number of calories, the calories from fat, and amounts of total fat, saturated fat, cholesterol, sodium, total carbohydrates, complex carbohydrates, sugars, dietary fiber, and total protein per serving.[21] FDA may require, by regulation, the listing of vitamins, minerals, and other nutrients, after determination that the information "will assist consumers in maintaining healthy dietary practices."[22]

FDA issued extensive new regulations in 1993* which completely dictate the format and contents of a "Nutrition Facts" box, including headings, type faces, spacing, type size, color, and layout. It concluded that vitamins A and C, calcium, and iron should be added to the mandatory declarations. Other nutrients, such as vitamins D or E, potassium, and soluble fiber, may be voluntarily declared, and must be declared if a claim related to them is made in labeling. Only nutrients specifically authorized by regulation may be declared in the nutrition facts box.[23]

Information for each nutrient must be based on the percent of its Daily Value (DV) provided by a serving of the food. The DV is based on the Daily Reference Value (DRV) for the macronutrients (e.g., fat) and the Reference Daily Intake (RDI) for micronutrients (e.g., vitamins) set by FDA.[24] Both parameters differ from the U.S. Recommended Dietary Allowances previously required by FDA and the NAS-NRC Food and Nutrition Board's Recommended Daily Dietary Allowances. FDA used a 2000-calorie daily diet for establishing the DVs, and the nutrition facts box must include a footnote to that effect.[25] Figure 20.1 illustrates a sample nutrition facts label.

The nutrition facts box currently appears on the vast majority of packaged food products and has reportedly been well accepted by consumers.

Congress treated raw agricultural commodities (along with raw fish) differently from other foods with respect to nutrition information in the NLEA. Rather than mandating nutrition labeling, the law required FDA to issue voluntary nutritional guidelines for retailers so they could provide consumers with nutrition information for the 20 varieties of vegetables and fruit most frequently consumed during a year, as determined by FDA.[26] FDA was directed to issue a regulation defining "substantial compliance" with the voluntary guidelines, and to report on the voluntary actions by food retailers within 30 months. If FDA concluded compliance was not substantial, it was to promulgate regulations requiring retailers to provide nutrition infor-

* FDA retained the section number (101.9) but completely revised the regulation.

Nutrition Facts			
Serving Size 1 Cup (228g)			
Servings Per Container 2			
Amount Per Serving			
Calories 260		Calories from Fat 120	
		% Daily Value*	
Total Fat 13 g			**20%**
Saturated Fat 5g			**25%**
Cholesterol 30mg			**10%**
Sodium 660mg			**28%**
Total Carbohydrate 31g			**10%**
Dietary Fiber 0g			**0%**
Sugars 5g			
Protein 5g			
Vitamin A 4%	•	Vitamin C 2%	
Calcium 15%	•	Iron 4%	

* Percent Daily Values are based on a 2,000 calorie diet. Your daily values may be higher or lower depending on your calorie needs:

	Calories	2,000	2,500
Total Fat	Less than	65g	80g
Sat Fat	Less than	20g	25g
Cholesterol	Less than	300mg	300mg
Sodium	Less than	2,400mg	2,400mg
Total Carbohydrate		300g	375g
Dietary Fiber		25g	30g

Calories per gram:
Fat 9 • Carbohydrate 4 • Protein 4

FIGURE 20.1 Sample nutrition facts label. (From Code of Federal Regulations, Vol. 21, Sec. 101.9(d)(12).)

mation. The regulations could allow posting of the information near the raw agricultural commodities, use of brochures, notebooks or leaflets, and communication of supplemental information by video, live demonstration, or other media.[27]

FDA identified the 20 most frequently consumed fruits to include bananas, apples, watermelons, oranges, cantaloupes, grapes, grapefruits, strawberries, peaches, pears, nectarines, honeydew melons, plums, avocadoes, lemons, pineapples, tangerines, sweet cherries, kiwi fruits, and limes.[28] The 20 vegetables are potatoes, iceberg lettuce, tomatoes, onions, carrots, celery, sweet corn, broccoli, green cabbage, cucumbers, bell peppers, cauliflower, leaf lettuce, sweet potatoes, mushrooms, green onions, green (snap) beans, radishes, summer squash, and asparagus.[29] FDA's guidelines recommend point-of-purchase displays if labels are not used, and permit media supplementation.[30] Requirements for stating serving sizes and nutrients are the same as for other foods, but the daily values were established by FDA as an appendix to the regulations.[31] Nutrition information may be supplied voluntarily for other fruits and vegetables, and is required if nutritional claims are made for them.

FDA defined "compliance" to require a food retailer to provide nutrition labeling for at least 90% of the listed raw agricultural commodities it sells,[32] and would find "substantial compliance" if at least 60% of a representative sample of 2,000 stores to be surveyed were in compliance.[33] FDA claims it conducts biennial surveys to determine substantial compliance by food retailers and apparently is satisfied to date. The final rules on voluntary lableing were published in August 1996.[34]

The NLEA authorized FDA to establish nutrition labeling for dietary supplements separately from other foods.[35] FDA's efforts to issue such regulations were first delayed by Congress, then superseded by enactment of the DSHEA, which expressly addressed nutrition labeling for dietary supplements.[36] FDA's regulations were to require nutrition information "appropriate for the product." Congress instructed that dietary ingredients not present in significant amounts need not be listed, ingredients included in the nutrition labeling need not be repeated in the ingredient list, and the nutrition labeling "may include the source of the dietary ingredient."[37]

FDA issued new regulations, effective in March 1999, establishing a "Supplement Facts" box containing nutrition information for dietary supplements.[38] See Figure 2 for an illustration of a supplement facts box for a multi-vitamin product.

There still remain significant compliance problems for small packages that contain multi-nutrient products.

20.4 NUTRIENT CONTENT CLAIMS

The NLEA for the first time authorized food labeling to include claims which "characterize the level of any nutrient" included in nutrition labeling, if it complies with regulations to be issued by FDA.[39] Congress gave FDA specific directions on certain aspects of nutrient content claims. For example, a claim "may not state the absence of a nutrient unless . . . it is usually present in the food . . . or . . . [it] would assist consumers in maintaining healthy dietary practices."[40] Congress was concerned about cholesterol, fat, and saturated fat levels, and prohibited nutrient content claims for foods with amounts of substances that FDA finds will increase the risk of disease or a health-related condition which is diet related.[41] Congress also instructed FDA to define in regulations the descriptors "free," "low," "light" or "lite," "reduced," "less," and "high," unless the agency found any of these terms to be misleading.[42]

FDA has published regulations authorizing nutrient content claims for foods with established DRVs or RDIs.[43] For example, a label may claim that a food is "high in," "rich in," or an "excellent source of" a vitamin or mineral for which FDA has established an RDI if the food provides 20% or more of the RDI per serving.[44] FDA regulations also authorize, with detailed requirements, claims for "good source," "more," "light" or "lite," caloric content, sodium content and fat, fatty acid, and cholesterol content.[45] Terms such as "fortified," "enriched," "added," "extra," and "plus" are considered to be "more" claims, requiring at least 10% more of the

Supplement Facts

Serving Size 1 Tablet

	Amount Per Serving	% Daily Value
Vitamin A (as retinyl acetate and 50% as beta-carotene)	5000 IU	100%
Vitamin C (as ascorbic acid)	60 mg	100%
Vitamin D (as cholecalciferol)	400 IU	100%
Vitamin E (as di-alpha tocopheryl acetate)	30 IU	100%
Thiamin (as thiamin mononitrate)	1.5 mg	100%
Riboflavin	1.7 mg	100%
Niacin (as niacinamide)	20 mg	100%
Vitamin B_6 (as pyridoxine hydrochloride)	2.0 mg	100%
Folate (as folic acid)	400 mcg	100%
Vitamin B_{12} (as cyanocobalamin)	6 mcg	100%
Biotin	30 mcg	10%
Pantothenic Acid (as calcium pantothenate)	10 mcg	100%

Other ingredients: Gelatin, lactose, magnesium stearate, microcrystalline cellulose, FD&C Yellow No. 6, propylene glycol, propylparaben, and sodium benzoate.

FIGURE 20.2 Sample supplement facts label. (From Code of Regulations, Vol. 21, Sec. 101.36(e)(10)(i).)

DV per serving "than an appropriate reference food." The regulations also require label disclosures of the reference food and the percentage or fractional difference.[46]

FDA addressed nutrient content claims for antioxidants, permitting claims only for nutrients that have established RDIs and have recognized antioxidant activity based on scientific evidence that the nutrients "inactivate free radicals or prevent fewer radical-initiated chemical reactions."[47] The agency also defined "healthy" as "an implied nutrient content claim" applicable only to a food low in fat and saturated fat, with limited amounts of sodium and cholesterol, that provides 10% of the DVs for vitamins A and C, calcium, iron, protein, or fiber (except for raw, frozen, or canned fruits and vegetables).[48]

Under the law, no nutrient content claim can be made for a food or nutrient for which no RDI or DRV and no FDA nutrient content claim regulation exists, even if it is truthful. For example, FDA has stated that a claim that a food or nutrient "contains lycopene" would be an unauthorized claim because lycopene does not have an RDI.[49] FDA would allow a label statement that the food provides a stated amount of lycopene per serving, so long as the claim does not suggest that the amount is substantial or otherwise characterize its level.

Under the NLEA, an interested party may petition FDA to issue a regulation that defines and permits a particular nutrient content claim, based on a showing that the proposed use of the nutrient "is of importance in human nutrition by virtue of its presence or absence at the levels that such claim would describe."[50] The petition and regulation process, however, is relatively time consuming and difficult.

The Food and Drug Administration Modernization Act of 1997 (FDAMA) amended the FDC Act to provide an alternative procedure for permitting a nutrient content claim in food labeling. A person seeking to use a claim can give FDA at least 120 days' advance notice, with a showing that the claim is based on a published authoritative statement by a scientific body of the United States government responsible for public health protection or research directly relating to human nutrition (such as the National Institutes of Health or the Centers for Disease Control and Prevention) or the National Academy of Sciences.[51] The notice must include the exact wording of the claim, a brief description of the basis for the claim, a copy of the authoritative statement, and a balanced representation of the relevant scientific literature. The claim must comply with the usual requirements and must accurately reflect the authoritative statement. The authoritative statement must be published by the scientific body. It cannot simply be a statement by an individual employee. FDA may halt use of the claim only by issuing a regulation or by seeking a court order based on the proponent's failure to meet the requirements.[52]

20.5 HEALTH-RELATED CLAIMS IN FOOD LABELING

Although FDA traditionally treated any health-related claim for food as a drug claim under the FDC Act, the agency came under pressure during the 1980s to revisit the subject. In 1984, the Kellogg Company began labeling and advertising its "All Bran" cereal product with the claim: "At last, some news about cancer you can live with. The National Cancer Institute believes a high fiber, low fat diet may reduce your risk of some kinds of cancer." The campaign received favorable comments from the NCI and the Federal Trade Commission. Although FDA initially objected, it took no regulatory action. Instead, with additional prodding from Congress, FDA in 1987 proposed a rule permitting health claims based on "publicly available . . . well-designed scientific . . . studies."[53] The overall scope and tone of the proposal were clearly intended to permit only limited health-related claims in food labeling. Although this was a major departure for FDA, it did not satisfy the food industry or Congress.

In 1990, in the NLEA, Congress amended the FDC Act expressly to allow food labeling to bear a claim that "characterizes the relationship of any substance to a disease or health-related condition."[54] However, a health claim was allowed only if authorized by FDA regulations. Congress again included certain disqualifying conditions, to be determined in FDA's regulations, that might increase "the risk of a disease or health-related condition which is diet related."[55] In addition, the statute required FDA to issue regulations only on a determination

> based on the totality of publicly available scientific evidence (including evidence from well-designed studies conducted in a manner which is consistent with generally recognized scientific procedures and principles), that there is significant scientific agreement, among experts qualified by scientific training and experience to evaluate such claims, that the claim is supported by such evidence.[56]

The "significant scientific agreement" standard has become a matter of controversy, arising from a lawsuit involving dietary supplements. The NLEA excluded dietary supplements from the general health claims provision, making them subject to a procedure and standard to be separately established by FDA regulation.[57] FDA simply treated dietary supplements and conventional foods the same way in its health claims regulation, applying the "significant scientific agreement" standard to both categories.[58] The agency then rejected several petitions for health claims for dietary supplements and the disappointed petitioners appealed to the court. The agency prevailed in the lower court, but the court of appeals overturned FDA's regulations, finding that the agency had failed to adequately explain the meaning of "significant scientific agreement" and, in addition, improperly refused to consider the use of disclaimers in health claims.[59] Following up its loss in court, FDA began an administrative proceeding to develop guidance clarifying the standard, establish rules for considering general health claims for dietary supplements, and reconsider the specific claims subject to the court's decision.[60] The matter is pending but will affect future health claims determinations.

As part of the NLEA, Congress instructed FDA to determine whether ten potential health claims for conventional foods and dietary supplements were appropriate, including the relationships between:

calcium and osteoporosis,
dietary fiber and cancer,
lipids and cardiovascular disease,
lipids and cancer,
sodium and hypertension,
dietary fiber and cardiovascular disease,
folic acid and neural tube defects,
antioxidant vitamins and cancer,
zinc and immune function in the elderly, and
omega-3 fatty acids and heart disease.[61]

FDA initially authorized eight health claims concerning (1) calcium and osteoporosis, (2) fat and cancer, (3) sodium and hypertension, (4) saturated fat/cholesterol and heart disease, (5) fiber-containing grains/fruits/vegetables and cancer, (6) the same fiber-containing substances and heart disease, (7) fruits/vegetables and cancer, and (8) folate and neural tube defects.[62]

More recently, FDA also issued health claims regulations for dietary sugars/alcohols and dental caries, soluble fiber (primarily oat bran) and coronary heart disease, and, in October 1999, for soy protein and coronary heart disease.[63]

Examples of "model health claims" recommended by FDA for fruits, vegetables, and herbs in relation to cancer and coronary heart disease include the following:

- Low fat diets rich in fiber-containing grain products, fruits, and vegetables may reduce the risk of some types of cancer, a disease associated with many factors.[64]

- Diets low in saturated fat and cholesterol and rich in fruits, vegetables, and grain products that contain some types of dietary fiber, particularly soluble fiber, may reduce the risk of heart disease, a disease associated with many factors.[65]
- Low fat diets rich in fruits and vegetables (foods that are low in fat and may contain dietary fiber, vitamin A, and vitamin C) may reduce the risk of some types of cancer, a disease associated with many factors. Broccoli is high in vitamins A and C, and it is a good source of dietary fiber.[66]
- 25 grams of soy protein a day, as part of a diet low in saturated fat and cholesterol, may reduce the risk of heart disease. A serving of [name of food] supplies __ grams of soy protein.[67]
- Diets low in saturated fat and cholesterol that include 25 grams of soy protein a day may reduce the risk of heart disease. One serving of [name of food] provides __ grams of soy protein.[68]

The model claims recommended by FDA are not particularly well designed for labeling and advertising, and they are not necessarily mandatory. However, FDA tries to encourage the use of fully developed statements.

As with nutrient content claims, the FDAMA added an alternative procedure for making health-related claims for foods. Thus, a claim may be made if it is the subject of a "published . . . authoritative statement, which is currently in effect," issued by a governmental scientific body or the National Academy of Sciences.[69] The proponent must give 120 days' notice to FDA, providing the text of the claim, the basis for the claim, the authoritative statement, and a balanced representation of the relevant scientific literature. There are disqualifying factors depending on the composition of the product, and the claim must not be "false and misleading in any particular," or fail to reveal facts that are material in the light of the claim.[70] FDA can still prevent the claim by issuing a regulation prohibiting or modifying the claim or by filing a lawsuit.

The desirability of health claims for foods, for industry and consumers, assures that their use will expand in the future.

20.6 STATEMENTS OF NUTRITIONAL SUPPORT

For dietary supplements, the DSHEA authorized health claims without FDA approval for four types of "statements of nutritional support" in labeling. These include a statement that:

- Claims a benefit related to a classical nutrient deficiency disease and discloses the prevalence of such disease in the United States;
- Describes the role of a nutrient or dietary ingredient intended to affect the structure or function in humans;
- Characterizes the documented mechanism by which a nutrient or dietary ingredient acts to maintain such structure or function; or
- Describes general well-being from consumption of a nutrient or dietary ingredient.[71]

The manufacturer must be able to prove that the statement is truthful and not misleading and must notify FDA within 30 days after first marketing the supplement with that statement. The product's labeling must contain the disclaimer: "This statement has not been evaluated by the Food and Drug Administration. This product is not intended to diagnose, treat, cure, or prevent any disease."[72] These so-called structure/function claims have been widely used in labeling and advertising for dietary supplements. Thousands of notifications have been submitted to FDA. If FDA believes a statement goes too far in making disease-related claims, the agency sends a letter (commonly known as a "courtesy letter") advising the notifier to consult with agency drug regulators and to comply with drug requirements.

FDA is trying to gain some control over these claims by promulgating a rule defining the types of statements that are appropriate structure/function claims for dietary supplements and establishing criteria for determining when a statement constitutes an impermissible disease claim.[73] The final rule lists ten criteria for identifying express or implied disease claims that would be impermissible for dietary supplements. These include obvious references to diseases, symptoms, or well known drug ingredients, use of references to scientific publications with diseases in their titles, use of pictures, vignettes or symbols, and claims of ability to substitute for disease therapies. In a compromise with industry critics, FDA decided that a claim for "an effect on an abnormal condition associated with a natural state or process" (e.g., pregnancy or menopause) would be a disease claim *except* for "common conditions associated with natural states or processes that do not cause significant or permanent harm." Thus, FDA agreed that hot flashes, morning sickness, mild memory problems, and hair loss associated with aging were acceptable structure/function claims but toxemia or acute psychosis of pregnancy were not. Controversy over the distinction between acceptable structure/function claims and unacceptable drug claims for dietary supplements is likely to continue.

FDA's final rule reversed its September 1997 position that a structure/function claim is acceptable for any food when the claim is derived from the nutritive value of the food.[74] FDA now asserts that structure/function claims based on "nutritive value" are permissible only for conventional foods; dietary supplements may make structure/function claims only in compliance with the notification and disclaimer requirements. FDA concludes that the DSHEA excludes dietary supplements from the provision which includes structure/function claims as part of the definition of food. This reversal, which seems likely to be challenged, would result in a very large increase in the number of notifications to FDA.

Finally, it is important to note that the provision for statements of nutritional support appears in the FDC Act as an exception to the requirement for FDA approval of health claims. Although this has not been fully explored by the agency or the courts, it is at least arguable that the disclaimer and notification provisions are not required if the structure/function claim would not be regarded as a health claim under the law.

In any event, dietary supplements are more often labeled with statements of nutritional support than with overt health claims.

20.7 FOOD FOR SPECIAL DIETARY USES

With the advent of the NLEA and DSHEA, the concept of foods for special dietary uses has become less important. However, the FDC Act still authorizes FDA to issue regulations requiring labeling information concerning vitamin, mineral, and other dietary properties of a food intended for special dietary uses.[75] FDA has published regulations that require information on hypoallergenic foods, infant foods, foods intended to be used to reduce or maintain body weight, foods for diabetics, and foods for regulating sodium intake.[76]

Special dietary food labeling regulations, however, are subject to the most onerous procedural requirements for developing final rules, including an opportunity for a formal evidentiary hearing.[77] Because these procedures are expensive and extremely time consuming, they have rarely been used in recent years. In any event, the changes in the law brought by NLEA and DSHEA effectively supersede most of the goals of the special dietary foods provision.

20.8 CLAIMS FOR MEDICAL FOODS

Over the years, FDA has recognized that certain foods are used in connection with the treatment of diseases. The so-called "medical foods" were expressly recognized by Congress in 1988 in legislation relating to orphan drugs. The measure is not part of the FDC Act but is subject to FDA jurisdiction.[78] As defined, a medical food must be used under the supervision of a physician for the specific dietary management of a disease or condition for which distinctive nutritional requirements, based on recognized scientific principles, are established by medical evaluation. Medical foods are permitted to bear labeling which overtly claims to have an effect on a disease or other medical condition. Medical foods are also exempt from FDA's regulations on nutrition labeling, health claims, and nutrient content claims.[79]

A medical food claim must not be false or misleading. It may not relate to the cure, mitigation, treatment, or prevention of disease and can refer only to the patient's special dietary needs that exist because of the disease. Although FDA would probably prefer that such products be restricted to sale on doctors' orders, nothing in the law or regulations prohibits the sale of over-the-counter medical foods, so long as they are labeled for use under the supervision of a physician. This category has received increased interest in recent years, but such products are still relatively rare. The medical food area may be expanded by marketers and become subject to greater scrutiny by FDA in the future.

20.9 CONCLUSION

As discussed, the law has been broadened in recent years to reflect the increased interests of consumers, industry, food scientists, health care professionals, and Congress in making more information available concerning the health benefits of food. The trend is clearly in favor of more, rather than less, freedom to provide truthful, nonmisleading health-related information in food labeling. There still remain legal and regulatory concerns over the need to distinguish between health claims for foods and therapeutic claims for drugs. The line between these kinds of claims may never be precisely drawn, and health claims will undoubtedly be the subject of regulatory attention over the next several years. Nevertheless, it seems clear that the use of health claims in labeling and advertising of foods will expand, to the public's benefit.

ACKNOWLEDGMENT

The valuable assistance of Kelly F. Merrill in preparing this chapter is gratefully acknowledged.

REFERENCES

1. Food, Drug, and Cosmetic Act, U.S. Code, vol. 21, sec. 301 et seq.
2. Nutrition Labeling and Education Act of 1990, U.S. Statutes at Large 104 (1990): 2353.
3. Dietary Supplement Health and Education Act of 1994, U.S. Statutes at Large 108 (1994): 4325.
4. Food and Drug Administration Modernization Act of 1997, U.S. Statutes at Large 111 (1997): 2296.
5. *Nutrilab, Inc. V. Schweiker,* 713 F. 2d 335 (7th Circuit 1983; *American Health Products Co. v. Hayes,* 574 F. Supp. 1498 (Southern District, New York 1983), affirmed 744 F. 2d 912 (2nd Circuit 1984).
6. Food, Drug, and Cosmetic Act, sec. 403(q)(1).
7. Dietary Supplement Health and Education Act of 1994, sec. 2(2) and 2(8).8.
8. Food, Drug, and Cosmetic Act, sec. 201(f).
9. Food, Drug, and Cosmetic Act, sec. 201(g)(1)(C).
10. Nutrilab, Inc., 713 F. 2d at 338.
11. Food, Drug, and Cosmetic Act, sec. 201(ff)(1).
12. Food, Drug, and Cosmetic Act, sec. 201(ff)(2).
13. Food, Drug, and Cosmetic Act, sec. 411(c)(3).
14. U.S. Code, vol. 21, sec. 360; Code of Federal Regulations, vol. 21, sec. 101.9(j)(8).
15. Food, Drug, and Cosmetic Act, sec. 201(g)(1).
16. Food, Drug, and Cosmetic Act, sec. 201(p) and sec. 505.
17. Code of Federal Regulations, vol. 21, sec. 101.9; Federal Register, vol. 38, p. 2125, January 17, 1973.
18. Food, Drug, and Cosmetic Act, sec. 201(n) and sec. 701(a).
19. Nutrition Labeling and Education Act of 1990, sec. 2; Food, Drug, and Cosmetic Act, sec. 403(q).
20. Food, Drug, and Cosmetic Act, sec. 403(q)(1)(A).
21. Food, Drug, and Cosmetic Act, sec. 403(q)(1)(C) and (D).
22. Food, Drug, and Cosmetic Act, sec. 403(q)(1)(E).
23. Code of Federal Regulations, vol. 21, sec. 101.9; Federal Register, vol. 58, p. 2175, January 6, 1993.
24. Code of Federal Regulations, vol. 21, sec. 101.9(c)(8) and (9).
25. Code of Federal Regulations, vol. 21, sec. 101.9(c)(9) and (d)(9).
26. Food, Drug, and Cosmetic Act, sec. 403(q)(4)(i)(I).
27. Food, Drug, and Cosmetic Act, sec. 403(q)(4)(D)(iii).
28. Code of Federal Regulations, vol. 21, sec. 101.44(a).
29. Code of Federal Regulations, vol. 21, sec. 101.44(b).
30. Code of Federal Regulations, vol. 21, sec. 101.45(a)(3).
31. Code of Federal Regulations, vol 21, part 101, appendix C.
32. Code of Federal Regulations, vol. 21, sec. 101.43(a).
33. Code of Federal Regulations, vol. 21, sec. 101.43(b) and (c).

34. Federal Register, vol. 61, p. 42742, August 16, 1996.
35. Food, Drug, and Cosmetic Act, sec. 403(q)(5)(E).
36. Food, Drug, and Cosmetic Act, sec. 403(q)(5)(F).
37. Food, Drug, and Cosmetic Act, sec. 403(q)(F)(5)(i) and (iii).
38. Code of Federal Regulations, vol. 21, sec. 101.36; Federal Register, vol. 62, page 49849, September 23, 1997.
39. Nutrition Labelling and Education Act of 1990, sec. 3(a); Food, Drug, and Cosmetic Act, sec. 403(r)(1)(A).
40. Food, Drug, and Cosmetic Act, sec. 403(r)(2)(A)(ii).
41. Food, Drug, and Cosmetic Act, sec. 403(r)(2)(A)(iii).
42. Nutrition Labelling and Education Act of 1990, sec. 3(b)(1)(A).
43. Code of Federal Regulations, vol. 21, sec, 101,13 and 101,54-101.69.
44. Code of Federal Regulations, vol. 21, sec. 101.54(b).
45. Code of Federal Regulations, vol. 21, sec. 101.54-101.62.
46. Code of Federal Regulations, vol. 21, sec. 101.54(e).
47. Code of Federal Regulations, vol. 21, sec. 101.54(g).
48. Code of Federal Regulations, vol. 21, sec. 101.65(d)(2).
49. Federal Register, vol. 62, pp. 49868 and 49873, September 23, 1997.
50. Code of Federal Regulations, vol. 21, sec. 101.69(m)(1)(B).
51. Food, Drug, and Cosmetic Act, sec. 403(r)(2)(G).
52. Food, Drug, and Cosmetic Act, sec. 403(r)(2)(H).
53. Federal Register, vol. 52, p. 28843, August 4, 1987.
54. Food, Drug, and Cosmetic Act, sec. 403(r)(1)(B).
55. Food, Drug, and Cosmetic Act, sec. 403(r)(3)(A).
56. Food, Drug, and Cosmetic Act, sec. 403(r)(3)(B)(i).
57. Food, Drug, and Cosmetic Act, sec. 403(r)(5)(D).
58. Federal Register, vol. 58, pp. 2478, 2507, 2533, January 6, 1993.
59. *Pearson v. Shalala,* 164 F. 2d 650 (D.C. Circuit 1999).
60. Federal Register, vol. 64, p. 67289, December 1, 1999; Federal Register, vol. 64, p. 71794, December 22, 1999.
61. Nutrition Labelling and Education Act of 1990, sec. 3(b)(1)(A)(vi) and (x).
62. Code of Federal Regulations, vol. 21, sec. 101.72-101.79.
63. Code of Federal Regulations, vol. 21, sec. 101.80-101.82.
64. Code of Federal Regulations, vol. 21, sec. 101.76(e)(1).
65. Code of Federal Regulations, vol. 21, sec. 101.77(e)(1).
66. Code of Federal Regulations, vol. 21, sec. 101.78(e)(1).
67. Code of Federal Regulations, vol. 21, sec. 101.82(e)(1).
68. Code of Federal Regulations, vol. 21, sec. 101.82(e)(2).
69. Food, Drug, and Cosmetic Act, sec. 403(r)(3)(C)(i).
70. Food, Drug, and Cosmetic Act, sec. 201(n) and 403(r)(3)(C)(iii).
71. Food, Drug, and Cosmetic Act, sec. 403(r)(6).
72. Food, Drug, and Cosmetic Act, sec. 403(r)(6)(B) and (C).
73. Code of Federal Regulations, vol. 21, sec. 101.93(f) and (g); Federal Register, vol. 65, p. 1000, Jan. 6, 2000.
74. Federal Register, vol. 65, p. 1033.
75. Food, Drug, and Cosmetic Act, sec. 403(j).
76. Code of Federal Regulations, vol. 21, part 105.
77. Food, Drug, and Cosmetic Act, sec. 701(e).
78. U.S. Code, vol. 21, sec. 350ee.
79. Code of Federal Regulations, vol. 21, sec. 101.9(j)(8), 101.13(q)(4)(ii), and 101.14(f)(2).

Index

F

G

H

I

K

L

M

N